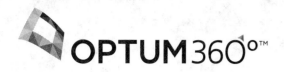 **OPTUM**360°™

 REFRE

MW00910671

SAVE UP TO 25%*

when you renew your coding essentials.

Buy 1–2 items, save 15%
Buy 3–5 items, save 20%
Buy 6+ items, save 25%

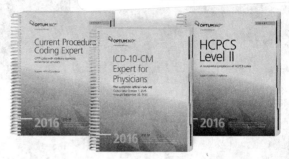

ITEM #	TITLE INDICATE THE ITEMS YOU WISH TO PURCHASE	QUANTITY	PRICE PER PRODUCT	TOTAL
			Subtotal	
	(AK, DE, HI, MT, NH & OR are exempt)		Sales Tax	
	1 item $10.95 • 2–4 items $12.95 • 5+ CALL		Shipping & Handling	
			TOTAL AMOUNT ENCLOSED	

Save up to 25% when you renew.

 Visit **optumcoding.com** and enter the promo code below.

Call **1-800-464-3649, option 1,** and mention the promo code below.

Fax this order form with purchase order to **1-801-982-4033.** *Optum360 no longer accepts credit cards by fax.*

PROMO CODE
FOBA16WA

Mail this order form with payment and/or purchase order to:
Optum360, PO Box 88050, Chicago, IL 60680-9920.
Optum360 no longer accepts credit cards by mail.

Name

Address

Customer Number   Contact Number

○ CHECK ENCLOSED (PAYABLE TO OPTUM360)

○ BILL ME   ○ P.O.#

(   )
Telephone
(   )
Fax

E-mail

Optum360 respects your right to privacy. We will not sell or rent your email address or fax number to anyone outside Optum360 and its business partners. If you would like to remove your name from Optum360 promotions, please call 1-800-464-3649, option 1.

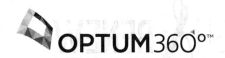

PIONEER
THE NEW FRONTIER OF CODING

WITH A TRUSTED, INDUSTRY LEADER BY YOUR SIDE.

Navigate the changing landscape of coding and move forward with confidence.

With Optum360 tools and resources at your fingertips, you can open a world of opportunities and help build the foundation for greater efficiencies, financial gains, and competitive advantages. For over 30 years, our print resources have remained trusted tools for coding professionals, and our 2016 editions offer the same quality and reliability you have come to expect from us.

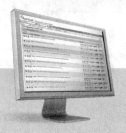

Eliminate roadblocks with web-based coding solutions.
ICD-10 will have 668 percent more codes than ICD-9. Web-based coding solutions can help you experience a smooth, successful transition with fast access to ICD-10 codes, data and mapping tools, and can easily be used in conjunction with our ICD-10 books. Learn more about EncoderPro.com and RevenueCyclePro.com today by visiting **optumcoding.com/transitions.**

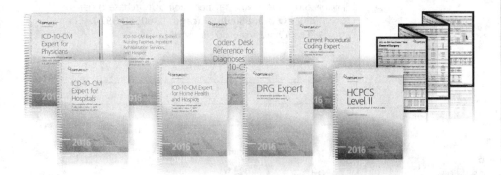

The new frontier of coding awaits.
Save up to 25% on the ICD-10, CPT®, and HCPCS coding resources you need.

 Visit OptumCoding.com and enter promo code **00000AD3** to save 25%

 Call 1.800.464.3649, option 1 and mention promo code **00000AD3** to save 20%

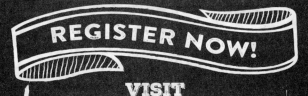
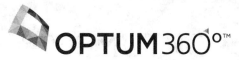

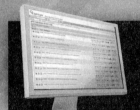
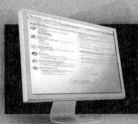

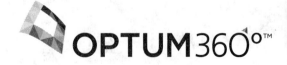

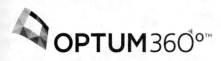
OPTUM 360°™

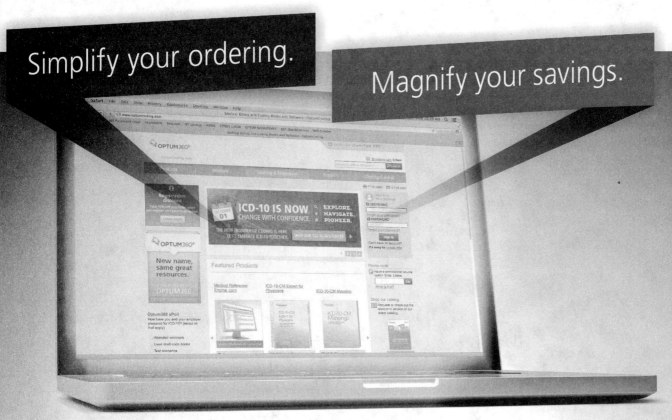

Simplify your ordering.

Magnify your savings.

---

1 Click.

Visit optumcoding.com

- Find the products you need quickly and easily.
- View all available formats and edition years on the same page.
- Chat live with a customer service representative.
- Visit Coding Central for expert resources including articles, *Inside Track to ICD-10* and coding scenarios to test your knowledge.
- View our catalog online. Utilize our interactive online catalog features to view product information quickly and easily.

2 Register.

By registering, you'll be able to:

- Enjoy special promotions, discounts and automatic rewards.
- Get recommendations based on your order history.
- Check on shipment status and tracking.
- View order and payment history.
- Pay invoices.
- Manage your address book and ship orders to multiple locations.
- Renew your order with a single click.
- Compile a wish list of the products you want and purchase when you're ready.

3 Save.

Get 15% off your next order

Register for an account and receive a coupon via email for 15% off your next order.

Plus, save even more with our no-cost eRewards program.

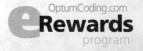
OptumCoding.com
eRewards
program

Register for an account and you're automatically enrolled in our eRewards program, where you'll get a $50 coupon for every $500 you spend*. When logged in at optumcoding.com, the eRewards meter keeps track of purchases toward your next reward.

Visit us at optumcoding.com to register today!

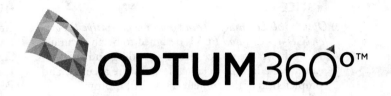

Optum360 Learning:
Coding from the Operative Report
for ICD-10-CM and PCS

2016

Fourth Edition

OUR COMMITMENT TO ACCURACY

Optum360 is committed to producing accurate and reliable materials.

To report corrections, please visit www.optumcoding.com/accuracy or email accuracy@optum.com. You can also reach customer service by calling 1.800.464.3649.

ACKNOWLEDGMENTS

Gregory A. Kemp, MA, *Product Manager*
Karen Schmidt, BSN, *Technical Director*
Stacy Perry, *Manager, Desktop Publishing*
Lisa Singley, *Project Manager*
Peggy Willard, CCS, AHIMA-Approved
 ICD-10-CM/PCS Trainer *Clinical/Technical Editor*
Anita Schmidt, BS, RHIT, AHIMA-Approved
 ICD-10-CM/PCS Trainer, *Clinical/Technical Editor*
Tracy Betzler, *Senior Desktop Publishing Specialist*
Hope M. Dunn, *Senior Desktop Publishing Specialist*
Katie Russell, *Desktop Publishing Specialist*
Kate Holden, *Editor*

ABOUT THE TECHNICAL EDITORS

Peggy Willard, CCS, AHIMA-Approved ICD-10-CM/PCS Trainer

Ms. Willard has several years of experience in Level I Adult and Pediatric Trauma hospital coding, specializing in ICD-9-CM, DRG, and CPT coding. She has been extensively trained in ICD-10-CM and PCS. Her recent experience includes in-depth analysis of medical record documentation, ICD-10-CM code assignment, and DRG shifts based on ICD-10-CM code assignment. Ms. Willard's expertise includes conducting coding audits, conducting coding training for coding staff and clinical documentation specialists, and creating internal ICD-10-CM coding guidelines/tips. Ms. Willard is an active member of the American Health Information Management Association (AHIMA) and the Minnesota Health Information Management Association (MHIMA).

Anita Schmidt, BS, RHIT, AHIMA-Approved ICD-10-CM/PCS Trainer

Ms. Schmidt has expertise in level I adult and pediatric trauma hospital coding, specializing in ICD-9-CM, DRG, and CPT coding. Her experience includes analysis of medical record documentation and assignment of ICD-9-CM codes and DRGs, and CPT code assignments for same-day surgery cases. She has conducted coding training and auditing including DRG validation, conducted electronic health record training, and worked with clinical documentation specialists to identify documentation needs and potential areas for physician education. Ms. Schmidt is an AHIMA-approved ICD-10-CM/PCS trainer, and is an active member of the American Health Information Management Association (AHIMA) and the Minnesota Health Information Management Association (MHIMA).

Contents

Chapter 1: History

The history of operative reports in medical record keeping runs parallel to the practice of medicine and surgery. As far back as 25,000 BC there are records of the method used to amputate fingers as depicted in drawings on caverns in Spain. Centuries later, in Egypt, Imhotep is credited with six papyri describing 48 cases of clinical surgery. According to a history of medical records in the book *Medical Record Management*, each case followed a definite form. There is evidence of the surgeon's operation, including the type of injury (e.g., penetrating wound to the head), exam, diagnosis (e.g., whether the wound is treatable), and treatment. Another early medical record attributed to Egyptian scribes, dated 500 years later in 1550 BC, is methodical in describing disease and the methods of treating individual cases.

EARLY RECORD KEEPING

While many of the early records of operations may be a far cry from present documentation, they do show the early interest in charting patient care and the methodology of record keeping. Evidence of early "hospital" record keeping is found in the names of patients, summaries of their cases, and treatment outcomes inscribed in columns in the ruins of temples in Egypt dedicated to the care of the sick, according to the book *Medical Record Management*. Hippocrates, the "Father of Medicine" born in 460 BC, supposedly drew upon the information from the columns to enhance his medical knowledge. The Hippocratic Oath that physicians pledge to contains language acknowledging the privacy that must exist between physician and patient. Hippocrates' detailed method of record keeping provides evidence of his clinical expertise and lends support to his medical theories.

HOSPITAL RECORDS

The origin of the word "hospital," from the Latin hospitalis, is found in writings about a hospital established in Rome some 700 years after the time of Hippocrates. During the Middle Ages, there is evidence of the first clinical notes derived from the work of Hippocrates. The preserved case histories of patients at St. Bartholomew's Hospital, built in Medieval times, indicate that records were kept on all patients from the start in 1137.

The reign of King Henry VIII during the Renaissance brought rules and regulations to hospitals, including those governing record keeping and privacy. The Belgian Monk Andreas Vesalius kept secret his anatomical sketches made of the bodies of criminals due to the Roman Catholic ban on human dissection, similar to the silencing of Leonardo DaVinci's portfolio of anatomical drawings in the Middle Ages. Soon after the death of King Henry VIII, a Papal decree in 1556 lead to legalized dissection that ultimately advanced the study of surgery. In 16th and 17th century Europe, the term medical record was beginning to mean more than a single case history. Physicians were required to write orders for inpatients that were maintained as part of the entire patient record.

RECORD KEEPING IN AMERICA

The availability of health care services in America was sporadic until 1751, when Benjamin Franklin founded the nation's first incorporated hospital, the Philadelphia Hospital. Benjamin Franklin was the hospital's secretary, keeping track of the patients' names, addresses, medical problems, and dates of hospitalization. The New York Hospital, which opened in 1771, has records dating back nearly two centuries that resemble the system for recording patient histories used presently by major medical institutions. The Massachusetts General Hospital carries the distinction of having a complete file of clinical cases dating back to Sept. 3, 1821, the day it opened.

Operative reporting was infrequent until the mid-1880's, prior to the advent of effective anesthesia, as surgery was performed only in dire emergencies. Surgery was considered a last resort, representing barely more than one case per month in major medical institutions during the early to mid 1800s. In 1846, the future of surgery changed dramatically when William T.G. Morton, a Boston dentist, administered an anesthetic to Gilbert Abbott for a vascular tumor on his jaw. John Collins, M.D., surgically removed the tumor. Upon wakening, Abbot informed his audience that he had no pain. News spread quickly as journals around the world proclaimed "We have conquered pain." Little more than 20 years later, in 1868, Joseph Lister made the connection between the infection on hospital wards and the effect on wound healing based upon Louis Pasteur's "germ theory" of disease. Lister's solution of steam-sprayed carbolic acid to sterilize instruments and the skin of the patient and surgeon diminished the incidence of infection.

STANDARDIZED RECORD KEEPING

By the turn of the 20th century, operative reports and medical record keeping had taken on new importance. The American Medical Association (AMA), in 1905, published an article about clinical charting in small hospitals from a presentation given at the association's 56th annual meeting. The American College of Surgeons (ACS), founded in 1913, required school candidates to submit case records of major surgeries they had performed on patients. Discrepancies in the information among the records lead to a standard in hospital programs that demanded "that accurate and complete case records be written for all patients and filed in an accessible manner in the hospital," according to the book *Health Information Management*.

Standardization gave way to the creation of specialty groups. The Association of Record Librarians of North America (ARLNA) was organized by medical record workers in 1928 during a Clinical Conference of the American College of Surgeons to "elevate the standards of clinical records in hospitals and other medical institutions." In 1938 the Association changed its name to the American Association of Medical Record Librarians (AAMRL) and, in 1970, to the American Medical Record Association. The Association changed its name in 1991 to the American Health Information Management Association (AHIMA).

THE JOINT COMMISSION (FORMERLY JOINT COMMISSION ON ACCREDITATION OF HEALTHCARE ORGANIZATIONS)

Education, exams to qualify for a national registry of medical record workers, and accreditation of medical record technicians followed. In 1951, the American College of Physicians, the American Hospital Association, the AMA, and the Canadian Medical Association joined with the ACS to create the Joint Commission on Accreditation of Hospitals. In 1952, the Joint Commission took over the job of establishing hospital standards, which extends to the quality of record keeping. In 1987, the Joint Commission changed its name to the Joint Commission on Accreditation of Healthcare Organizations (JCAHO). In 2008, JCAHO changed its name to the Joint Commission. Over the years, the commission has extended its accreditation to include ambulatory health care, health care networks, long-term care, home care, mental health, chemical dependency, disabilities services, and pathology and clinical laboratory services.

The Joint Commission accreditation is a standard in the Medicare program for allocating federal funds to hospitals (generally through fiscal intermediaries).

The Joint Commission surveys most hospitals every three years and its accredited hospitals are not subject to the Medicare survey and certification process, though eligible for Medicare funding. Any hospital that meets the following requirements may apply for a Joint Commission accreditation survey under current hospital standards:

- The hospital operates in the United States or its territories, or is run by the U. S. government or under a charter of Congress if outside the United States.

- The hospital assesses and improves the quality of its services, including a review of care by clinicians.

- The hospital identifies the services it offers, indicating which it provides directly, under contract, or through some other arrangement.

- The hospital provides services covered by Joint Commission's standards.

The Joint Commission publishes the *Comprehensive Accreditation Manual for Hospitals: The Official Handbook* (CAMH), which explains the accreditation process, identifies and describes the standards, and explains the scoring of compliance with the standards.

SUMMARY

The process of keeping records of a patient encounter regardless of the location of service has evolved from the days of earliest recorded medical care to the present. Current guidelines affect what is required and when it should be recorded. These guidelines affect care in a hospital, clinic, and even private practice across all medical specialties.

Chapter 2: Documentation

Medical documentation is performed to establish and maintain a lasting record of a patient's encounters with health care professionals and services. It is chronological written evidence of what happened to a patient's health during single, multiple, or a lifetime of encounters. The written record at one time can be as simple as a short written note or at another time as complicated as an operative report.

Documentation in the medical record must contain information to justify that the admission and continued hospitalization, the encounter or visit, and the services performed for a patient are medically necessary. It must describe the patient's progress and response to therapies and surgeries while at the same time allowing continued care of the patient by other health care professionals. A chart that is comprehensive, well-organized, and accurate enables the physician and other health care professionals to quickly access needed information and is essential in providing quality patient care. To meet all of these needs, record documentation must have several characteristics present to reflect the adequacy and type of care received by the patient.

CONTENT

Hospitals, outpatient facilities, and providers are required to keep a medical record of every patient admitted or seen in an encounter or visit. A complete medical record generally includes the following components depending on where the service was rendered:

- Consent to treatment statement (when applicable)
- Consultations and reports
- Discharge summary (when applicable)
- Discharge/transfer instructions (when applicable)
- History and physical (when applicable)
- Laboratory and pathology tests and results
- Radiology procedures (results and notes)
- Other services performed (e.g., pulmonary, respiratory, physical, occupational therapy, dietary)
- Medication records
- Nursing assessments or services
- Visits and examinations
- Operative/procedural consent to treatment statement
- Operative reports
- Physician's orders
- Progress notes

The Joint Commission has developed guidelines that govern documentation and medical records. According to the guidelines, inpatient medical records must contain the following:

- Patient's name, address, date of birth, and next of kin
- Patient's medical history including the chief complaint, details of the present illness, relevant past, social, and family histories and an inventory of body systems
- Any known allergies
- A medical history completed within the first 24 hours of admission to inpatient services
- A physical examination completed within 24 hours of admission
- A conclusion drawn from the admission history and physical examination
- A statement of the course of action planned for the patient while in the hospital
- Diagnostic and therapeutic orders
- Progress notes made by the medical staff
- Consultation reports
- Nursing notes and entries by nonphysicians
- Reports of procedures, tests, and their results
- Reports of pathology and clinical laboratory examinations, radiology and nuclear medicine examinations or treatment
- Conclusions at the termination of hospitalization

TIMELINESS

Hospitals must pay particular attention to the timeliness of health record documentation if, for no other reason, to meet standards developed by the Joint Commission. Meeting deadlines also helps to support the need for ongoing patient care and hastens reimbursement by third-party payers. Documentation standards for operative reports include:

- History and physical written within 30 days prior to surgery
- Signed informed consent to surgery obtained prior to the procedure (excluding emergencies)
- Operative progress note written immediately after surgery if the operative report is not placed in the record immediately after surgery
- Status report for patient requiring additional surgery

In November 2008, the Joint Commission clarified its policy regarding reports of operative and other invasive procedures, tests, and their results:

1. An organization's policy, based on state law, would define the time frame for dictation and placement in the medical record. The most important issue is that there needs to be enough information in the record immediately after surgery in order to manage the patient throughout the postoperative period. This information could be entered as the operative report or as a hand-written operative progress note.

2. If the operative report is not placed in the medical record immediately after surgery due to transcription or filing delay, then an operative progress note should be entered in the medical record immediately after surgery to provide pertinent information for anyone required to attend to the patient. This operative progress note should contain at a minimum comparable operative report information. These elements include; name of primary surgeon and assistants, findings, technical procedures performed, specimens removed, and postoperative diagnosis as well as estimated blood loss.

3. Immediately after surgery is defined as "upon completion of surgery, before the patient is transferred to the next level of care, for example the post anesthesia care unit." This is to ensure that pertinent information is available to the next caregiver.

OPERATIVE REPORTS

A major part of the medical record is the section devoted to the operative report. However, the operative report must do more than contribute to the development of surgery or provide mortality and morbidity information to statisticians. An operative report must outline the logic used in treating a patient and document why the particular type of surgery was performed, the steps involved, and the outcome. An adequate operative record provides pre- and postoperative information, as well as consent to treat forms and status reports when additional surgery is required after the initial surgery was performed. It serves as the basis for reimbursing the surgeon, surgical team, and inpatient or outpatient facility and as the official record for claims involving malpractice, worker's compensation, accidental trauma, or medical hardship.

Despite regulations, however, operative reports are seldom easy to interpret and code. Regardless of the physician's specificity about how a service was performed, coders must understand:

- How operative reports and notes are organized
- Availability of standard forms for recording information either in a written or electronic format
- The documentation required in the health record for each episode of care (e.g., diagnostic or therapeutic surgical care or procedural care)

Organization

Organization of the health record (including operative reports) is determined by the hospital unless specified by accrediting agencies. However, the classification system used in organizing data is common among hospitals.

Legal and Administrative Data

Administrative data belonging at the front of the health record include billing information specifying Medicare, Medicaid, and any supplemental insurance. Legal data generally cover specific patient orders such as signed conditions of participation (CoP), refusals of any specified procedures, living wills, and power of attorney.

 KEY POINT

According to Medicare's conditions of participation (CoP), a hospital must inform each patient, or when appropriate, the patient's representative (as allowed under HIPAA or state law), of the patient's rights, in advance of furnishing or discontinuing patient care whenever possible. A signed consent form must be in the patient's record prior to each surgery. CoP requires hospitals to develop policies that ensure each patient is informed of his or her rights in language that the patient understands (e.g., hospital must provide interpretation for those who speak a language aside from English or, for other reasons, require alternative methods of communication). The policies must cover any state or federal regulation notice regarding patient rights, including the right to an advance directive and notice of noncoverage.

KEY POINT

Most health care facilities now use a digital version of the patient's paper chart, called an electronic health record (EHR). An EHR contains the patient's medical history, diagnosis, and treatment history, including allergies, immunization records, and radiology and laboratory test results. These can be shared by various providers involved with the patient's care across a health care organization or even outside the organization.

KEY POINT

An operative progress note summarizing each procedure performed must be included in the patient record.

A technical description should be documented to aid in code selection, especially when eponyms are used.

Those who are authorized to make entries in the medical record should use only those abbreviations approved by the provider/facility. This aids in consistency and allows coders and others to correctly interpret the records.

Inpatient

The section devoted to inpatient admissions should be organized by episode of care usually filed in chronological order. Some hospitals actually file in reverse chronological order, so it is important to make sure of the facility's policy on chart organization. Information from the individual encounters should be grouped together. Documentation for each surgical encounter should include the following:

- Clinical data:
    - for each episode of care should include dates of admission and discharge, medical history to establish a diagnosis for the basis of treatment, physical exam, records of medications, physician orders, clinical assessments, and ancillary reports (e.g., pathology, radiology)
- Preoperative diagnosis:
    - not always required, but serves as a quick reference when documenting the procedure
- Anesthesia:
    - preanesthesia evaluations
    - postanesthesia evaluations
- Joint Commission requires at least one postanesthesia report describing any anesthesia-related complication:
    - reasons for terminating surgery prior to or after administering anesthesia, when applicable
- Operative session
- Findings, organs examined, sutures, packing, duration, and time of completion
- Blood transfusions/IV infusions
- Complications
- Recovery:
    - patient condition upon arrival and transfer from the recovery room
- Nursing data:
    - objective information such as amount of fluids taken and subjective data regarding the patient's response to therapy

The primary surgeon is responsible for any documentation regarding the findings, the procedures used, biopsy (if any), and the postoperative diagnosis. Any assistants participating in the surgery should be listed in addition to the primary surgeon.

The operative progress note summarizing each procedure must be included in the patient record. If eponyms are used, a technical description should be documented to aid in the selection of the ICD-10-CM diagnosis or ICD-10-PCS procedure codes. In addition to the basic elements, the summary should contain the following items:

- Pre- and postoperative diagnoses
- Title of procedure
- Surgeon, cosurgeon, assistant surgeon
- Anesthetic and anesthesiologist

- Summary of procedure

- Complications and unusual services

- Immediate postoperative condition

- Estimate of blood loss and replacement

- Fluids given and invasive tubes, drains, and catheters used

- Hardware or foreign bodies intentionally left in the operative site

While all elements may not be necessary, the importance of each element increases with the complexity of the procedure. For example, a biopsy does not require the same level of detail as an open laparotomy procedure.

Each clinical event should be documented as soon as possible after its occurrence. The records of discharged patients must be completed within 30 days following discharge.

Outpatient

Documentation of operations and procedures performed in outpatient hospitals, short-stay surgery facilities, physician offices, and group practices generally follow the requirements of accrediting agencies and site specific internal guidelines. Major differences may be found in the type of forms used to document the information and the type of information required by each facility.

Accuracy

The importance of the accuracy of documentation cannot be overstated.

Documentation is the foundation for reimbursement and its accuracy can make and sustain decisions in cases of appeal. Inadequate documentation leads to improper reimbursement and inconsistent determinations, delays in the appeals process, and reversals at higher appellate levels. The elements of accuracy in the operative report include:

- Approved abbreviations understood by anyone authorized to make entries in the record and the coders and others required to interpret the records

- Legibility

- Proper correction of errors—standard is a line through the error and the note "wrong record" followed by the recording of the correct information

- Explanations for accidental omissions and out-of-sequence data

SUMMARY

Documentation has evolved into an extensive set of guidelines. Again, a chart that is comprehensive, well organized, and accurate enables the physician and other health care professionals to quickly access needed information and is essential in providing quality patient care. All services and procedures a patient receives must be documented. The documentation is used to provide patient care, communicate between providers, and support the treatment or service billed to the payer or payers.

Chapter 3: Coding

It is a reality in today's modern medical science that the codes within ICD-9-CM fall short of our ever-changing medical reporting needs. The ninth revision of the International Classification of Diseases (ICD) was released more than 30 years ago as a modern and expansive system that was then only partially filled. Thousands of codes have been added to ICD-9-CM to classify new procedures and diseases over the years, and today the remaining space in ICD-9-CM procedure and diagnosis coding systems cannot accommodate our new technologies or our new understanding of diseases. An overhaul of our coding systems was needed.

Through the World Health Organization (WHO), ICD-10 was created and adopted in 1994. This is the system upon which the 10th revision of ICD that is used as the U.S. diagnosis coding system (ICD-10-CM) is based. Concurrent to the clinical modification of ICD-10 by the National Center for Health Statistics (NCHS), the Centers for Medicare and Medicaid Services (CMS) commissioned 3M Health Information Systems to develop a new procedure coding system to replace volume 3 of ICD-9-CM, used for inpatient procedure coding.

After the coding systems were drafted and modified, they needed only to be implemented; but progress was slow. The government was moving cautiously toward implementation, partly because: (1) the medical reimbursement industry has been adjusting to the impact of the Health Insurance Portability and Accountability Act (HIPAA) of 1996; (2) the scope of change is massive and will have a profound effect upon all care providers, payers, and government agencies; and (3) the change is big enough and costly enough to carry considerable political impact.

Two important events occurred late in 2002 that affected ICD-10-CM and ICD-10-PCS and their implementation. First, a subcommittee on coding for the National Committee on Vital and Health Statistics (NCVHS) forwarded a recommendation to the full committee that ICD-10-CM and ICD-10-PCS be adopted by the secretary of Health and Human Services (HHS). ICD-10-CM and ICD-10-PCS took one step closer to national rule making, which opened up a formal public comment period. The second event was the posting of a near-final draft of ICD-10-CM on the CMS website. While an earlier draft included only the tabular section of ICD-10-CM, the 2002 draft included the index as well.

In June 2003, NCHS posted a pre-release draft of ICD-10-CM on the NCHS website. That pre-release draft contained both index and tabular sections and a table of drugs and chemicals, which could be downloaded from the NCHS website. Since that time, Optum360 has published updated versions of the complete text.

On August 22, 2008, HHS published a notice of proposed rule making (NPRM) to adopt the ICD-10 coding systems (ICD-10-CM and ICD-10-PCS) to replace ICD-9-CM in transactions under HIPAA.

Proposed rule NPRM CMS-0013-P called for updated versions of HIPAA electronic transaction standards. Specifically, the rule urged adoption of version 5010 to facilitate electronic health care transactions to accommodate the ICD-10 code sets. This NPRM also proposed implementing ICD-10-CM for diagnosis coding and ICD-10-PCS for inpatient hospital procedure coding, effective October 1,

 DEFINITIONS

CMS. Centers for Medicare and Medicaid Services. Federal agency that administers the public health programs.

NCHS. National Center for Health Statistics. Division of the Centers for Disease Control and Prevention that compiles statistical information used to guide actions and policies to improve the public health of U.S. citizens. The NCHS maintains the ICD-9-CM diagnosis coding system.

WHO. World Health Organization. International agency comprising UN members to promote the physical, mental, and emotional health of the people of the world and to track morbidity and mortality statistics worldwide. WHO maintains the International Classification of Diseases (ICD) medical code set.

2011. The comment period for this proposed rule was closed on October 21, 2008.

On January 16, 2009, HHS published a final rule in the *Federal Register*, 45 CFR, part 162, "HIPAA Administrative Simplification: Modifications to Medical Data Code Set Standards to Adopt ICD-10-CM and ICD-10-PCS." This rule may be downloaded at http://edocket.access.gpo.gov/2009/pdf/E9-743.pdf.

This final rule adopted modifications to standard medical data code sets for coding diagnoses and inpatient hospital procedures by adopting ICD-10-CM for diagnosis coding, including the *ICD-10-CM Official Guidelines for Coding and Reporting*, and ICD-10-PCS for inpatient hospital procedure coding, effective October 1, 2013. In August 2012 CMS released a final rule to extend the implementation date by a year, to October 1, 2014.

On April 1, 2014, the Protecting Access to Medicare Act of 2014 (PAMA) (Pub. L. 113-93) was enacted with a provision stipulating that the secretary of the Department of Health and Human Services could not adopt ICD-10 prior to October 1, 2015.

HHS issued an interim final rule on August 4, 2014, finalizing October 1, 2015, as the new ICD-10 compliance date. This rule will also require HIPAA covered entities to continue to use ICD-9-CM through September 30, 2015. This interim final rule may be viewed at http://www.gpo.gov/fdsys/pkg/FR-2014-08-04/pdf/2014-18347.pdf.

A successful transition from ICD-9-CM to the ICD-10 coding systems will require focused training for individuals and organizations. The first step in transitioning to the new coding system is to develop a firm foundation in understanding the coding conventions and guidelines in ICD-10 to prepare the medical office, practice, department, facility, or organization for the significant changes that the new coding system will bring. Nearly everyone will be affected: human resources staff, accountants, information systems staff, physicians—just to name a few. ICD-10 provides tremendous opportunities for disease and procedure tracking, but also creates enormous challenges.

 KEY POINT

NCHS is responsible for developing the diagnostic portion of the ICD-10 coding system, ICD-10-CM. CMS is responsible for developing the procedure portion of the ICD-10 coding system, ICD-10-PCS.

HISTORY OF MODIFICATIONS TO ICD

The original intent of the World Health Organization for ICD was as a statistical tool for the international exchange of mortality data. A subsequent revision was expanded to accommodate data collection for morbidity statistics. An eventual seventh revision, published by WHO in 1955, was clinically modified for use in the United States based upon a joint study on the efficiency of hospital diseases indexing by the American Hospital Association (AHA) and the American Association of Medical Record Librarians (AAMRL). Results of that study led to the 1959 publication of the *International Classification of Diseases, Adapted for Indexing Hospital Records (ICDA)*, by the federal Public Health Service. The ICDA uniformly modified ICD-7, and it gave the United States a way to classify operations and treatments.

Hospitals were initially slow in their acceptance of ICDA, though momentum picked up. An eighth edition of ICD, published by WHO in 1965, initially lacked the depth of clinical data required for America's emerging health care system. In 1968, two widely accepted modifications were published in the United States: the Eighth Revision International Classification of Diseases, Adapted (ICDA-8), and the Hospital Adaptation of ICDA (H-ICDA). Hospitals used either of these two systems through the latter years of the next decade.

ICD-9 and ICD-9-CM

The ninth revision by WHO in 1975 prompted the typical American response: clinical modification. This time, the impetus flowed from a process initiated in 1977 by NCHS to modify ICD-9 for hospital indexing and retrieving case data for clinical studies. The NCHS and the newly created Council on Clinical Classifications modified ICD-9 according to U.S. clinical standard, and developed a companion procedural classification. This classification, published as volume 3 of ICD-9-CM, revised a portion of WHO's International Classification of Procedure Modification (ICPM). In 1978, the three-volume set was published in the United States for use one year later. There were no further changes in the direction to ICD-9-CM until the October 1983 implementation of diagnosis related groups (DRG), which gave ICD-9-CM a new significance. After more than 30 years since ICD's arrival in the United States, the classification system proves indispensable to hospitals interested in payment schedules for health care services.

ICD-10-CM

The evolution of ICD took another turn in 1994 when WHO published ICD-10. Again, the NCHS wanted to modify the latest revision, but with an emphasis on problems that had been identified in the current ICD-9-CM and resolved by the improvements to ICD-10 for classifying mortality and morbidity data. The Center for Health Policy Studies (CHPS) was awarded the NCHS contract to analyze ICD-10 and to develop the appropriate clinical modifications.

Phase I provided the analysis for clinical modification. According to CHPS, ICD-10 had to be modified to do the following:

- Return the level of specificity found in ICD-9-CM

- Facilitate an alphabetic index to assign codes

- Provide code titles and language that complement accepted clinical practice

- Remove codes unique to mortality coding

Phase II followed protocol. CHPS developed modifications based on the analysis, including the following:

- Increasing the five-character structure to six (eventually seven) characters

- Incorporating common fourth-, fifth-, and eventually sixth-digit subclassifications

- Creating laterality

- Combining certain codes

- Adding trimesters to obstetric codes

- Creating combined diagnosis/symptoms codes

- Deactivating procedure codes

Also, in the second phase, CHPS expanded the codes for alcohol/drug abuse, diabetes mellitus, and injuries.

A draft of ICD-10-CM for public comment was released at the conclusion of phase II. Since that time, the drafts have been revised and updated concurrent with the

KEY POINT

WHO's seventh edition of ICD was the first edition modified by the United States. Two versions of a modified ICD-8 were published in 1968. A procedure classification was created by the U.S. government and accompanied the clinical modification of ICD-9, which was published in 1978.

DEFINITIONS

morbidity. Diseased condition or state.

mortality. Condition of being mortal (subject to death).

changes in ICD-9-CM, and to accommodate classification needs as they have been identified. The final version was based on an analysis of the comments by NCHS and phase III reviewers.

ICD-10-PCS

The original ICD-9-CM, volume 3, was developed in the mid-1970s when the National Center for Health Statistics (NCHS) and the Council on Clinical Classifications modified the World Health Organization (WHO) version of ICD-9 according to the U.S. clinical standard. As a part of that work, a companion procedure classification (volume 3) was developed. Since that time, the Centers for Medicare and Medicaid Services (CMS) has been responsible for updating and maintaining the ICD-9-CM procedure system. In place since 1979, the system is inadequate to keep up with 30 years of technical advances and the corresponding need for new codes. This is increasingly important when assessing and tracking the quality of medical processes and outcomes, and compiling statistics that are valuable tools for research. ICD-10-PCS has unique, precise codes to differentiate body parts, surgical approaches, and devices used. It can be used to identify resource consumption differences and outcomes for different procedures, and describes precisely what was done to the patient.

REGULATORY PROCESS

This section outlines the regulatory process as defined by HIPAA for adoption of a new standard code set. Recently, legislation has been introduced in both houses of Congress that address national health information issues. A few bills that have been introduced include provisions for adopting ICD-10. Both the House and Senate must approve legislation before the bill advances to the president for signature. The inclusion of ICD-10 adoption provisions within current legislation is separate from the process outlined in HIPAA. Should a bill pass both the House and Senate and be signed by the president, the regulatory process outlined here must still take place.

Background

On Wednesday, November 5, 2003, the National Committee on Vital and Health Statistics (NCVHS) voted to recommend that the secretary of HHS take steps toward national adoption of ICD-10-CM and ICD-10-PCS as replacements under HIPAA standards for the current uses of ICD-9-CM, volumes 1, 2, and 3.

Administrative Simplification

Congress addressed the need for a consistent framework for electronic transactions and other administrative simplification issues in HIPAA, which became part of the Social Security Act titled "Administrative Simplification." Sections 1171 through 1179 require any standard adopted by the secretary of HHS (including the standard code sets):

- To be developed, adopted, or modified by a standard-setting organization

- To adopt code standards applicable to health plans, health care clearinghouses, and health care providers who transmit any health information in electronic form

- To adopt transaction standards and data elements for the electronic exchange of health information for certain health care transactions

 KEY POINT

The following websites post updated versions of the ICD-10-CM code set, guidelines, and mappings:

- The 2016 release of ICD-10-CM is available on the NCHS website at: http://www.cdc.gov/nchs/icd/icd10cm.htm.

- The 2016 release of ICD-10-PCS is available on the CMS website at: https://www.cms.gov/Medicare/Coding/ICD10/2016-ICD-10-PCS-and-GEMs.html.

- To ensure that procedures exist for the routine maintenance, testing, enhancement, and expansion of code sets

- To set a compliance date not later than 24 months after the date on which an initial standard or implementation specification is adopted for all covered entities except small health plans

The transactions and code sets final rule (2000) adopted a number of standard medical data code sets for use in those transactions, including:

- ICD-9-CM, volumes 1 and 2, for coding and reporting diseases, injuries, impairments, other health problems and their manifestations, and causes of injury, disease, impairment, or other health problems

- ICD-9-CM, volume 3, for the following procedures reported by hospitals: prevention, diagnosis, treatment, and management

- CPT codes for physician services and all other health care services

- HCPCS codes for other substances, equipment, supplies, and other items used in health care

The rule also included adoption of a procedure for maintaining existing standards, adopting modifications to existing standards, and adopting new standards.

Process

The committee formulated a letter of recommendation requesting that the secretary of HHS initiate the regulatory process for the concurrent national adoption of the two classification systems with an implementation period of at least two years following issuance of a final rule.

The NCVHS recommendation was the first step of the regulatory process. The next step was the acceptance of the recommendation by the secretary of Health and Human Services. In the meantime, American Health Information Management Association (AHIMA) had urged the secretary to issue a notice of proposed rule making (NPRM).

On August 22, 2008, the NPRM was published in the *Federal Register* with a proposed implementation date of October 1 of 2011. A two-year implementation period after establishment of the final rule is required under the HIPAA two-year window for compliance.

The comment period for the NPRM closed on October 21, 2008. However, a final rule was not published at that time.

Upon publishing the ICD-10 and version 5010/NCPDP[1] version D.0 (electronic transaction standards) final rules, both CMS and the industry will begin documenting the requirements for both ICD-10 and version 5010 system changes, initiate and/or complete any gap analyses, and then undertake design and system changes. Version 5010 is progressing first, based on the need to have this transaction standard in place prior to ICD-10 implementation to accommodate the increase in the size of the fields for the ICD-10 code sets.

---

1. National Council for Prescription Drug Programs

In the United States, the clinical modification of the code set is maintained by the ICD-10-CM Coordination and Maintenance Committee (NCHS, CMS, AHA, and AHIMA). However, the code set standard is approved by legislative process.

The administrative simplification provision of HIPAA encourages the development of health care information systems by establishing standards, including code sets for each data element for health care services. HIPAA requires the secretary of HHS to adopt the code set standards. The secretary then tasked the NCVHS with studying and recommending the standard code sets. These impact studies have been completed, and reports have been made to Congress and HHS.

In summary, the necessary steps to implementation include:

1. Development of recommendations for standards to be adopted by HHS/NCVHS (November 2003)

2. Publication of the proposed rule in the *Federal Register* with a 60-day public comment period (August 2008)

3. Analysis of the public comments and publication of the final rule in the *Federal Register* with the effective date of the rule being 60 days after publication (October 2008)

4. Distribution of standards and coordinated preparation and distribution of implementation guidelines and crosswalks. Implementation is 24 months from the effective date, excluding small health plans (fewer than 50 participants), which have 36 months to comply.

Step 1 of this process ended up lasting until 2008. Cost/benefit analyses were performed. According to the regulatory process, implementation was no sooner · than October 1, 2009. However, the NPRM was not released before May 1, 2007, making the 2009 implementation date impossible.

On August 22, 2008, HHS published an NPRM to adopt the ICD-10 coding systems (ICD-10-CM and ICD-10-PCS) to replace ICD-9-CM in HIPAA transactions.

Proposed rule NPRM CMS-0013-P called for updated versions of HIPAA electronic transaction standards. Specifically, the rule urged adoption of version 5010 to facilitate electronic health care transactions to accommodate the ICD-10 code sets. This NPRM also proposed implementing ICD-10-CM for diagnosis coding and ICD-10-PCS for inpatient hospital procedure coding, effective October 1, 2011. The comment period for this proposed rule was closed on October 21, 2008.

On January 16, 2009, HHS published a final rule in the *Federal Register*, 45 CFR, part 162, "HIPAA Administrative Simplification: Modifications to Medical Data Code Set Standards to Adopt ICD-10-CM and ICD-10-PCS." This final rule adopts modifications to standard medical data code sets for coding diagnoses and inpatient hospital procedures by adopting ICD-10-CM for diagnosis coding, including the "ICD-10-CM Official Guidelines for Coding and Reporting," and ICD-10-PCS for inpatient hospital procedure coding, effective October 1, 2013.

On August 24, 2012, HHS published a final rule to delay the implementation date of ICD-10 until October 1, 2014.

On April 2, 2014, Congress enacted the Protecting Access to Medicare Act of 2014, which contained a provision to delay the implementation of ICD-10

CM/PCS by at least a year. The act prohibited HHS from adopting the ICD-10 CM/PCS code sets as the mandatory standard until at least October 1, 2015.

HHS subsequently issued an interim final rule on August 4, 2014, finalizing October 1, 2015, as the new ICD-10 compliance date.

DOCUMENTATION

The ICD-10 classification and coding systems are constructed with future reporting needs in mind. Their architecture has been constructed on a grand scale. The documentation principles and concepts apply to documentation considerations created by the impact of both systems. There are thousands more codes in the ICD-10 coding systems than in ICD-9.

This greater level of detail, called "granularity," is good news for the nosologists and government researchers tracking disease in the United States. Do not underestimate the importance of this work; their statistics help drive health care reform, research, payment systems, and social programs. The granularity of ICD-10 does indeed provide benefits for everyone in our society.

DOCUMENTATION NEEDS

ICD-10 poses certain significant challenges to coders in both physician and facility settings.

As additional detail is to be reported with ICD-10, more detail will be required in the medical records from which the data for coding are extracted. For coders who are already facing these challenges on a daily basis, the increased specificity required to report ICD-10 may seem daunting.

The data granularity of ICD-10 in comparison to ICD-9-CM requires education of medical staff members in order to ensure adequate documentation from which to assign appropriately descriptive codes. Documentation improvement audits are useful tools in determining the need for improvement. Focused in-services that address changes in the coding components and documentation requirements for conditions often encountered within certain specialties may prove to be an effective method of ensuring that provider documentation meets the demands of the ICD-10 system.

 DEFINITIONS

data granularity. Degree or detail contained in data; the fineness in which data fields are subdivided.

nosologist. One who studies the classification of diseases.

DOCUMENTATION AND THE REIMBURSEMENT PROCESS

Documentation plays an integral role in the reimbursement process. Without it, bottlenecks that delay billing and payment can ensue.

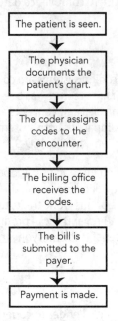

The resulting blockage occurs because of the increased granularity and documentation requirements of ICD-10 and is most likely to happen in the early steps of the process. The coder will be the first to recognize that important information is missing. A query is then generated for the doctor in order to gather more information. The doctor must then ensure that the necessary information is included in the medical record before the coding piece of the process can proceed.

It is therefore essential to disseminate information about ICD-10 granularity and the accompanying documentation requirements. By studying the differences in coding components and adjusting documentation habits now, future paperwork hurdles can be minimized.

A certain amount of "documentation chasing" is a normal expectation within the course of business; however, billing delays during the implementation phase of ICD-10 will not remain a constant. As the learning curve is conquered, the time spent on these steps should return to the usual, pre-implementation operating levels.

ADVANTAGES OF ICD-10 WITHIN THE REIMBURSEMENT PROCESS

There are also some definite advantages to using ICD-10 within the reimbursement cycle that occur at the coding stage and beyond. The data granularity of the classification system is likely to reduce time associated with the manual process of choosing the most appropriate codes. Coders are also much more likely to choose the correct code on the first attempt, since there is much less ambiguity in ICD-10. For payers, the clarity afforded by the ICD-10 coding system is likely to greatly enhance and assist in supporting medical necessity.

☞ KEY POINT

Providers should start by auditing their medical records to assess whether current documentation practices will support the level of detail required to code in the new systems. Provide medical staff with examples of where their current practices fall short, and inform them of the resultant backlogs in the deficiency process and revenue cycles.

With ICD-10, the diagnosis gives a more complete description of the condition, thereby leaving less room for denials.

Increased Granularity

The primary reason for creating a coding system that assigns a number to the diagnosis or condition is simply to record and retrieve information in an efficient way. One of the main purposes we use this for is—and always has been—to gather data for research and statistics.

Nosologists, medical researchers, and epidemiologists are constantly tracking disease in the United States based on the coded data. A coding system for documenting and reporting cases allows the researchers, the statisticians, and the epidemiologists to gather the information upon which many important health care decisions are made. As such, the integrity of statistics and research findings are extremely important. Data drives health care reform, supports decisions regarding most effective and appropriate treatments, determines which clinical research endeavors to pursue, and aids in structuring and funding social programs concerned with health and well-being.

Data affects outcomes. Good data can help change the health care delivery system for the better. Coders are literally building the database that drives our future every time they choose the codes that are used for painting our statistical pictures and conducting research.

The increased granularity, or in other words, the greater level of detail afforded by ICD-10 provides the quality data needed to support improved clinical outcomes and more cost-effective disease management.

Chapter 4: Reimbursement

MEDICARE

CMS administers Medicare, a federal health insurance program for people 65 years or older, people with certain disabilities, and those with permanent kidney failure treated with dialysis or a transplant. Medicare has four parts—Part A for hospital insurance, Part B for medical insurance, Part C Medicare Advantage for managed care/HMO programs, and Part D for prescription drug coverage effective January 1, 2006.

Part A

Part A payment covers all nonphysician services delivered to an inpatient of a hospital (except pneumococcal vaccine and its administration and hepatitis B vaccine and its administration). Part A is available to anyone meeting eligibility requirements who has worked at least 10 years in Medicare covered employment.

Factors considered when admitting patients include:

- Severity of the signs and symptoms exhibited by the patient

- Medical predictability of something adverse happening to the patient

- Need for diagnostic studies that appropriately are outpatient services (e.g., their performance does not ordinarily require the patient to remain at the hospital for 24 hours or more) to assist in assessing whether the patient should be admitted

- Availability of diagnostic procedures at the time when and at the location where the patient presents

- Admissions of particular patients are not covered or noncovered solely on the basis of the length of time the patient actually spends in the hospital

The CMS internet-only manuals (IOM), Pub 100-4, chapters 3 and 4, cover payment of inpatient hospital services and is available online at http://www.cms.gov/Regulations-and-Guidance/Guidance/Manuals/Internet-Only-Manuals-IOMs-Items/CMS018912.html.

Part B

Medicare Part B helps pay for physician services, outpatient hospital care, blood, medical equipment and some home health services. Part B also pays for other medical services such as lab tests and physical and occupational therapy. Some preventive services such as mammograms and flu shots are also covered.

Medicare Part B covers hospital inpatient services, but only if payment cannot be made under Part A (e.g., the patient has exhausted Part A coverage) and the patient is entitled to Part B benefits. The services covered under Part B are:

- Diagnostic x-ray tests, diagnostic laboratory tests, and other diagnostic tests

- X-ray, radium, and radioactive isotope therapy, including materials and services of technicians

 DEFINITIONS

medical necessity. Medically appropriate and necessary to meet basic health needs; consistent with the diagnosis or condition and rendered in a cost-effective manner; consistent with national medical practice guidelines regarding type, frequency, and duration of treatment.

 KEY POINT

Part B covers the following hospital inpatient services, regardless of the beneficiary's eligibility for Part A coverage:

- Physicians' services
- Pneumococcal vaccine and its administration
- Hepatitis B vaccine and its administration

However, Medicare (Part A or Part B) requires that any nonphysician service for a hospital inpatient must be provided directly or arranged for by the hospital.

- Surgical dressings, and splints, casts, and other devices used for reduction of fractures and dislocations

- Prosthetic devices (other than dental) which replace all or part of an internal body organ (including contiguous tissue), or all or part of the function of a permanently inoperative or malfunctioning internal body organ, including replacement or repairs of such devices

- Leg, arm, back, and neck braces, trusses, and artificial legs, arms, and eyes, including adjustments, repairs, and replacements required because of breakage, wear, loss, or a change in the patient's physical condition

- Outpatient physical therapy, outpatient occupational therapy, and outpatient speech pathology services

- Ambulance services

Part C

Medicare Part C, or Medicare Advantage, was developed as part of the Balanced Budget Act of 1997 and provides an alternative for Medicare beneficiaries. These HMO/managed care plans provide lower-cost health care that is especially attractive to low-income beneficiaries. A beneficiary must be eligible for Part A and be enrolled in Part B to be eligible to switch to Part C coverage. Part C offers more benefits and lower out-of-pocket costs than Part A and B. For many plans there is low or no monthly premium to be covered by Medicare Advantage. For beneficiaries with a Medicare Advantage plan, the facility and physician components are still determined and reported using the same coding systems and billing documents as Part A and Part B.

Part D

Medicare Part D, known as the prescription drug coverage plan, became effective January 2006. This program has a great impact on the individual beneficiary. Providers must be familiar with the basics of the Part D program. However, this plan varies in cost of the individual medications from payer to payer, and beneficiaries should carefully consider all options before deciding which plan is best for them.

PAYMENT SYSTEMS

Inpatient

Medicare Severity-Diagnosis Related Groups

The Social Security Amendment of 1983 (Public Law 98-21) established the initial inpatient prospective payment system (IPPS) for hospital services provided to Medicare beneficiaries in short-term acute care facilities. Under the IPPS system, a hospital is paid a fixed amount for each patient discharged in a particular diagnosis or treatment category or diagnosis-related group (DRG). This fixed amount is intended to cover the cost of treating a typical patient for a particular DRG; the DRGs group patients with similar clinical conditions and similar treatments. To address the issue of clinical severity, CMS established new severity refined DRGs, called Medicare Severity-DRGs (MS-DRGs), in October 2007. These DRGs function in the same way as traditional CMS DRGs but comprise more than 750 groups and differentiate many more conditions based on severity of illness. In addition, the criteria used to designate diagnosis codes that are complications/comorbidities were completely revised.

The MS-DRG system relies on accurate diagnosis and procedure code assignment. Each case is assigned to a DRG. Each DRG has a relative weight assigned to it that is the same for all hospitals throughout the country and is updated each year. This relative weight is based on the complexity of the services expected to be required to treat that particular case. The DRG's relative weight is multiplied by the hospital's specific base rate, which is calculated based on several factors, including the wage index for that geographic area. The calculation of DRG relative weight times the hospital base rate determines the specific reimbursement rate for the case.

The DRG is determined by five variables:

1. The patient's principal diagnosis
2. The patient's secondary diagnoses, which include complication/comorbidities
3. Surgical and other invasive procedures
4. Sex of the patient
5. Discharge status

A hospital's Medicare population case complexity is measured by calculating the case-mix index, which is an average of all MS-DRG relative weights for the facility during a given period of time. The higher the case-mix index, the more complex the patient population and the higher the required level of resources used. Since severity is such an essential component of MS-DRG assignment and case-mix index calculation, documentation and code assignment to the highest degree of accuracy and specificity are of the utmost importance.

Review the following steps for accurate MS-DRG assignment:

Step 1
Assign the principal diagnosis based on the UHDDS definition: "That condition established after study to be chiefly responsible for occasioning the admission of the patient to the hospital for care." If the diagnosis documented at the time of discharge is qualified as "possible," "probable," "suspected," "likely," "questionable," "still to be ruled out," or other similar terms indicating uncertainty, code the condition as if it existed or was established.

Step 2
Assign diagnosis codes for secondary conditions, defined as those conditions that required: clinical evaluation, therapeutic treatment, diagnostic procedures, extended length of hospital stay, or increased nursing care and/or monitoring. Conditions that are designated as MCCs or CCs should be sequenced directly following the principal diagnosis.

Step 3
Assign procedure codes for all surgical procedures performed, as well as for other invasive procedures that may not have been performed in an operating room. For example, services provided in interventional radiology suites, cardiac catheterization rooms, or even provided at bedside may be designated as "valid non-OR procedures" and will affect MS-DRG assignment.

Step 4
Consider all required information (diagnosis and procedure codes, patient sex, and discharge status) when grouping the DRG. Note the medical diagnostic category (MDC) and MS-DRG initially grouped. Ensure that the MDC and MS-DRG

KEY POINT

Medicare Severity-DRGs, enacted in October 2007, improve by 9.41 percent the explanation of variance of hospital resources used over the previous version of DRGs.

KEY POINT

Under the MS-DRG system, physician documentation in the medical record must be specific because many chronic conditions are no longer designated as CCs. It is only when an acute exacerbation or an acute form of the disease process is documented and coded that the condition may be considered an MCC or CC and affect MS-DRG assignment.

match the type of case coded and that any case with a coded surgical procedure is assigned to a surgical MS-DRG.

Step 5

If the MS-DRG indicates "without CC/MCC," re-review the medical record to ensure that all conditions meeting the definition of secondary diagnosis have been coded appropriately. If any documentation is missing or ambiguous, query the physician for clarification.

Note: Steps 1 through 4 may be performed by software called a "grouper."

Outpatient

Hospitals provide two distinct types of services to outpatients:

- Services that are diagnostic in nature
- Services the physician requires to treat the patient

Both the diagnostic and the therapeutic services furnished by hospitals to outpatients are covered under Part B.

Medicare Physician Fee Schedule

The MPFS covers Part B services through the application of relative value units (RVUs) of the Resource Based Relative Value Scale (RBRVS). The relative value scale is a coded listing of procedures with unit values that indicate the relative value of the various services performed, taking into account the time, skill, and overhead cost required for each service. Each procedure (HCPCS Level I and II codes) provided by a physician is assigned an RVU. Each RVU is valued in terms of physician work, practice expense, and malpractice insurance. The initial physician work RVUs were produced from Harvard University studies under a cooperative agreement with CMS. Revisions and allocations for new codes have been made based upon the work required and recommendations from the Relative Value Update Committee (RUC). The practice expense and malpractice RVUs were developed by applying practice expense percentages to a base allowed charge for each service taken from historical Medicare charges. Practice expense and malpractice expense have been refined in recent years to reflect the actual cost of providing the services, including those provided in a hospital or other facility versus the physician's office.

Ambulatory Payment Classification

The Balanced Budget Act of 1997 changed Medicare outpatient reimbursement from a cost-based system to a PPS that pays hospitals specific rates for outpatient services. The PPS includes most hospital outpatient services and Medicare Part B services provided to hospital inpatients lacking Part A coverage. The physicians' fee schedule still applies to physical, occupational, and speech therapies; durable medical equipment; clinical diagnostic laboratory services; and nonimplantable orthotics and prosthetics.

Outpatient prospective payment system (OPPS) payments are based on the APC system, which divides all outpatient services into groups. The services within each group are clinically similar and require comparable resources. Each APC is assigned a relative payment weight based on the median cost of the services within the APC. The rates actually paid to hospitals vary, depending on the area's wage level. Some incidental items and services will be packaged into the APC payment for the services, including anesthesia, certain drugs, supplies, and recovery room and observation services. A hospital may furnish a number of

DEFINITIONS

Major Diagnostic Category (MDC). Classification of diagnoses typically grouped by body system. Used in diagnosis-related group (DRG) reimbursement.

services to a beneficiary on the same day and receive an APC payment for each service. The system went into effect on August 1, 2000. CMS final rule was published in the *Federal Register* on April 7, 2000 (65 FR 18434). Annual updates and changes are made to the OPPS and published in the *Federal Register*.

MEDICARE CLAIMS

All claims submitted to Medicare require diagnostic and procedure codes. Code selection is important since claims for certain services, especially when local policy has been established, may be denied due to the diagnosis.

The Administrative Simplification provision of the Health Insurance Portability and Accountability Act (HIPAA) requires that payers have the capability of receiving claims electronically to reduce costs and administrative functions of health care tracking and reimbursement. The provision applies to all payers and providers and affects all health claims and equivalent encounter information (professional, institutional, and dental). Health care providers, physicians, and suppliers of medical equipment must complete an Electronic Data Interchange (EDI) Enrollment Form prior to submitting claims electronically. Completed and signed EDI forms may be submitted to local carriers or fiscal intermediaries or regional contractors.

Hospital Claims

Inpatient and outpatient hospital claims are grouped into one of the DRGs or one or more of the APCs and submitted for reimbursement using electronic format 837i or paper form CMS-1450 (UB-04 claim form). The electronic format 837i includes all the fields from the CMS-1450 and was developed by a national Workgroup for Electronic Data Interchange (WEDI) that followed guidelines of the American National Standards Institutes (ANSI). The paper UB-04 is neither a government printed form nor distributed by CMS. The National Uniform Billing Committee is responsible for the form's design.

Other Outpatient Claims

Providers (non-institutional) and medical suppliers bill Medicare Part B covered services using the electronic format 837p or paper CMS-1500 form. It is used for billing several Medicaid covered services. The current version of CMS-1500 (08/05) was revised to accommodate the reporting of the National Provider Identifier (NPI). For Medicare claims, the 08-05 version must be submitted. Outpatient physician procedures are coded using HCPCS Level I (CPT) codes and Level II national codes. Follow CPT rules and append Medicare and CPT modifiers as appropriate.

SUMMARY

Medicare and other government and private health care plans pay only for services that are "reasonable and necessary." Upon request, a facility or provider office should be able to furnish medical record documentation, such as diagnostic information and operative reports or notes that support a service as being medically necessary.

It is important for the coder and biller to know the rules and guidelines for government payers and private payers. Although many private payers follow both Medicare and/or Medicaid guidelines, they may alter them to meet internal

 FOR MORE INFO

The CMS-1500 and the UB-04 are available online at:
http://www.cms.hhs.gov/CMSForms/

The website includes the forms and step-by-step instructions.

Medicare Contractors
Contact the U.S. Government Printing Office at (202) 512-1800 or your local Medicare contractor. For a list of local Medicare contractors, including their telephone number, go to http://www.cms.gov/medicare-cover age-database/indexes/contacts-contractor-websites-index.aspx

A copy of place of service (POS) codes is available at:
https://www.cms.gov/Medicare/ Coding/place-of-service-codes/ Place_of_Service_Code_Set.html.

An electronic data interchange (EDI) enrollment form that must be completed and signed prior to submitting a Medicare form is available at:
http://www.cms.gov/Medicare ProviderSupEnroll/.

guidelines. Private payers have different coverage guidelines and may pay for items not covered by government payers. It is also important to know which payers require electronic submission of claims and which request paper claims.

Chapter 5: Fraud and Abuse

The federal government and several of the states have laws governing health care claims. Physicians or facilities found in violation of the laws can be denied payment, banned from federal programs, or sued. In extreme cases, a physician may be charged with mail and wire fraud for mailing or filing the fraudulent claims.

FRAUD

Fraud is defined as an intentional false statement or representation of material facts made by a person to obtain some benefit or payment when none exists. Fraud may be committed either for the person's own benefit or for the benefit of some other party. It is necessary to prove that fraudulent acts were performed knowingly and willfully.

Examples of fraud include:

- Billing for services not furnished

- Soliciting, offering, or receiving a kickback, bribe, or rebate

- Violating the physician self-referral ("Stark") prohibition

- Using an incorrect provider identifier in order to be paid

- Selling, sharing, or purchasing Medicare Health Insurance Claim numbers in order to bill false claims to the Medicare program

- Offering incentives to Medicare patients that are not offered to other patients (e.g., routinely waiving or discounting Medicare deductibles, coinsurance, or copayments)

- Falsifying information on applications, certification forms, medical records, billing statements, cost reports, or on any statement filed with the government

- Using inappropriate procedure or diagnosis codes to misrepresent the medical necessity or coverage status of the services furnished

- Consistently using procedure codes that describe more extensive services than those actually performed (upcoding)

Four elements must be in place to prosecute for fraud. These elements are as follows:

- Intentionally misrepresents the truth about an important event or fact

- The misrepresentation is believed by the victim (the organization or person to whom the misrepresentation was made)

- The victim relies upon and acts upon misrepresentation

- The victim suffers loss of money and/or property as a result of relying upon and acting upon the misrepresentation

 DEFINITIONS

abuse. In medical reimbursement, an incident that is inconsistent with accepted medical, business, or fiscal practices and directly or indirectly results in unnecessary costs to the Medicare program, improper reimbursement, or reimbursement for services that do not meet professionally recognized standards of care or that are medically unnecessary.

fraud. Intentional deception or misrepresentation that is known to be false and could result in an unauthorized benefit. Fraud arises from a false statement or misrepresentation that affects payments under the Medicare program.

ABUSE

Abuse describes practices that, either directly or indirectly, result in unnecessary costs to the Medicare program. Abuse is similar to fraud except that in fraud cases it must be proven that acts were committed knowingly and willfully.

Examples of abuse include:

- Billing for services/items in excess of those needed by the patient
- Providing medically unnecessary services (lack of medical necessity documentation)
- Routinely filing duplicate claims (even if it does not result in duplicate payment)
- Collecting in excess of the deductible or coinsurance amounts due from a patient
- Unbundling or "exploding" charges (e.g., reporting a series of codes when there is one specific code that describes and includes payment for all components of the series of codes).

 DEFINITIONS

compliance program. A program put in place by a health care entity to protect itself from liability. Compliance programs are typically built upon the seven elements of a compliance program as detailed in the U.S. Sentencing Guidelines. By following these guidelines, the facility will not only help to protect itself from fraud, waste, and abuse, but also create a more efficient and effective work environment.

SANCTIONS

It is a crime to defraud the United States government. Those found guilty may be sent to prison, fined, or both. Criminal convictions usually include restitution and significant penalties. Civil monetary penalties (CMPs) can be as high as $10,000 per claim, and the government can collect three times the amount of actual damages caused by the defendant. A conviction can result in mandatory exclusion from federal and state health programs. In absence of a conviction the Office of Inspector General may exclude providers for other violations within the scope of those statutes designed to protect the Medicare program. A criminal conviction could result in exclusion from Medicare for a period of five years or more. A provider can be excluded for any of the actions listed as examples under the prior section defining "fraud."

COMPLIANCE

An established compliance program can minimize sanctions, penalties, and exclusions by showing a good faith attempt to detect and avoid misconduct within the organization. The AHA recently reported that 96 percent of surveyed hospitals either had a compliance program in effect or were planning to initiate one.

Compliance issues are important to the general good management of patients, as well as important for expedient and accurate reimbursement. When looking at compliance issues, consider current patient data, physician signatures, signed consent forms, Medicare limitation of liability waiver, and insurance forms.

Compliance Programs

The federal government's push to fight fraud and abuse in Medicare and Medicaid has prompted the development of compliance programs. Not only can a plan demonstrate mistakes are inadvertent, but a plan in place prior to any investigation may mitigate liability and help reduce any penalties. Components of a compliance plan include the following:

- Written standards of conduct and written policies and procedures that promote the physician and/or practice to compliance

- Designation of a chief compliance officer and/or a corporate compliance committee

- Development and implementation of educational and training programs for all employees involved in health care delivery and the reimbursement process

- Maintenance of a process to receive complaints (hotline), including the adoption of procedures to protect the anonymity of complainants and to protect whistleblowers from retaliation

- Investigation and correction of identified systemic problems and the development of policies addressing the non-employment or retention of sanctioned employees

- Development of a system to reply to allegations of improper or illegal activities and the enforcement of appropriate disciplinary action against employees who have violated internal compliance policies or governmental health care program regulations

- Monitoring of compliance by auditing and/or other examination methods to regulate compliance and reduce problems or potential problems

Office of Inspector General

Compliance Program for Hospitals

In February 1998, the OIG issued its "Compliance Program Guidance for Hospitals." According to the guidelines, with respect to reimbursement claims, a hospital's written policies and procedures must follow federal and state statutes and regulations regarding claims submission and Medicare cost reports. Policies and procedures should:

- Provide for proper and timely documentation of all physician and other professional services prior to billing to ensure that only accurate and properly documented services are billed

- Emphasize that claims must be submitted with documentation that supports the claims. Documentation, which may include patient records, must record the length of time spent in conducting the activity leading to the record entry, and the identity of the individual providing the service. The hospital should consult with its medical staff to establish other appropriate documentation guidelines

- State that, consistent with appropriate guidance from medical staff, physician and hospital records and medical notes used as a basis for a claim submission must be organized in a legible form so they can be audited and reviewed

- Indicate that the diagnosis and procedures reported on the reimbursement claim are based on the medical record and other documentation, and that the documentation necessary for accurate code assignment is available to coding staff

 KEY POINT

Following is an excerpt from the OIG letter published to announce the development of government compliance programs:

"...While compliance programs are not a novel idea, they are becoming increasingly popular as affirmative steps toward promoting a high level of ethical and lawful corporate conduct. Numerous providers have expressed interest in better protecting their operations from fraud through the adoption of compliance programs. Many companies already have a program or are in the process of developing one either in-house or with the assistance of outside consultants. When fraud is discovered, both the Department of Justice and my office look at the entity to see if reasonable efforts have been made by management to avoid and detect any misbehavior that occurs within their operations. We use this analysis to determine the level of sanctions, penalties and exclusions that will be imposed upon the provider. To my knowledge, this is the first time the government is revealing the elements upon which we base those judgments..."

- Show that compensation for coders and billing consultants does not give financial incentive to improperly upcoded claims

In addition, the guidelines recommend paying particular attention to issues of medical necessity, appropriate diagnosis codes, DRG coding, individual Medicare Part B claims (including evaluation and management coding) and the use of patient discharge status codes.

The OIG released "Supplemental Compliance Program Guidance for Hospitals" in January 2005. These additional guidelines emphasize additional areas of concern. They also reference the penalties associated with incorrect billing and failure to follow a compliance plan.

- Submission of accurate claims and information must be complete, accurate, and reflect reasonable and necessary services. Hospitals are also required to disclose and return overpayments from claims submission errors. Particularly important are:
  - outpatient procedure coding and the outpatient prospective payment system (OPPS)
  - admissions and discharges, billing for the patient status correctly
  - supplemental payment considerations
  - use of information technology as sources of errors such as submitting duplicate claims, outdated charge description masters (CDMs), circumventing multiple procedure discounting rules
- Referral statutes, the physician self-referral law, antikickback statute, and compensation arrangements with physicians
- Payments to reduce or limit services, gainsharing arrangements
- Emergency Medical Treatment and Labor Act (EMTALA)
- Substandard care including supplies and other services
- Relationships with federal health care beneficiaries such as patient copay waivers or reimbursement to the beneficiary, gifts, transportation services
- HIPAA privacy and security rules
- Billing substantially higher than usual charges
- Areas of general interest:
  - discounts to uninsured patients
  - preventive care services
  - professional courtesy, including insurance-only billing

Draft Compliance Plan for Individual and Small Group Physician Practices

The draft compliance program guidance for individual and small group physician practices contains seven elements the OIG has determined are fundamental to an effective compliance program. The elements are not mandatory or binding, nor does the guidance plan exclude internal requirements particular to the individual and small group physician practice.

Seven elements are recommended:

1. Implementing written policies that include:
   - Code of conduct that establishes the practice's expectations with respect to billing and coding, patient care, documentation, and payer relationships
   - Policies and procedures to prevent fraudulent or erroneous conduct in their practices. The OIG has developed a list of potential risk areas affecting physician providers. These risk areas include: (a) coding and billing; (b) reasonable and necessary services; (c) documentation and (d) improper inducements, kickbacks and self-referrals.

2. Designating a compliance officer/contact

3. Conducting comprehensive training and education

4. Developing accessible lines of communication

5. Conducting internal monitoring and auditing

6. Enforcing standards through well-publicized disciplinary guidelines

7. Responding promptly to detected offenses and undertaking corrective action

The OIG recommends, as a first step, a good faith commitment to compliance. Smaller practices should consider addressing each of the elements in a manner that best suits the practice. By contrast, larger practices should address the elements in a more systematic manner. For example, larger practices can use both this guidance and the "Third-Party Medical Billing Compliance Program Guidance" to create a compliance program unique to the practice.

The OIG does consider an effective compliance program that pre-dates any governmental investigation when addressing administrative sanctions. However, the burden is on the physician practice to demonstrate the effectiveness of the compliance program. In addition, an effective compliance plan in place at the time of the criminal offense may mitigate criminal sanctions.

Compliance Program Guidance for Third-Party Medical Billing Companies

Billing companies have become a vital piece of national health care. Providers rely on them to submit claims in accordance with state and federal guidelines. In addition, practices are turning to third-party billing companies for guidance on insurance reimbursement, contracting, and credentialing, as well as overall business decision making.

The compliance program elements proposed by the OIG in December 1998 are similar to those of the clinical laboratory model compliance program and the hospital compliance program. These elements offer guidance that can be modified to fit the needs and financial aspects of a specific billing company, regardless of size and services provided. The seven elements recommended include:

1. Written standards of conduct and written policies and procedures

   Code of conduct to include a commitment to compliance by managers and employees with respect to billing and coding, claims submission processes, code gaming, and financial incentives with providers.

2. Designation of a compliance officer or committee

   This individual or group must report directly to the governing body of the billing company and is charged with operating and monitoring the compliance program

3. Education and training programs for all employees

4. Hotline or process to receive complaints and a procedure to protect anonymity

5. System of enforcement and disciplinary action for violators

6. Implementation of audits and/or risk reduction techniques

7. Process for correcting systemic problems and policies addressing nonemployment of sanctioned individuals

SUMMARY

Fraud and abuse in the medical community have been the focus of government investigation and even news headlines. This has resulted in emphasis on being compliant with the federal and local guidelines. All health care service providers, from facility and physician to coder and biller, are responsible for being compliant. Correctly coding and billing for services and procedures will ensure compliance and is a safeguard against charges of fraud and abuse.

Chapter 6:
Operative Report Coding

As part of the medical record, the operative report plays many roles in the overall scheme of health care. The chief role of the operative report is for the current and continuing care of inpatient services. The operative report may also be used for the billing and reporting of services to the government and other payers and to track information for studies and statistics.

For documented services to be readily available for various health care, financial, and other needs, someone—usually a coder—must change the written word into a more user-friendly system. The coder converts the written word into numeric and alphanumeric codes that can be entered and later retrieved from computers and their associated databases.

It is in this modifying of data that the medical records coder has become an integral part of today's health care environment. Information incorporated into codes must be accurate if it is to be used by health care entities. Because codes are also used for reimbursement accuracy, coding is indispensable to the operation and continued fiscal health of a hospital, surgery center, or physician's practice.

In all coding and coding systems, there are many different facets that come into play. Accurate coding is of premier importance. However, to accurately code for operative and procedural services it is necessary to understand other issues, such as how the reports are organized, the forms that are used, and the documentation required (see the documentation chapter). A coder must also know how to code from the operative report by extracting the information necessary to code a service. Required skills include the following:

- Being able to understand names and terms used in operative reports
- Retrieving information from documentation in the operative report
- Identifying underdocumented or incorrect information (and knowing where to find the correct information)
- Understanding code selection (simplifying the search)
- Knowing when to seek clarification or additional information from the physician

NAMES AND TERMS THAT DESCRIBE OPERATIVE REPORTS

The first step in coding from an operative report is understanding the various names that are used to define the documentation recorded for a surgical or treatment session. The operative report and the operative progress, procedure, and treatment note contain both diagnostic and procedural information. Generally, the terms fall into the following categories:

- Operative report
- Operative or procedure progress note
- Treatment report or note

Operative Report

An operative report is a formal way of presenting detailed information about what occurred and what procedures were performed for a patient in the operating room.

A formal operative report generally includes four distinct elements:

1. Heading

The section heading summarizes the operative encounter. The heading includes:

- Facility specific information
- Patient specific information
- Date of operation or surgery
- Operation specific information
- Operation(s) or procedure(s) performed

Depending on the type of operation and the course of surgery, other information may be listed in the heading such as:

- Hardware
- Component
- Grafts
- Complications
- Drains
- Tourniquet time
- Other material left in place (e.g., mesh)

Facility Specific Information

Hospital specific information lists:

- Name of the facility
- Address of facility
- Patient's medical record or other number used to track the patient
- Admit date

Patient Specific Information

Patient specific information lists:

- Name
- Date of birth and/or age
- Sex

Date of Operation or Surgery

- E.g., 01/02/07

Diagnostic Information

- Preoperative diagnoses
- Postoperative diagnoses

KEY POINT

A formal operative report generally includes four distinct elements:

1. Heading
2. History or indication for surgery
3. Body (the operation(s)/ procedure(s) in detail)
4. Findings

KEY POINT

Standards of the requirements for operative report documentation and time frames are found in JCAHO standard manual IM.6.30, CMS CoP §482.51 (b) (6), facility accreditation standards, and federal and state licensure regulations and payer policies along with professional practice standards.

Operation Specific Information
- Attending surgeon*
- Cosurgeon*
- Resident surgeon*
- Surgery assistants*
- Anesthetic (e.g., general, regional, local)
- Anesthesiologist/CRNA/Provider of anesthesia
- Operating microscope
- Other special equipment or robotics
- Complications
- Estimated blood loss

Responsibility for documentation by the surgeon, cosurgeon, resident, or assistant-at-surgery

All surgeons involved with the procedure should be listed, including the primary surgeon and any cosurgeons and assistant surgeons. For surgical procedures with more than one surgeon, the primary surgeon is responsible for the procedural note. A resident or intern may dictate the note, but the primary surgeon must indicate agreement by reading, correcting, and signing the documentation. Cosurgeons called in to handle a situation demanding a particular area of expertise share responsibility in the procedure and must record their involvement. Assistant surgeons only provide assistance when needed and do not have their own primary operative responsibilities and do not dictate any part of the report. The report should clearly indicate the portion(s) of the procedure performed by each physician when more than one surgeon participates in the procedure.

Operation(s) or Procedure Performed
- This section depends on the specific case (e.g., removal of foreign body posterior neck, cholecystectomy)

2. History or Indication for Surgery
This section provides a brief history or indication concerning why a surgery course of treatment is being followed.

3. Body of the Operative Report
This section provides detailed description of the operation(s) from the prepping and draping of the patient to the closure of the wound and dressings applied at the end of the surgery.

Additional information that can be found in the body of the operative report includes:

- Name and serial number where appropriate of grafts, hardware, and devices used in performing the procedure
- Intraoperative robotic assistance
- Intraoperative testing
- Intraoperative neurological stimulation or monitoring
- Specimens sent to pathology

- Preliminary report of frozen section or other intraoperative pathology review
- Portions of the procedure performed and documented by a separate physician

4. Findings

This section provides a synopsis of what was found during the operation.

Some of the above-mentioned information, which is standard in an operative report, is unnecessary to include in the sample reports included here.

OPERATIVE REPORT CODING GUIDELINES

It is important that the coder completely read the operative report before assigning diagnosis or procedure codes. Although the name of the procedure should be listed in the header information, the procedure must be documented in the body of the operative report. It is important to read the operative report to be able to accurately report all the procedures performed. Sometimes a physician may forget to list a component of the procedure in the header but describe it completely in the body of the operative report. The coder may determine upon reading the body of the report that a more extensive procedure was performed and subsequently report a more inclusive code. Or a procedure may be in the header and not be described at all in the body of the report, necessitating that the physician be asked whether the procedure was performed.

For example, a procedure report may state that an EGD with biopsy was performed and the procedure identifies no abnormalities seen, findings do not indicate any lesions or polyps. The operative report did not indicate that specimens were sent to the pathology department and a pathology report is not in the chart. The coder can send an inquiry to the physician to determine if lesions were biopsied, destroyed, or not found. The physician can amend the documentation according to the facility guidelines or write or dictate an addendum.

Reading the complete operative or procedure report and not relying on the heading information may also affect diagnosis coding. The findings section of the report may identify conditions not listed in the pre- or post-procedure or operative report diagnosis. Comorbidities or complications may be identified; additional or different diagnosis codes would then be assigned.

THE OPERATIVE OR PROCEDURE PROGRESS NOTE

Inpatient and Outpatient Setting

In an inpatient and outpatient facility setting an operative progress note is written to allow a continuum of patient care. Less formal than an operative report, a progress note is a hand written abbreviated account that gives the most pertinent details of the procedures. The operative progress note follows the chronological order of the progress (staff) notes. It should be written or dictated immediately or before transfer to the next level of care. It is generally written for three purposes:

☼ CODING AXIOM

ICD-10-PCS Official Guidelines for Coding and Reporting Section A11:

Many of the terms used to construct PCS codes are defined within the system. It is the coder's responsibility to determine what the documentation in the medical record equates to in the PCS definitions. The physician is not expected to use the terms used in PCS code descriptions, nor is the coder required to query the physician when the correlation between the documentation and the defined PCS terms is clear.

☞ KEY POINT

Coders should use all available information when coding operative reports. Reviewing information such as the operative report in its entirety, progress note, and any other supporting documentation (e.g., anesthesia report/notes) ensures more accurate coding.

- To inform other health care professionals of what occurred in the operating room while awaiting a transcription of the dictated report

- To meet accreditation standards

- As a cross reference to remind the surgeon and alert other health care professionals about the operation

The operative or progress note includes:

- Date of service

- Attending surgeon

- Cosurgeon

- Resident surgeon

- Surgery assistants

- Anesthetic (e.g., general, regional, local)

- Anesthesiologist/CRNA/Provider of anesthesia

- Estimated blood loss and replacement

- Pre- and postoperative diagnoses

- Complications and unusual services

- Title of procedure(s) performed

- Complications and unusual services

- Brief summary of findings

- Immediate postoperative condition

- Fluids given and invasive tubes, drains, and catheters used

- Hardware or foreign bodies intentionally left in the operative site

The name of the patient and the medical record number should be listed on the progress/staff note and depending on the facility or office, the referring physician may be listed.

As with the sample operative reports, not all of the above-mentioned information is included in sample progress notes in *Optum360 Learning: Coding from the Operative Report for ICD-10-CM and PCS.*

 KEY POINT

Any intraoperative misadventure should be summarized in the complications section in the heading of the operative report and in the operative progress note. Specific information about the complication and the steps taken to handle the complication are documented in the body of the operative report. The same information may be discussed in the operative progress note.

KEY POINT

Codes for complications that occur during (intraoperative) or after (postoperative) surgery may be used to substantiate medical necessity for additional procedures or services performed.

KEY POINT

A treatment can be medical or surgical. The term "treatment" as it applies to a note or report generally is used to document a type of therapy to correct a problem or condition. A treatment refers to a more conservative approach to a problem than invasive surgery (e.g., burn treatment).

RETRIEVING INFORMATION FROM DOCUMENTATION IN THE OPERATIVE REPORT

It is important to look at all documentation regarding an operation, procedure, or treatment for information. For example, information may be found in the body of the operative report or the progress note that was not mentioned in the heading of the operative report. Coding should never rely on the information listed in the heading of an operative report. Information from one source of documentation (e.g., operative progress note) may support or even contradict information listed in another source (e.g., operative report).

Documentation in the medical record that could influence, add to, or change coding assignments should also be reviewed. This documentation includes:

- Progress/staff notes
- Physician orders
- Pathology reports
- Device serial number and/or packing information
- Discharge summaries
- History and physicals
- Emergency department reports
- Ventilator documentation forms
- Anesthesiology reports/forms
- Recovery room course and information
- Complications (intraoperative/postoperative)
- Ambulance services
- Consultants' reports

Coders should never attempt to code an operative report, note, or other services without all of the proper documentation present. Do not code only from the operative report or an operative progress note if other supplemental documentation is available. Use all documentation in tandem to determine code assignments.

Methods for Retrieving Information

1. Read the complete operative report
2. Note any differences or questions that arise between the documentation in the heading and in the history or indication for surgery, body, or findings listed in the report
3. Answer the questions by reviewing the operative report documentation against documentation listed in other areas of the chart (listed above)
4. When questions cannot be resolved by documentation in the medical record seek additional information from the physician

Where Other Operative Information Can Be Found

Documentation can be found in several locations, including:

- Progress/staff notes in chronological order beginning with the earlier dates of service

- Other forms or reports filed in separate sections, depending on protocol established by the facility or physician's office

For example, a pathology report may clarify the type of tumor found in an operative session (e.g., benign or malignant) or further specify the nature of a condition. Confirm specimens (whether neoplastic tumors or not) excised with the pathology reports to ensure diagnostic specificity. Many payers take issue with nonspecific codes. Making diagnostic specificity a standard practice is an excellent preparation for ICD-10, in which the granularity of data required to code is further refined.

UNDERDOCUMENTED OR INCORRECT INFORMATION

Information in the medical record can be underdocumented or incorrect as evidenced in a report where the operative report body does not agree with the heading or other chart documentation. Finding underdocumented or incorrect information requires the coder to seek information from outside of the operative report proper whether in an inpatient or outpatient setting.

Underdocumented

Example:
- The operative progress note states a procedure was performed although the procedure is not listed in the heading of the operative report but detailed in the body of the report.

Incorrect

Example:
- The operative report heading specifies the patient was a male and a hysterectomy was performed.

- The operative report states a female had a skiing accident, though the face sheet says a male was admitted to the hospital.

- The heading of the operative report indicates a procedure was performed on the left leg and the body of the operative report states the procedure was performed on the right leg.

When conflicts exist in the documentation of a medical record that may affect coding assignment and accuracy of the document, ask others in the office. Seek information from the medical records director, office manager, or other entity about when to request additional information from the surgeon. Coders should also seek guidance regarding the conditions necessary for an addendum to the medical record.

Physician office coders should make sure to receive a copy of any hospital record addendum that has been documented. A system must be in place when the document is received by the surgeon to prevent important information being filed without the coder's knowledge.

CODE SELECTION

Although pre- and postoperative diagnoses and procedures are listed in the heading of the operative report, they alone may not contain the information

 KEY POINT

Room assignment can be used to look for complications or other conditions that may affect code assignment. One should ask, for example, why a patient was in an intermediate care or intensive care room. Are these rooms the only ones available, or are there other conditions present?

When there are conflicts in the documentation that may affect coding assignment and accuracy of the document, ask others in the office. Seek information from the medical records director, office manager, or other entity about when to request additional information from the surgeon. Coders should also seek guidance regarding the conditions necessary for an addendum to the medical record.

necessary to accurately code an operative report. Abstract information should be available from all documentation before assigning the correct code. For example, compare the following information listed in an operative report heading, against the information listed in the body of the operative report and the operative progress note:

Heading of the Operative Report

- Preoperative diagnosis: Cholelithiasis
- Postoperative diagnosis: Same
- Procedure: Cholecystectomy

Body of the Operative Report

- "The laparoscope was introduced through a periumbilical incision."
- "The gallbladder was acutely inflamed."
- "An intraoperative cholangiogram showed stone in the duct."

Operative Progress Note

- Preoperative diagnosis: Cholelithiasis
- Postoperative diagnosis: Cholecystitis with choledocholithasis
- Procedure: Laparoscopic cholecystectomy with intraoperative cholangiograms

WHEN TO SEEK CLARIFICATION OR ADDITIONAL INFORMATION FROM THE PHYSICIAN

Coders frequently seek clarification or additional information from the physician responsible for the service provided. However, coders should consider the time it takes from their schedule and the physician's schedule when deciding whether to seek clarification. For example, there are times when it is essential to make a request:

- When a review of the documentation does not resolve contradictory or conflicting information
- When the coder suspects a complication occurred yet there is no clear documentation to support the coder's suspicion. For example, in the body of the operative report the coder notes that the bowel was repaired during an operation on another close anatomical site and the reason why the bowel was repaired is not apparent.

Once coded, the operative report and other sources of documented information are changed from the written word into numeric or alpha-numeric codes. Complete and accurate coding presents an accurate picture of what happened.

Hospital Versus Outpatient Documents

The operative progress note can be advantageous to hospital coders because the note presents a complete record of services performed for the patient. The same may not be true for a physician's office that simply receives a copy of the discharge summary and the operative report from the hospital. It may take time before the documents are received and the hospital coder has the time to look at

 KEY POINT

Failure to comply with correct coding that matches documentation may result in fraud and abuse action against the facility or practice. This could ultimately result in fines and sanctions against the organization and, in the event of fraud, imprisonment.

the information concurrently soon after discharge when transcription is complete.

Physician offices should have protocol in place to ensure the coder has all of the information necessary to accurately code services provided by the surgeon, cosurgeon, or assistant surgeon.

Coding and Documentation Scrutinized by Auditors

Auditors may compare the operative report documentation and the reported codes to determine the legitimacy of a claims request or other issues regarding fraud, abuse, and compliance. Coding accuracy is important. Failure to comply with correct coding that matches documentation may result in fraud and abuse action against the practice. These types of actions could ultimately result in fines and sanctions against the facility or practice and, in instances of proven fraudulent behavior, imprisonment.

Operative Reports, Progress, Procedure, and Treatment Notes

In the following chapters we will present information by Major Diagnostic Category (MDC) using actual operative reports, progress, procedure, and treatment notes. The chapters are designed to show coders how to distinguish among similar codes and code sets as well as familiarize coders with coding-related issues.

Please note that the case scenarios that follow are grouped using the most current ICD-10 MS-DRG version available, version 33.

 DEFINITIONS

medical auditor: A professional who evaluates a provider's utilization, quality of care, or level of reimbursement.

Chapter 7: Operative Reports

Pre-MDC

Operative Report Pre-MDC—#1

Preoperative diagnosis:
Need for long-term ventilation

Postoperative diagnosis:
Same

Procedure performed:
Tracheostomy

Indications:
This 57-year-old male patient was admitted due to severe alcohol withdrawal. He subsequently developed acute respiratory distress syndrome due to the withdrawal and has been on mechanical ventilation for a week. The patient has failed multiple attempts at weaning and therefore needs a tracheostomy for long-term ventilation purposes.

Procedure description:
The patient was brought directly from the ICU to the operating room. The patient was given moderate sedation. The area over the neck was prepped and draped in a sterile fashion. Lidocaine 1% with epinephrine was injected into the skin and subcutaneous tissue for further anesthetic purposes. A transverse incision was made above the suprasternal notch, and dissection was performed down to the strap muscles, which were divided in the midline. Dissection was further carried down using Bovie electrocautery to the level of the trachea. The second tracheal ring was identified. A #11 scalpel was then used to create a box-type incision in the second tracheal ring, and the trachea was opened. The existing endotracheal tube was backed out, and dense secretions were aspirated. A #6 low-pressure cuff Shiley tracheostomy tube was successfully inserted into the trachea, and tidal CO_2 was confirmed when it was connected to the circuit. The tracheostomy tube was secured to the skin using 3-0 Prolene suture. Hemostasis was maintained throughout the case. Sterile dressing was applied. The patient was moved back to the intensive care unit directly in critical but stable condition.

Code all relevant ICD-10-CM diagnosis and ICD-10-PCS procedure codes in accordance with official guidelines and coding conventions.

Diagnosis Codes (at discharge):

_____

_____

Procedure Codes:

_____

_____

MS-DRG:

_____

_____

Answers and Rationale

Preoperative diagnosis:
Need for long-term ventilation

Postoperative diagnosis:
Same

Procedure performed:
Tracheostomy

Indications:
This 57-year-old male patient was admitted due to severe alcohol withdrawal.[1] He subsequently developed acute respiratory distress syndrome[2] due to the withdrawal and has been on mechanical ventilation for a week.[4] The patient has failed multiple attempts at weaning and therefore needs a tracheostomy for long-term ventilation purposes.

Procedure description:
The patient was brought directly from the ICU to the operating room. The patient was given moderate sedation. The area over the neck was prepped and draped in a sterile fashion. Lidocaine 1% with epinephrine was injected into the skin and subcutaneous tissue for further anesthetic purposes. A transverse incision was made[3] above the suprasternal notch, and dissection was performed down to the strap muscles, which were divided in the midline. Dissection was further carried down using Bovie electrocautery to the level of the trachea.[3] The second tracheal ring was identified. A #11 scalpel was then used to create a box-type incision in the second tracheal ring, and the trachea was opened. The existing endotracheal tube was backed out, and dense secretions were aspirated. A #6 low-pressure cuff Shiley tracheostomy tube was successfully inserted into the trachea[3], and tidal CO2 was confirmed when it was connected to the circuit. The tracheostomy tube was secured to the skin using 3-0 Prolene suture. Hemostasis was maintained throughout the case. Sterile dressing was applied. The patient was moved back to the intensive care unit directly in critical but stable condition.

Diagnosis Codes (at discharge)

F1Ø.239   **Alcohol dependence with withdrawal, unspecified**[1]

J8Ø   **Acute respiratory distress syndrome**[2]

Rationale for Diagnosis Codes
In this case, the withdrawal is sequenced first as that was the reason for admission. The patient then developed the acute respiratory distress syndrome, making it appropriate as a secondary diagnosis. Under "Withdrawal" in the ICD-10-CM index, the coder is instructed to see "Dependence," which leads to the code above.

Procedure Codes

ØB11ØF4   **Bypass Trachea to Cutaneous with Tracheostomy Device, Open Approach**[3]

5A1955Z   **Respiratory Ventilation, Greater than 96 Consecutive Hours**[4]

Rationale for Procedure Codes
The ICD-10-PCS index entry for the tracheostomy procedure suggests the root operation *Bypass*. This root operation coincides with the procedure's objective. It is important to note that the procedure was performed using an open approach, as noted by the mention of dissection down to the trachea, and that the device inserted was a tracheostomy device (sixth character of F). Last, a seventh character of 4 indicates that the bypass is to the skin of the neck or cutaneous tissue. To ensure accurate reimbursement, it is important that the procedure codes also reflect the week on the ventilator. To determine the appropriate code for the ventilator in ICD-10-PCS, locate "Mechanical ventilation" in the index, which instructs the coder to see "Performance, Respiratory 5A19." At this point, given that the specific table containing the code is referenced, the coder may refer to the given terms in the index or go straight to the 5A1 table. In either instance, the code selection depends on the amount of time the patient was on the ventilator, in this case greater than 96 hours (four days).

MS-DRG

004   **Tracheostomy with Mechanical Ventilation 96+ Hours or   RW 10.9458 Principal Diagnosis Except Face, Mouth and Neck without Major O.R.**

CODING AXIOM

ICD-10-PCS Official Guidelines for Coding and Reporting Section B3.6a:

Bypass procedures are coded by identifying the body part bypassed "from" and the body part bypassed "to." The fourth-character body part specifies the body part bypassed from, and the qualifier specifies the body part bypassed to.

OPERATIVE REPORT PRE-MDC—#2

Preoperative diagnosis:
Hepatocellular carcinoma

Postoperative diagnosis:
Hepatocellular carcinoma

Procedure performed:
Liver transplant

Indications:
This 36-year-old female has hepatocellular carcinoma and meets the Milan criteria for liver transplant. She was evaluated by our multidisciplinary transplant committee, and a transplant was recommended.

Procedure description:
The patient was brought to the operating room, and monitoring devices and infusion lines were placed by anesthesia. Then general anesthesia was induced. A bilateral subcostal incision was made to enter the peritoneal cavity. The hepatic artery was identified and divided, as were the right and left hepatic arteries, individually. The portal limb was identified and was noted to be extremely small and had very little blood flow within it. It was carefully dissected free up to the bifurcation and divided. The attachments of the liver to the retroperitoneum were then divided. The caudate lobe encircled the vena cava; therefore it was not possible to remove the liver without interrupting the vena cava. At this point, surgical clamps were placed on the vein above and below the liver, and the liver was dissected free and removed. Due to the abnormalities of the portal limb, the decision was made to use the vena cava as the venous inflow. The donor liver was then placed using 5-0 Prolene for the suprahepatic anastomosis and 7-0 Prolene for the hepatic artery anastomosis. The portal vein of the donor liver was then connected to the inferior vena cava using 6-0 Prolene. The infrahepatic cava of the donor was oversewn with 4-0 Prolene. The clamps were released. The liver was then flushed and inspected. It achieved a satisfactory appearance and began to make bile. There was a strong palpable pulse in the hepatic artery. There was no tension on the portal vein anastomosis demonstrated by the infusion of the biliary catheter with saline with no evidence of leakage. The abdomen was irrigated with warm saline and was closed with running 2-0 Prolene. The patient tolerated the procedure well.

Code all relevant ICD-10-CM diagnosis and ICD-10-PCS procedure codes in accordance with official guidelines and coding conventions.

Diagnosis Codes:

_____

_____

Procedure Codes:

_____

_____

MS-DRG:

_____

KEY POINT

The Milan criteria:

- One lesion smaller than 5cm.
- Up to three lesions smaller than 3 cm
- No extrahepatic manifestations
- No vascular invasion

Answers and Rationale

Preoperative diagnosis:
Hepatocellular carcinoma

Postoperative diagnosis:
Hepatocellular carcinoma[1]

Procedure performed:
Liver transplant[2]

Indications:
This 36-year-old female has hepatocellular carcinoma and meets the Milan criteria for liver transplant. She was evaluated by our multidisciplinary transplant committee, and a transplant was recommended.

Procedure description:
The patient was brought to the operating room, and monitoring devices and infusion lines were placed by anesthesia. Then general anesthesia was induced. A bilateral subcostal incision was made to enter the peritoneal cavity.[2] The hepatic artery was identified and divided, as were the right and left hepatic arteries, individually. The portal limb was identified and was noted to be extremely small and had very little blood flow within it. It was carefully dissected free up to the bifurcation and divided. The attachments of the liver to the retroperitoneum were then divided. The caudate lobe encircled the vena cava; therefore it was not possible to remove the liver without interrupting the vena cava. At this point, surgical clamps were placed on the vein above and below the liver, and the liver was dissected free and removed.[2] Due to the abnormalities of the portal limb, the decision was made to use the vena cava as the venous inflow. The donor liver was then placed[2] using 5-0 Prolene for the suprahepatic anastomosis and 7-0 Prolene for the hepatic artery anastomosis. The portal vein of the donor liver was then connected to the inferior vena cava using 6-0 Prolene. The infrahepatic cava of the donor was oversewn with 4-0 Prolene. The clamps were released. The liver was then flushed and inspected. It achieved a satisfactory appearance and began to make bile. There was a strong palpable pulse in the hepatic artery. There was no tension on the portal vein anastomosis demonstrated by the infusion of the biliary catheter with saline with no evidence of leakage. The abdomen was irrigated with warm saline and was closed with running 2-0 Prolene. The patient tolerated the procedure well.

Diagnosis Codes

C22.0   **Liver cell carcinoma[1]**

Rationale for Diagnosis Codes

Hepatocellular carcinoma is one of the few malignant neoplasm diagnoses automatically assigned to a primary malignancy site of the liver. In most cases, liver neoplasms are considered and assumed to be metastatic sites. The ICD-10-CM Alphabetic Index and Tabular List confirm the assignment of C22.0 for hepatocellular carcinoma not further specified.

Procedure Codes

0FY00Z0   **Transplantation of Liver, Allogeneic, Open Approach[2]**

Rationale for Procedure Codes

When a whole functioning body part is inserted in lieu of the patient's diseased organ, the root operation is *Transplant*. In this case, the transplant was of the liver. Since the replacement is referred to as the *donor* liver, the coder can assume the transplanted organ is donated by a human and would therefore be considered allogeneic, with a seventh-character value of 0.

MS-DRG

006   **Liver Transplant without MCC**   **RW 4.8330**

🕯 **CODING AXIOM**

ICD-10-CM Official Guidelines for Coding and Reporting Section I.C.2:

The Neoplasm Table in the Alphabetic Index should be referenced first. However, if the histological term (hepatocellular carcinoma) is documented, that term should be referenced first, rather than going immediately to the Neoplasm Table, to determine which column in the table is appropriate.

MDC 1 Diseases and Disorders of the Nervous System

OPERATIVE REPORT MDC 1—#1

Preoperative diagnosis:
Left progressive acoustic neuroma

Postoperative diagnosis:
Left progressive acoustic neuroma

Procedure performed:
Gamma-knife resection of the neuroma

Indications:
A 46-year-old male patient with chronic benign HTN and rheumatoid arthritis presented a month ago with new onset symptoms of hearing loss on the left side, tinnitus, headache, and balance problems. MRI showed an enhancing mass in the left cerebellopontine (CP) angle cistern and left internal auditory canal. The mass measured 2.8 cm in length with the left CP angle cistern component measuring 1.6 cm in transverse diameter. Due to the complexity of the mass location, the patient opted to have gamma knife surgery.

Procedure description:
The patient was taken to the gamma knife suite, and after some sedation, the Leksell stereotactic frame was applied to the head and attached. Then the localizing frame was applied, and the patient was taken to the MR suite where a volume acquisition MRI with gadolinium was obtained. All this information was transferred to the working station in the gamma knife area where all the images that revealed the mass were viewed. After the skull measurements were entered, dose planning began by applying multiple shots to conform to the shape of the mass. This required complex planning to minimize the amount of radiation to the cranial nerves and the brain stem. After the dose plan was achieved, the patient was taken to the gamma knife unit, and all the shots were applied without any complication. The patient was taken to the recovery area where the frame was removed. The patient tolerated the procedure well, and there were no complications.

Code all relevant ICD-10-CM diagnosis and ICD-10-PCS procedure codes in accordance with official guidelines and coding conventions.

Diagnosis Codes:

_____

_____

Procedure Codes:

_____

_____

MS-DRG:

_____

_____

Answers and Rationale

Preoperative diagnosis:
Left progressive acoustic neuroma

Postoperative diagnosis:
Left progressive acoustic neuroma[1]

Procedure performed:
Gamma-knife[4] resection of the neuroma

Indications:
A 46-year-old male patient with chronic benign HTN[2] and rheumatoid arthritis[3] presented a month ago with new onset symptoms of hearing loss on the left side, tinnitus, headache, and balance problems. MRI showed an enhancing mass in the left cerebellopontine (CP) angle cistern and left internal auditory canal. The mass measured 2.8 cm in length with the left CP angle cistern component measuring 1.6 cm in transverse diameter. Due to the complexity of the mass location, the patient opted to have gamma knife surgery.

Procedure description:
The patient was taken to the gamma knife suite, and after some sedation, the Leksell stereotactic frame was applied to the head and attached. Then the localizing frame was applied, and the patient was taken to the MR suite where a volume acquisition MRI with gadolinium was obtained. All this information was transferred to the working station in the gamma knife area where all the images that revealed the mass were viewed. After the skull measurements were entered, dose planning began by applying multiple shots to conform to the shape of the mass. This required complex planning to minimize the amount of radiation to the cranial nerves and the brain stem. After the dose plan was achieved, the patient was taken to the gamma knife unit, and all the shots were applied without any complication.[4] The patient was taken to the recovery area where the frame was removed. The patient tolerated the procedure well, and there were no complications.

Diagnosis Codes

D33.3	Benign neoplasm of cranial nerves[1]
I1Ø	Essential (primary) hypertension[2]
MØ6.9	Rheumatoid arthritis, unspecified[3]

Rationale for Diagnosis Codes
The diagnoses as stated provide straightforward terms to reference in the ICD-10-CM index. The hearing loss, tinnitus, headache, and balance problems would not be reported as secondary diagnoses, as these are symptoms that are routinely associated with an acoustic neuroma.

Procedure Codes

DØ2ØJZZ	Stereotactic Gamma Beam Radiosurgery of Brain[4]

Rationale for Procedure Codes
To locate the appropriate table for this procedure, the coder must consider first the procedure's objective and second the method. In this instance, the neuroma is being resected via gamma knife surgery, which is noninvasive and uses radiation to destroy tumors and other abnormalities of the brain. Due to the use of radiation, the surgery is located in the *Radiation Therapy* section of ICD-10-PCS, table DØ2 Central and Peripheral Nervous System/Stereotactic Radiosurgery.

MS-DRG

042	Peripheral/Cranial Nerve and Other Nervous System Procedures without CC/MCC	RW 1.9242

If an open excision of the acoustic nerve is incorrectly reported rather than DØ2ØJZZ, the MS-DRG is higher-weighted 027 Craniotomy and Endovascular Intracranial Procedures without CC/MCC (RW 2.2835).

🕯 **CODING AXIOM**

ICD-10-CM Official Guidelines for Coding and Reporting Section I.B.5:

Signs and symptoms that are associated routinely with a disease process should not be assigned as additional codes, unless otherwise instructed by the classification.

OPERATIVE REPORT MDC 1—#2

Preoperative diagnosis:
Suspected ventriculoperitoneal shunt malfunction, post-traumatic hydrocephalus

Procedure performed:
Shunt tap, adjustment of Medtronic Strata Valve

Procedure description:
After proper patient identification and appropriate preprocedure informed consent were obtained, the patient was positioned in a lateral decubitus partially prone position with right posterior region of his head uppermost to optimize access to the shunt valve. The patient's right parieto-occipital region was cleansed with alcohol, and the patient was then prepped with Betadine solution and sterilely draped in the usual fashion. The shunt valve was accessed with a 23-gauge Angiocath with satisfactory CSF egress noted. The Angiocath was connected to a manometer with findings as noted below.

Findings:
Satisfactory proximal outflow was noted from the shunt valve with opening pressure questionably approximately 12-15. The CSF was grossly clear in appearance. Runoff appeared satisfactory. After completion of the shunt tap, the patient's Strata shunt valve was checked. The pressure appeared to be level 0.5. The prior operative note had reported a setting of 1.5; therefore, this was reprogrammed externally to 1.5.

Code all relevant ICD-10-CM diagnosis and ICD-10-PCS procedure codes in accordance with official guidelines and coding conventions.

Diagnosis Codes:

_____

_____

Procedure Codes:

_____

_____

MS-DRG:

_____

_____

Answers and Rationale

Preoperative diagnosis:
Suspected ventriculoperitoneal shunt malfunction, post-traumatic hydrocephalus[2]

Procedure performed:
Shunt tap, adjustment of Medtronic Strata Valve

Procedure description:
After proper patient identification and appropriate preprocedure informed consent were obtained, the patient was positioned in a lateral decubitus partially-prone position with right posterior region of his head uppermost to optimize access to the shunt valve. The patient's right parieto-occipital region was cleansed with alcohol, and the patient was the prepped with Betadine solution and sterilely draped in the usual fashion. The shunt valve was accessed with a 23-gauge Angiocath with satisfactory CSF egress noted.[1,3] The Angiocath was connected to a manometer with findings as noted below.[4]

Findings:
Satisfactory proximal outflow was noted from the shunt valve with opening pressure questionably approximately 12-15. The CSF was grossly clear in appearance. Runoff appeared satisfactory. After completion of the shunt tap,[3] the patient's Strata shunt valve was checked. The pressure appeared to be level 0.5.[4] The prior operative note had reported a setting of 1.5; therefore, this was reprogrammed externally to 1.5.

Diagnosis Codes

Z45.41   **Encounter for adjustment and management of cerebrospinal fluid drainage device**[1]

G91.9   **Hydrocephalus, unspecified**[2]

Rationale for Diagnosis Codes
Although the original diagnosis is suspected malfunction of the ventriculoperitoneal (VP) shunt, the procedure did not demonstrate a problem in the device's function other than the valve needed to be readjusted. This is not considered a complication but instead routine adjustment of the shunt, and therefore a code for the encounter for adjustment and management would be more appropriate than a complication code. The hydrocephalus is still present (requiring a VP shunt) and should also be reported.

Procedure Codes

8C01X6J   **Collection of Cerebrospinal Fluid from Indwelling Device in Nervous System**[3]

4A003BD   **Measurement of Intracranial Pressure, Percutaneous Approach**[4]

Rationale for Procedure Codes
Code 8C01X6J should be reported for the shunt tap, which aspirates small amounts of fluid to check for adequate drainage.

The catheter was then connected to a manometer to measure the intraventricular pressure. This type of procedure can be found in the "Measurement and Monitoring" section of ICD-10-PCS. The routine adjustment of the pressure setting of the shunt was performed externally. This is not reported with root operation *Revision* as the device itself was functioning correctly and in correct position and it was not revised; only the settings were adjusted.

MS-DRG

092	**Other Disorders of Nervous System with CC**	RW 0.9075

⚗ CODING AXIOM

ICD-10-CM Official Guidelines for Coding and Reporting Section I.C.21.c.7:

- Aftercare visit codes cover situations when the initial treatment of a disease has been performed and the patient requires continued care during the healing or recovery phase, or for the long-term consequences of the disease. The aftercare Z code should not be used if treatment is directed at a current, acute disease. The diagnosis code is to be used in these cases.

- The aftercare Z codes also should not be used for injury aftercare. For aftercare of an injury, assign the acute injury code with the appropriate seventh character (for subsequent encounter).

- The aftercare codes are generally first-listed to explain the specific reason for the encounter.

- Aftercare codes should be used in conjunction with other aftercare codes or diagnosis codes to provide better detail on the specifics of an aftercare encounter visit, unless otherwise directed by the classification.

- Certain aftercare Z code categories need a secondary diagnosis code to describe the resolving condition or sequelae. For others, the condition is included in the code title.

OPERATIVE REPORT MDC 1—#3

Preoperative diagnosis:
Cerebral hemorrhage

Postoperative diagnosis:
Cerebral arteriovenous malformation with hemorrhage

Procedure performed:
Endovascular coil embolization

Indications:
The patient is a 35-year-old male who presented to the ED with severe headache of three-day duration and diplopia. Imaging revealed an arteriovenous malformation with a pin sized hole that was leaking slowly. The patient was brought to the catheterization suite for emergent AVM embolization.

Procedure description:
The patient was sedated using IV Versed. The right thigh area above the femoral artery was prepped and draped in the usual sterile fashion, and the area was infiltrated with 1% lidocaine for local anesthesia. Once it was established that adequate sedation had been achieved, a small incision was made over the femoral artery and a catheter was inserted into the vessel. The catheter was manipulated using fluoroscopic guidance through the vascular system to the site of the AVM. A HydroCoil 14 was then threaded through the catheter and into the AVM. The coil continued to be introduced into the defect until the entire defect was filled and confirmed under fluoroscopy. An injection of contrast was applied and it was ensured that the coiling was successful in blocking the blood flow to the AVM entirely, thereby closing the site of the hemorrhage. The catheter was removed. Pressure was applied to the incision site until hemostasis was obtained. The patient was then taken to the recovery room in hemodynamically stable condition.

Code all relevant ICD-10-CM diagnosis and ICD-10-PCS procedure codes in accordance with official guidelines and coding conventions.

Diagnosis Codes:

_____

_____

Procedure Codes:

_____

_____

MS-DRG:

_____

_____

Answers and Rationale

Preoperative diagnosis:
Cerebral hemorrhage

Postoperative diagnosis:
Cerebral arteriovenous malformation with hemorrhage[1]

Procedure performed:
Endovascular coil embolization

Indications:
The patient is a 35-year-old male who presented to the ED with severe headache of three-day duration and diplopia. Imaging revealed an arteriovenous malformation with a pin sized hole that was leaking slowly. The patient was brought to the catheterization suite for emergent AVM embolization.

Procedure description:
The patient was sedated using IV Versed. The right thigh area above the femoral artery was prepped and draped in the usual sterile fashion, and the area was infiltrated with 1% lidocaine for local anesthesia. Once it was established that adequate sedation had been achieved, a small incision was made over the femoral artery and a catheter was inserted into the vessel.[2] The catheter was manipulated using fluoroscopic guidance through the vascular system to the site of the AVM. A HydroCoil 14 was then threaded through the catheter and into the AVM. A total of six coils were introduced into the defect until the entire defect was filled[2] and confirmed under fluoroscopy. An injection of contrast applied and it was ensured that the coiling was successful in blocking the blood flow to the AVM entirely, thereby closing the site of the hemorrhage. The catheter was removed. Pressure was applied to the incision site until hemostasis was obtained. The patient was then taken to the recovery room in hemodynamically stable condition.

Diagnosis Codes

I60.8   Other nontraumatic subarachnoid hemorrhage[1]

Rationale for Diagnosis Codes
The terms "Malformation, arteriovenous, cerebral" in the ICD-10-CM index lead the coder to Q28.2. However, this is not the correct code for reporting a ruptured arteriovenous malformation (AVM), according to the Excludes 1 note under category Q28. The correct code according to the tabular instructional notes is I60.8, which is confirmed by the inclusion note that states "rupture of cerebral arteriovenous malformation."

Procedure Codes

Ø3LG3DZ   Occlusion of Intracranial Artery with Intraluminal Device, Percutaneous Approach[2]

Rationale for Procedure Codes
The procedure described completely closed off the AVM from the rest of the vascular system using six coils. This coincides with the ICD-10-PCS root operation *Occlusion*. The intent of endovascular coil embolization is to completely block off the abnormal arterial blood flow into the vein with coils inserted via a catheter guided through the femoral artery into the feeding artery of the brain AVM. This procedure is reported with a code originating from the "Upper Artery" tables. The artery is specified as intracranial, and the procedure is performed percutaneously under fluoroscopic guidance, which is reported using the fifth-character value of 3. HydroCoil endovascular coils are intraluminal devices, but they are not bioactive, making the correct device character value D.

MS-DRG

022   Intracranial Vascular Procedures with Principal Diagnosis   RW 4.9977
         of Hemorrhage without CC/MCC

If the AVM is reported incorrectly using code Q28.2, the MS-DRG groups to lower-weighted MS-DRG 027 Craniotomy and Endovascular Intracranial Procedures without CC/MCC (RW 2.2835).

CODING AXIOM

ICD-10-CM Official Guidelines for Coding and Reporting Section I.A.12.a:

A type 1 excludes note is a pure excludes note. It means "NOT CODED HERE!" An Excludes 1 note indicates that the code excluded should never be used at the same time as the code above the Excludes 1 note. This note is used when two conditions cannot occur together, such as a congenital form versus an acquired form of the same condition.

DEFINITIONS

occlusion. ICD-10-PCS root operation value L. Completely closing an orifice or the lumen of a tubular body part. The orifice can be natural or artificially created.

percutaneous. ICD-10-PCS approach value 3. Entry, by puncture or minor incision, of instrumentation through the skin or mucous membrane and any other body layers necessary to reach the site of the procedure.

OPERATIVE REPORT MDC 1—#4

Preoperative diagnosis:
Laceration, digital nerve

Postoperative diagnosis:
Laceration, right index finger, digital nerve injury

Procedure performed:
Wound exploration with repair of radial digital nerve of the right index finger

Indications:
Patient sustained the above-noted injury while replacing a piece of glass in the front door of her house that had broken. There is numbness in the radial aspect of the index finger. Procedure is indicated to repair the nerve and explore the wound for tendon damage.

Procedure description:
Under general anesthesia with the patient orally intubated, she was prepped and draped in the usual fashion. Under ischemic technique, I proceeded with extension of the wound for access. The flexor digitorum profunda was intact, and the superficialis has a very superficial cut of the radial aspect and therefore no repair is needed. I proceeded then to explore the radial neurovascular bundle. The radial digital nerve of the index finger was dissected proximally and distally. With the aid of a microscope, I proceeded with repair of the nerve with 9-0 Nylon. Since there was good vascular supply to the index finger, no vascular repair was attempted. I proceeded then to close the wound with 4-0 Nylon. The wound was dressed with Xeroform 4 x 4s, Kerlix, Webril, and a volar and dorsal splint in safe position. The patient was awakened in the operating room and taken to the recovery room in stable condition.

Code all relevant ICD-10-CM diagnosis and ICD-10-PCS procedure codes in accordance with official guidelines and coding conventions.

Diagnosis Codes:

_____

_____

Procedure Codes:

_____

_____

MS-DRG:

_____

_____

Answers and Rationale

Preoperative diagnosis:
Laceration, digital nerve

Postoperative diagnosis:
Laceration, right index finger, digital nerve injury[1]

Procedure performed:
Wound exploration with repair of radial digital nerve of the right index finger[1,6]

Indications:
Patient sustained the above-noted injury while replacing a piece of glass[2] in the front door of her house that had broken.[3-5] There is numbness in the radial aspect of the index finger. Procedure is indicated to repair the nerve and explore the wound for tendon damage.

Procedure description:
Under general anesthesia with the patient orally intubated, she was prepped and draped in the usual fashion. Under ischemic technique, I proceeded with extension of the wound for access.[6] The flexor digitorum profunda was intact, and the superficialis has a very superficial cut of the radial aspect and therefore no repair is needed.[7] I proceeded then to explore the radial neurovascular bundle. The radial digital nerve of the index finger was dissected proximally and distally. With the aid of a microscope, I proceeded with repair of the nerve with 9-0 Nylon.[6] Since there was good vascular supply to the index finger, no vascular repair was attempted. I proceeded then to close the wound with 4-0 Nylon. The wound was dressed with Xeroform 4 x 4s, Kerlix, Webril, and a volar and dorsal splint in safe position. The patient was awakened in the operating room and taken to the recovery room in stable condition.

Diagnosis Codes

S64.49ØA Injury of digital nerve of right index finger, initial encounter[1]

S61.21ØA Laceration without foreign body of right index finger without damage to nail, initial encounter[1]

W25.XXXA Contact with sharp glass, initial encounter[2]

Y92.Ø18 Other place in single-family (private) house as the place of occurrence of the external cause[3]

Y93.H9 Activity, other involving exterior property and land maintenance, building and construction[4]

Y99.8 Other external cause status[5]

Rationale for Diagnosis Codes
The terms "Laceration, Nerve" in the ICD-10-CM index instruct the coder to see "Injury, Nerve." Under this section, the nerve injuries are divided by anatomical site; in this case, the site was the radial digital nerve of the right index finger, which is identified by the code from category S64. Category S64 has a note to code also the open wound associated with the nerve injury using a code from category S61. When an injury is documented, an external cause code should be reported in addition to the injury code to give a complete picture of how an injury occurred. In addition, codes for place of occurrence, activity, and status should also be reported on the initial encounter when documented.

Procedure Codes

Ø1Q5ØZZ Repair Median Nerve, Open Approach[6]

ØLJXØZZ Inspection of Upper Tendon, Open Approach[7]

Rationale for Procedure Codes
The objective of the procedure is also the root operation in this scenario, the repair of the injured nerve. ICD-10-PCS does not provide a specific body part character value for digital nerves nor is there a specific reference for the median nerve in the "Body Part" key. Therefore, the coder must determine which larger nerve with a character value assigned could have the radial digital nerve of the index finger as an extension. Anatomy illustrations show that this nerve is a branch of the median nerve, making the appropriate character value 5. The wound was extended for access, which by definition is an open approach. There was no device used in the repair and no qualifier is needed. The exploration of the tendon is reported separately as it is not part of the approach and was done aside from the nerve repair to evaluate the tendon. *Coding Clinic*, second quarter 2013, page 36, directs that "if a separate inspection is carried out, it is coded."

MS-DRG

042	Peripheral/Cranial Nerve and Other Nervous System Procedures without CC/MCC	RW 1.9242

OPERATIVE REPORT MDC 1—#5

Preoperative diagnosis:
Facet arthropathy with facet joint mediated pain, L2-L3, L3-L4, and L4-L5 bilaterally.

Postoperative diagnosis:
Same

Procedure performed:
Radiofrequency rhizotomy

Indication:
The patient is a 70-year-old male referred for chronic low back pain due to his osteoarthritis of four years' duration. He has undergone successful diagnostic direct facet injections, which have provided significant relief from his pain. The patient presents today for fluoroscopically guided radiofrequency facet joint denervation of L2-L3, L3-L4, and L4-L5.

Procedure description:
The patient was transported to the operating room and placed in the prone position. The lumbar area was prepped and draped in the usual manner. Lidocaine 0.5% was injected over both sacral notches and over the superior junction of L4 and L5. Deep anesthesia was produced at these sites with 2% lidocaine. At each location a 16 gauge 2 ¼ inch Jelco IV catheter was introduced and used a "gun sight" to fluoroscopically direct a 10 cm 20 gauge Racz needle with 10 mm active tip onto the inferomedial portion of each sacral notch and the superior junction of each transverse process with its corresponding vertebral body. Each needle location was confirmed in the AP and lateral views by fluoroscopy, and no needle location encroached on any neural foramen. No CSF or blood was aspirated, and no paresthesias were elicited.

Local anesthesia was produced at each needle location with 0.5 ml of a 50:50 mixture of 2% lidocaine and 0.5 Bupivacaine with 5 mg of Depo Medrol per 3 ml of total solution. A radiofrequency thermal lesion was produced at each needle location to a temperature of 80 degrees centigrade for duration of 90 seconds. The patient tolerated the procedure well. The patient received a total of 2 mg of intravenous midazolam for sedation. Patient was returned to his room in satisfactory condition. The patient will follow up in three weeks.

Code all relevant ICD-10-CM diagnosis and ICD-10-PCS procedure codes in accordance with official guidelines and coding conventions.

Diagnosis Codes:
_____

_____

Procedure Codes:
_____

_____

MS-DRG:
_____

CODING AXIOM

ICD-10-CM Official Guidelines for Coding and Reporting Section I.C.6.b.1.a-b:

a. Category G89 codes are acceptable as principal diagnosis or the first-listed code:

- When pain control or pain management is the reason for the admission/encounter (e.g., a patient with displaced intervertebral disc, nerve impingement and severe back pain presents for injection of steroid into the spinal canal). The underlying cause of the pain should be reported as an additional diagnosis, if known.

- When a patient is admitted for the insertion of a neurostimulator for pain control, assign the appropriate pain code as the principal or first-listed diagnosis. When an admission or encounter is for a procedure aimed at treating the underlying condition and a neurostimulator is inserted for pain control during the same admission/encounter, a code for the underlying condition should be assigned as the principal diagnosis and the appropriate pain code should be assigned as a secondary diagnosis.

b. Category G89 codes can be used in conjunction with site-specific pain codes

- If the site-specific pain code does not fully describe whether the pain is acute or chronic, then both codes should be assigned.

- The sequencing of the G89 code with site-specific codes depends on the circumstances of admission. If the encounter is for pain control or management, code the G89 code first. If the encounter is for any other reason and a related definitive diagnosis has not been established by the provider, assign the code for the specific site first, followed by the G89 code.

Answers and Rationale

Preoperative diagnosis:
Facet arthropathy with facet joint mediated pain, L2-L3, L3-L4, and L4-L5 bilaterally.[2]

Postoperative diagnosis:
Same

Procedure performed:
Radiofrequency rhizotomy

Indication:
The patient is a 70-year-old male referred for chronic low back pain[1] due to his osteoarthritis[2] of four years' duration. He has undergone successful diagnostic direct facet injections, which have provided significant relief from his pain. The patient presents today for fluoroscopically guided radiofrequency facet joint denervation of L2-L3, L3-L4, and L4-L5.[3]

Procedure description:
The patient was transported to the operating room and placed in the prone position. The lumbar area was prepped and draped in the usual manner. Lidocaine 0.5% was injected over both sacral notches and over the superior junction of L4 and L5. Deep anesthesia was produced at these sites with 2% lidocaine. At each location a 16 gauge 2 ¼ inch Jelco IV catheter was introduced and used a "gun sight" to fluoroscopically direct a 10 cm 20 gauge Racz needle with 10 mm active tip onto the inferomedial portion of each sacral notch and the superior junction of each transverse process with its corresponding vertebral body. Each needle location was confirmed in the AP and lateral views by fluoroscopy, and no needle location encroached on any neural foramen. No CSF or blood was aspirated, and no paresthesias were elicited.

Local anesthesia was produced at each needle location with 0.5 ml of a 50:50 mixture of 2% lidocaine and 0.5 Bupivacaine with 5 mg of Depo Medrol per 3 ml of total solution. A radiofrequency thermal lesion was produced at each needle location to a temperature of 80 degrees centigrade for duration of 90 seconds. [3] The patient tolerated the procedure well. The patient received a total of 2 mg of intravenous midazolam for sedation. Patient was returned to his room in satisfactory condition. The patient will follow up in three weeks.

Diagnosis Codes

G89.29	**Other chronic pain**[1]
M54.5	**Low back pain**[1]
M47.816	**Spondylosis without myelopathy or radiculopathy, lumbar region**[2]

Rationale for Diagnosis Codes

The pain is specified as chronic low back pain and the encounter is for treatment of the chronic pain rather than the underlying condition. Therefore, according to coding guidelines, a code from G89.2 (Chronic pain, not elsewhere classified) should be reported as the principal diagnosis. Report the codes for the site-specific pain and underlying condition as secondary diagnoses. In this case, the term "Arthropathy" in the index refers the coder to "*see also* Arthritis." Under the entry for "Arthritis," the note "meaning osteoarthritis – *see* Osteoarthritis" should be noted since the physician uses osteoarthritis and facet arthropathy interchangeably in the "Indications" section. Once "Osteoarthritis" is referenced, the coder is led to "Spondylosis" and the code representing the lumbar area of the spine.

Procedure Codes

Ø15B3ZZ	**Destruction of Lumbar Nerve, Percutaneous Approach**[3]

Rationale for Procedure Codes

The objective of the radiofrequency denervation (rhizotomy) is to destroy the nerves in the bilateral L2-L5 vertebrae using radiofrequencies. This objective coincides with the root operation *Destruction*. The procedure code is coded only once, according to *AHA Coding Clinic for ICD-10-CM and ICD-10-PCS* (second quarter 2015, page 19), which clarifies that the vertebral-level designations along the spinal cord, such as L2, L3, L4 and L5, do not constitute separate and distinct body parts anatomically. Therefore, the multiple procedures guideline, B3.2b, cannot be applied.

MS-DRG

093	**Other Disorders of Nervous System without CC/MCC**	**RW 0.6981**

There are multiple risks to the MS-DRG assignment in this case, all of which result in higher-weighted, yet incorrect, MS-DRGs. The first is if the arthropathy is reported as the principal diagnosis, the DRG would then group to an MS-DRG from MDC 8 Diseases and Disorders of the Musculoskeletal System and Connective Tissue. The second is if the nerve destruction is reported using either an open or percutaneous endoscopic approach rather than percutaneous. This is due to the percutaneous approach not being considered an O.R. procedure and therefore not grouping to MS-DRG 030 Spinal Procedures without CC/MCC (RW 1.7982).

 CODING AXIOM

ICD-10-PCS Official Guidelines for Coding and Reporting Section B3.2b:

During the same operative episode, multiple procedures are coded if: The same root operation is repeated in multiple body parts, and those body parts are separate and distinct body parts classified to a single ICD-10-PCS body part value.

MDC 2 Diseases and Disorders of the Eye

OPERATIVE REPORT MDC 2—#1

Preoperative diagnoses:
Diabetic retinopathy with macular edema and retinal detachment

Postoperative diagnoses:
Diabetic retinopathy and macular edema and traction retinal detachment

Procedure description:
Vitrectomy with endolaser panretinal photocoagulation and scleral buckling

History of presenting illness:
A 76-year-old diabetic female presented with retinopathy and macular edema. Indirect ophthalmoscopy revealed severe traction retinal detachment.

Procedure details:
With the patient under general anesthesia, pars plana vitrectomy was performed in the left eye with concomitant endolaser panretinal photocoagulation. Cryocoagulation was performed to areas superior and inferior to the macula that were suspicious for retinal tears. The vitrectomy was then extended as far as visualization allowed and endolaser panretinal photocoagulation was used. Temporary silicone oil tamponade was used, and encircling scleral buckles were placed by suturing a silicone band around the scleral bed and securing it. Paracentesis was performed to remove residual subretinal fluid. The retina was again inspected with indirect ophthalmoscopy, and no retinal tears, subretinal fluid, or hemorrhages were found.

Code all relevant ICD-10-CM diagnosis and ICD-10-PCS procedure codes in accordance with official guidelines and coding conventions.

Diagnosis Codes:

_____

_____

Procedure Codes:

_____

_____

MS-DRG:

_____

_____

DEFINITIONS

concomitant. Occurring at the same time, accompanying.

Answers and Rationale

Preoperative diagnoses:
Diabetic retinopathy with macular edema and retinal detachment

Postoperative diagnoses:
Diabetic retinopathy and macular edema[1] and traction retinal detachment[2]

Procedure description:
Vitrectomy with endolaser panretinal photocoagulation and scleral buckling

History of presenting illness:
A 76-year-old diabetic female presented with retinopathy and macular edema. Indirect ophthalmoscopy revealed severe traction retinal detachment.

Procedure details:
With the patient under general anesthesia, pars plana vitrectomy was performed in the left eye[3] with concomitant endolaser panretinal photocoagulation. Cryocoagulation was performed to areas superior and inferior to the macula that were suspicious for retinal tears. The vitrectomy was then extended as far as visualization allowed [3] and endolaser panretinal photocoagulation was used. Temporary silicone oil tamponade was used, and encircling scleral buckles were placed by suturing a silicone band around the scleral bed[4] and securing it. Paracentesis was performed to remove residual subretinal fluid. The retina was again inspected with indirect ophthalmoscopy, and no retinal tears, subretinal fluid, or hemorrhages were found.

Diagnosis Codes

E11.311   **Type 2 diabetes mellitus with unspecified diabetic retinopathy with macular edema[1]**

H33.42   **Traction detachment of retina, left eye[2]**

Rationale for Diagnosis Codes
Diabetic tractional retinal detachment is a severe complication in diabetic retinopathy. When the retina detaches, vision is lost. The retinopathy, edema, and detachment are all considered complications of the diabetes per the documentation and associated coding conventions. Coding guidelines section I.C.4.a.2 specifies that when the type of diabetes is not specified, the default is type 2.

Procedure Codes

Ø8B53ZZ   **Excision of Vitreous, Left Eye, Percutaneous Approach[3]**

Ø8U13JZ   **Supplement of Left Eye with Synthetic Substitute, Percutaneous Approach[4]**

Rationale for Procedure Codes
The term "Vitrectomy" in the ICD-10-PCS index gives the coder a choice between the root operations of *Excision* and *Resection*. Based on the documentation noting that the vitreous humor was removed to the extent that the physician could see, the coder cannot assume that the entire vitreous was removed, which means that the root operation is *Excision*. The term "Photocoagulation" leads to the root operations of either *Destruction* or *Repair*, according to the index. In this case, the laser was being used to repair the retinal damage. Although the photocoagulation procedure did occur, it occurred in conjunction with the insertion of scleral buckles, which would be classified as the root operation *Supplement*. It is important at this point to note that procedural steps that are components of another procedure are not coded separately, according to *ICD-10-PCS Official Guidelines for Coding and Reporting* section B3.1b. In this case, the photocoagulation occurs as a part of the placement of the scleral buckles and is therefore not coded separately.

MS-DRG:

115   **Extraocular Procedures Except Orbit**   **RW 1.3151**

It is important to note that the code H33.42 would serve as a complication/comorbidity (CC) for this MS-DRG. Not sequencing the diagnoses correctly results in a higher-weighted but incorrect, and therefore at-risk, MS-DRG.

CODING AXIOM

ICD-10-CM Official Guidelines for Coding and Reporting Section I.C.4.a:

The diabetes mellitus codes are combination codes that include the type of diabetes mellitus, the body system affected, and the complications affecting that body system. As many codes within a particular category as are necessary to describe all of the complications of the disease may be used. They should be sequenced based on the reason for a particular encounter. Assign as many codes from categories EØ8–E13 as needed to identify all of the associated conditions that the patient has.

DEFINITIONS

congenital. Present at birth, occurring through heredity or an influence during gestation up to the moment of birth.

epiphora. Overflow of tears down the cheeks due to a stricture in the lacrimal passages.

OPERATIVE REPORT MDC 2—#2

Preoperative diagnosis:
Bilateral congenital obstruction nasolacrimal ducts, right side greater than left

Postoperative diagnosis:
Same

Procedure performed:
Probing of nasolacrimal duct, bilateral

Indications:
This 14-month-old baby girl presents for nasolacrimal duct probing and dilation. The child has a history since birth of epiphora of both eyes, with worsening of the condition when she has a cold or is out on windy days. Besides tearing, she has crusting and drainage around the eyes. She was recently on antibiotics for conjunctivitis and increased mucus in the eye. Her parents have tried warm compresses and massage of the lacrimal sac, but that has not been helpful.

Procedure description:
The child was brought to the operating room and placed in the supine position on the operating table. General anesthesia was induced. A nasal speculum was used to examine the nose bilaterally. After dilation of the punctum on the left side, the left nasolacrimal system was probed. Methylene blue solution was injected through the nasolacrimal system and suctioned through the nose and noted to be patent. Attention was then turned to the right side. The right nasolacrimal system was dilated using a punctual dilator. Next, a 000 probe was inserted, followed by successively larger probes until the nasolacrimal system was noted to be open. Methylene blue solution was injected through the right nasolacrimal system and suctioned through the nose and noted to be patent. Maxitrol ophthalmic solution was injected into the right punctum and noted to irrigate cleanly through the system. The child was discharged to the post-anesthesia care unit in good condition.

Code all relevant ICD-10-CM diagnosis and ICD-10-PCS procedure codes in accordance with official guidelines and coding conventions.

Diagnosis Codes:

_____

_____

Procedure Codes:

_____

_____

MS-DRG:

_____

_____

Answers and Rationale

Preoperative diagnosis:
Bilateral congenital obstruction nasolacrimal ducts, right side greater than left[1]

Postoperative diagnosis:
Same

Procedure performed:
Probing of nasolacrimal duct, bilateral

Indications:
This 14-month-old baby girl presents for nasolacrimal duct probing and dilation. The child has a history since birth of epiphora of both eyes,[2] with worsening of the condition when she has a cold or is out on windy days. Besides tearing, she has crusting and drainage around the eyes. She was recently on antibiotics for conjunctivitis and increased mucous in the eye. Her parents have tried warm compresses and massage of the lacrimal sac, but that has not been helpful.

Procedure description:
The child was brought to the operating room and placed in the supine position on the operating table. General anesthesia was induced. A nasal speculum was used to examine the nose bilaterally. After dilation of the punctum on the left side, the left nasolacrimal system was probed.[3] Methylene blue solution was injected through the nasolacrimal system and suctioned through the nose and noted to be patent. Attention was then turned to the right side. The right nasolacrimal system was dilated using a punctual dilator. Next, a 000 probe was inserted, followed by successively larger probes until the nasolacrimal system was noted to be open.[4] Methylene blue solution was injected through the right nasolacrimal system and suctioned through the nose and noted to be patent. Maxitrol ophthalmic solution was injected into the right punctum and noted to irrigate cleanly through the system. The child was discharged to the post-anesthesia care unit in good condition.

Diagnosis Codes

Q10.5   **Congenital stenosis and stricture of lacrimal duct[1]**

H04.203   **Unspecified epiphora, bilateral lacrimal glands[2]**

Rationale for Diagnosis Codes
The documentation states that the obstruction is congenital and is present with epiphora. Because ICD-10-CM does not classify epiphora as a congenital anomaly, a code from chapter 17, "Congenital Malformations, Deformations and Chromosomal Abnormalities," should be reported first.

Procedure Codes

087Y7ZZ   **Dilation of Left Lacrimal Duct, Via Natural or Artificial Opening[3]**

087X7ZZ   **Dilation of Right Lacrimal Duct, Via Natural or Artificial Opening[4]**

Rationale for Procedure Codes
The root operation of a procedure must coincide with the objective of the procedure. Although the documentation states that the objective is lacrimal probing and it appears that the punctal dilation is part of the approach, the objective is to dilate and remove the obstruction of the lacrimal ducts. This makes the correct root operation *Dilation* rather than *Inspection*.

MS-DRG

115   **Extraocular Procedures Except Orbit**   **RW 1.3151**

☼ CODING AXIOM

ICD-10-CM Official Guidelines for Coding and Reporting Section I.C.17:

When a malformation/deformation/or chromosomal abnormality does not have a unique code assignment, assign additional code(s) for any manifestations that may be present.

OPERATIVE REPORT MDC 2—#3

Preoperative diagnosis:
Lazy left eye

Postoperative diagnosis:
Lazy left eye

Indications:
The patient is a 3-year-old with history of lazy eye for the past two years. Patient has been treated with alternative methods without success. The risks and benefits of surgery have been explained to the parents, and after careful consideration the parents have consented to surgical treatment.

Procedure description:
The patient was taken to the operating suite. After induction of general anesthesia, the patient was prepped and draped. A speculum was placed in the left eye. An incision was made in the conjunctiva at the limbus. The medial rectus muscle was isolated with a muscle hook and resected. The muscle was reattached to the sclera by adjustable sutures. Attention was then turned to the lateral rectus muscle. The procedure was repeated. A single 10-0 Nylon suture was placed. TobraDex ointment was instilled into the left conjunctival sac and a firm patch placed on the left eye. The patient tolerated the procedure well and was sent to recovery in satisfactory condition.

Code all relevant ICD-10-CM diagnosis and ICD-10-PCS procedure codes in accordance with official guidelines and coding conventions.

Diagnosis Codes:

_____

_____

Procedure Codes:

_____

_____

MS-DRG:

_____

_____

Answers and Rationale

Preoperative diagnosis:
Lazy left eye

Postoperative diagnosis:
Lazy left eye[1]

Indications:
The patient is a 3-year-old with history of lazy eye for the past two years. Patient has been treated with alternative methods without success. The risks and benefits of surgery have been explained to the parents, and after careful consideration the parents have consented to surgical treatment.

Procedure description:
The patient was taken to the operating suite. After induction of general anesthesia, the patient was prepped and draped. A speculum was placed in the left eye. An incision was made in the conjunctiva at the limbus.[2,3] The medial rectus muscle was isolated with a muscle hook and resected. The muscle was reattached to the sclera by adjustable sutures.[2] Attention was then turned to the lateral rectus muscle. The procedure was repeated.[3] A single 10-0 Nylon suture was placed. TobraDex ointment was instilled into the left conjunctival sac and a firm patch placed on the left eye. The patient tolerated the procedure well and was sent to recovery in satisfactory condition.

Diagnosis Codes

H53.002   Unspecified amblyopia, left eye[1]

Rationale for Diagnosis Codes
Lazy eye is also known as amblyopia ex anopsia. ICD-10-CM does not have an entry in the index for lazy eye.

Procedure Codes

08SM0ZZ   Reposition Left Extraocular Muscle, Open Approach[2]

08SM0ZZ   Reposition Left Extraocular Muscle, Open Approach[3]

Rationale for Procedure Codes
Both the medial rectus and lateral rectus muscles were divided and reattached to the sclera to correct the positioning of the eye. This procedure coincides with the definition of the root operation *Reposition*. Another key to code assignment in this case is that these muscles are two of the four extraocular muscles and thus are found in the *Eye* section of ICD-10-PCS rather than the *Muscles* section. It is appropriate for code 08SM0ZZ to be reported twice according to coding guideline section B3.2b.

MS-DRG

115   Extraocular Procedures Except Orbit   RW 1.3151

 DEFINITIONS

amblyopia. Diminished sight in one eye without alteration in structure.

lazy eye. Decreased or impaired vision in one or both eyes without detectable anatomic damage to the retina or visual pathways, brought on by disuse, often as a result of esotropia. Lazy eye is usually not correctable by eyeglasses or contact lenses.

CODING AXIOM

ICD-10-PCS Official Guidelines for Coding and Reporting Section B3.2b:

During the same operative episode, multiple procedures are coded if: The same root operation is repeated in multiple body parts, and those body parts are separate and distinct body parts classified to a single ICD-10-PCS body part value.

OPERATIVE REPORT MDC 2—#4

Preoperative diagnosis:
Nuclear sclerotic senile cataract

Postoperative diagnosis:
Same

Procedure performed:
Phacoemulsification with implantation of posterior chamber intraocular lens, right eye

Procedure description:
Following instillation of dilating and antibiotic eye drops, the patient was brought to the operating room, where anesthesia was induced. A retrobulbar block of 5 cc of a 50:50 mixture of 2% lidocaine with Wydase and 0.75% Marcaine was given. The Honan balloon was then applied to the right eye at 40 mmHg for 5 minutes. The patient was prepared and draped as usual. A lid speculum was placed between the lids of the right eye. A conjunctival flap was formed when a clear-cornea incision was made. Hydrodissection of the lens nucleus was performed. The lens nucleus was then removed using the phacoemulsification handpiece. The remaining cortex was removed using the I/A handpiece. The posterior chamber intraocular lens was inspected and irrigated. Using a smooth lens forceps, the lens was folded and placed in the appropriate position. It was noted to be well centered and well positioned. Miochol was injected, and the wound was closed with interrupted 10-0 Vicryl suture. Ancef and Decadron were injected, and the lid speculum was removed. A patch and shield were applied. There were no complications, and the patient was transported from the operating room in good condition.

Code all relevant ICD-10-CM diagnosis and ICD-10-PCS procedure codes in accordance with official guidelines and coding conventions.

Diagnosis Codes:

_____

_____

Procedure Codes:

_____

_____

MS-DRG:

_____

_____

Answers and Rationale

Preoperative diagnosis:
Nuclear sclerotic senile cataract[1]

Postoperative diagnosis:
Same

Procedure performed:
Phacoemulsification with implantation of posterior chamber intraocular lens, right eye[1,2]

Procedure description:
Following instillation of dilating and antibiotic eye drops, the patient was brought to the operating room, where anesthesia was induced. A retrobulbar block of 5 cc of a 50:50 mixture of 2% lidocaine with Wydase and 0.75% Marcaine was given. The Honan balloon was then applied to the right eye at 40 mmHg for 5 minutes. The patient was prepared and draped as usual. A lid speculum was placed between the lids of the right eye. A conjunctival flap was formed when a clear-cornea incision was made. Hydrodissection of the lens nucleus was performed. The lens nucleus was then removed using the phacoemulsification handpiece.[2] The remaining cortex was removed using the I/A handpiece. The posterior chamber intraocular lens was inspected and irrigated. Using a smooth lens forceps, the lens was folded and placed in the appropriate position.[2] It was noted to be well centered and well positioned. Miochol was injected, and the wound was closed with interrupted 10-0 Vicryl suture. Ancef and Decadron were injected, and the lid speculum was removed. A patch and shield were applied. There were no complications, and the patient was transported from the operating room in good condition.

Diagnosis Codes

H25.11   **Age-related nuclear cataract, right eye[1]**

Rationale for Diagnosis Codes
The terms "Cataract, Nuclear, Sclerotic" in the ICD-10-CM index direct the coder to see "Cataract, Senile, Nuclear," which leads to code H25.1. The fifth character of 1 is added to complete the code and distinguish that the cataract is of the right eye.

Procedure Codes

Ø8RJ3JZ   **Replacement of Right Lens with Synthetic Substitute, Percutaneous Approach[2]**

Rationale for Procedure Codes
Because the lens is removed and then a prosthetic lens is placed, ICD-10-PCS considers this a *Replacement* root operation. This is confirmed by the index, which divides the term "Phacoemulsification" by whether or not there is a lens insertion done at the same time. The resection and insertion would not be reported separately as they are both included in the root operation "Replacement."

MS-DRG

117   **Intraocular Procedures without CC/MCC**   **RW 0.8340**

 DEFINITIONS

replacement. ICD-10-PCS root operation value R. Putting in or on biological or synthetic material that physically takes the place and/or function of all or a portion of a body part. The body part may have been taken out or replaced, or may be taken out, physically eradicated, or rendered nonfunctional during the "replacement" procedure. A "removal" procedure is coded for taking out the device used in a previous "replacement" procedure.

DEFINITIONS

blepharochalasis. Loss of elasticity and relaxation of skin of the eyelid, thickened or indurated skin on the eyelid associated with recurrent episodes of edema, and intracellular atrophy.

blepharoplasty. Plastic surgery of the eyelids to remove excess fat and redundant skin weighting down the lid. The eyelid is pulled tight and sutured to support sagging muscles.

OPERATIVE REPORT MDC 2—#5

PREOPERATIVE DIAGNOSIS:
Visual field defects

Postoperative diagnosis:
Blepharochalasis

Procedure performed:
Upper and lower blepharoplasties

Procedure description:
Under general anesthesia the patient was prepped and draped in the usual fashion and marked following instillation of Xylocaine with epinephrine in the four eyelids. I proceeded with the right upper blepharoplasty. A skin and muscle excision was done as marked by incising the skin and creating the entire upper eyelid flap as designed, skin and muscle. The fat was then identified and removed bipolar in the usual fashion. I proceeded then with the left side upper eyelid surgery, incising the upper eyelid as designed and excising skin and muscle, removing the medial fat pad on the contralateral side. Hemostasis was accomplished on both sides with a Bovie as needed and the wound closed with 5-0 Prolene subcuticular closure.

We proceeded then with the left lower eyelid surgery. A lateral incision was made just inferior to the canthus and prolonged in a subsidiary fashion. Generous undermining was done at the subcutaneous level, a band of hypertrophic muscle was excised along the ciliary margin, and the medial fat pad excised. Hemostasis was accomplished with bipolar Bovie as needed, the skin flap was reflected superiorly and laterally, the excess was excised, and the wound was closed with 6-0 Prolene sutures. We then proceeded with the right lower eyelid surgery. Again the skin was incised just inferior to the lateral canthal area and continued in a subiciliary fashion. A generous skin flap was raised and the hypertrophic orbicularis excised, followed by excision of the medial fat pad. Hemostasis was accomplished with the bipolar as needed. The skin flap reflected superiorly and laterally, the excess excised accommodating to the incision, and the wound was then closed with 6-0 Prolene. Once this was accomplished, the wounds were dressed with cold compresses. The patient was awakened in the operating room and taken to the recovery room in stable condition.

Code all relevant ICD-10-CM diagnosis and ICD-10-PCS procedure codes in accordance with official guidelines and coding conventions.

Diagnosis Codes:

_____

_____

Procedure Codes:

_____

_____

MS-DRG:

_____

_____

Answers and Rationale

Preoperative diagnosis:
Visual field defects[5]

Postoperative diagnosis:
Blepharochalasis[1-4]

Procedure performed:
Upper and lower blepharoplasties

Procedure description:
Under general anesthesia the patient was prepped and draped in the usual fashion and marked following instillation of Xylocaine with epinephrine in the four eyelids.[1-4] I proceeded with the right upper blepharoplasty. A skin and muscle excision was done as marked by incising the skin and creating the entire upper eyelid flap as designed, skin and muscle. The fat was then identified and removed bipolar in the usual fashion.[6] I proceeded then with the left side upper eyelid surgery, incising the upper eyelid as designed, removing the medial fat pad on the contralateral side.[7] Hemostasis was accomplished on both sides with a Bovie as needed and the wound closed with 5-0 Prolene subcuticular closure.

We proceeded then with the left lower eyelid surgery. A lateral incision was made just inferior to the canthus and prolonged in a subsidiary fashion. Generous undermining was done at the subcutaneous level, a band of hypertrophic muscle was excised along the ciliary margin, and the medial fat pad excised. Hemostasis was accomplished with bipolar Bovie as needed, the skin flap was reflected superiorly and laterally, the excess was excised, and the wound was closed with 6-0 Prolene sutures.[9] We then proceeded with the right lower eyelid surgery. Again the skin was incised just inferior to the lateral canthal area and continued in a subciliary fashion. A generous skin flap was raised and the hypertrophic orbicularis excised, followed by excision of the medial fat pad. Hemostasis was accomplished with the bipolar as needed. The skin flap reflected superiorly and laterally, the excess excised accommodating to the incision, and the wound was then closed with 6-0 Prolene.[8] Once this was accomplished, the wounds were dressed with cold compresses. The patient was awakened in the operating room and taken to the recovery room in stable condition.

Diagnosis Codes

H02.31	**Blepharochalasis right upper eyelid**[1]
H02.32	**Blepharochalasis right lower eyelid**[2]
H02.34	**Blepharochalasis left upper eyelid**[3]
H02.35	**Blepharochalasis left lower eyelid**[4]
H53.453	**Other localized visual field defect, bilateral**[5]

Rationale for Diagnosis Codes

The blepharochalasis is not specified as being of the right and left, upper and lower eyelids, but it can be assumed based on the procedure performed on both the upper and lower eyelids of bilateral eyes. Report any documented visual field defect to indicate the clinical impact of the blepharochalasis.

Procedure Codes

08SN0ZZ	**Reposition Right Upper Eyelid, Open Approach**[6]
08SP0ZZ	**Reposition Left Upper Eyelid, Open Approach**[7]
08SQ0ZZ	**Reposition Right Lower Eyelid, Open Approach**[8]
08SR0ZZ	**Reposition Left Lower Eyelid, Open Approach**[9]

Rationale for Procedure Codes

Although it seems that multiple root operations were performed during this procedure, such as excision of fat, repair of the eyelids, etc., before assigning any codes, the coder must determine the procedure's objective. The various procedures were performed with the single objective of moving the eyelids out of the visual field. This objective coincides with the ICD-10-PCS root operation *Reposition*, and therefore all of the individual procedures are encompassed within this root operation. Because there is no body part character value that combines the eyelids, a code should be reported for each eyelid, resulting in four separate procedure codes. The documentation reflects that the operation was performed via an incision, making the approach character value 0, or *Open*.

MS-DRG

115	Extraocular Procedures Except Orbit	RW 1.3151

MDC 3 Diseases and Disorders of the Ear, Nose, Mouth and Throat

OPERATIVE REPORT MDC 3—#1

Preoperative diagnosis:
1. Suspected supraglottic cancer to left anterior neck
2. Lymphadenopathy

Postoperative diagnosis:
1. Supraglottic cancer to left anterior neck

Procedure performed:
1. Microdirect laryngoscopy with biopsy
2. Tru-Cut needle biopsy of left anterior neck lymph node

Indications:
The patient initially presented with persistent dysphagia and hoarseness and recently discovered a left anterior neck mass. He has been a heavy smoker for the past 30+ years and carries a diagnosis of long-standing COPD.

Procedure description:
The patient was brought into the operating room and identified, and general endotracheal anesthesia was induced. The patient was then sterilely prepped and draped in the usual manner. The lingual mobile tongue was without evidence of lesions, and there was no evidence of lesions in the oral cavity. The tongue base was normal appearing. A vallecula laryngoscope was then carefully inserted in the oral cavity and the tongue retracted anteriorly. The vallecula was then examined and noted to be without evidence of obvious lesions. The area of epiglottic folds and arytenoid regions were noted to be markedly edematous. There was noted to be greater fullness of the left tip of the epiglottis on the lingual surface as well as the left arytenoid. There was no obvious friability of the mucosa. The true vocal cords were visualized and noted to be of normal appearance. Photo documentation with 5 mm rigid telescope was then performed. The vallecula scope was then placed into suspension, and multiple biopsies were taken of the vallecula and the tip of the epiglottis, the left area epiglottic fold, and laryngeal surface of the epiglottis. Hemostasis was obtained with adrenaline-soaked pledgets. No further evidence of bleeding was noted. The vallecula scope was removed, and the patient tolerated the procedure well.

Next, the left neck was sterilely prepped with Betadine. A Tru-Cut needle biopsy was then carried out through the skin and subcutaneous tissue to a palpable left anterior neck mass just below the hyoid bone. This lymph node was greater than a centimeter in size and firm to palpation. Multiple passes with the Tru-Cut needle were then performed, and this tissue was sent for pathologic examination. Hemostasis was obtained with a pressure type dressing on the anterior neck. The patient was then safely awakened from general anesthesia and transferred to the recovery room in stable condition.

Operative report addendum:
Pathology report (gross & microscopic) was viewed by myself (surgeon) and indicated supraglottic squamous cell carcinoma; the Tru-Cut biopsies of the neck lymph node also involved metastatic disease of the same tumor.

Code all relevant ICD-10-CM diagnosis and ICD-10-PCS procedure codes in accordance with official guidelines and coding conventions.

Diagnosis Codes:

_____

_____

Procedure Codes:

_____

_____

MS-DRG:

_____

_____

Answers and Rationale

Preoperative diagnosis:

1. Suspected supraglottic cancer to left anterior neck

2. Lymphadenopathy

Postoperative diagnosis:

1. Supraglottic cancer to left anterior neck[1]

Procedure performed:

1. Microdirect laryngoscopy with biopsy[5]

2. Tru-Cut needle biopsy of left anterior neck lymph node[6]

Indications:

The patient initially presented with persistent dysphagia and hoarseness and recently discovered a left anterior neck mass. He has been a heavy smoker for the past 30+ years[3] and carries a diagnosis of long-standing COPD.[4]

Procedure description:

The patient was brought into the operating room and identified, and general endotracheal anesthesia was induced. The patient was then sterilely prepped and draped in the usual manner. The lingual mobile tongue was without evidence of lesions, and there was no evidence of lesions in the oral cavity. The tongue base was normal appearing.[7] A vallecula laryngoscope was then carefully inserted in the oral cavity and the tongue retracted anteriorly.[5] The vallecula was then examined and noted to be without evidence of obvious lesions. The area of epiglottic folds and arytenoid regions were noted to be markedly edematous. There was noted to be greater fullness of the left tip of the epiglottis on the lingual surface as well as the left arytenoid. There was no obvious friability of the mucosa. The true vocal cords were visualized and noted to be of normal appearance. Photo documentation with 5 mm rigid telescope was then performed. The vallecula scope was then placed into suspension, and multiple biopsies were taken of the vallecula and the tip of the epiglottis, the left area epiglottic fold, and laryngeal surface of the epiglottis. [5]Hemostasis was obtained with adrenaline-soaked pledgets. No further evidence of bleeding was noted. The vallecula scope was removed, [6] and the patient tolerated the procedure well.

Next, the left neck was sterilely prepped with Betadine. A Tru-Cut needle biopsy was then carried out through the skin and subcutaneous tissue[6] to a palpable left anterior neck mass just below the hyoid bone. This lymph node was greater than a centimeter in size and firm to palpation. Multiple passes with the Tru-Cut needle were then performed, and this tissue was sent for pathologic examination.[6] Hemostasis was obtained with a pressure type dressing on the anterior neck. The patient was then safely awakened from general anesthesia and transferred to the recovery room in stable condition.

Operative report addendum:

Pathology report (gross & microscopic) was viewed by myself (surgeon) and indicated supraglottic squamous cell carcinoma; the Tru-Cut biopsies of the neck lymph node also involved metastatic disease of the same tumor. [2]

Diagnosis Codes

C32.1 **Malignant neoplasm of supraglottis[1]**

C77.Ø **Secondary and unspecified malignant neoplasm of lymph nodes of head, face and neck[2]**

F17.21Ø **Nicotine dependence, cigarettes, uncomplicated[3]**

J44.9 **Chronic obstructive pulmonary disease, unspecified[4]**

Rationale for Diagnosis Codes

The postoperative diagnosis and the operative report addendum confirm the malignant neoplasm of the supraglottis. The addendum also documents that the mass excised from the neck was a lymph node affected by metastatic carcinoma. The indications section indicates that the patient has been dependent on cigarettes for more than 30 years and also carries a diagnosis of COPD. The "code also" note under category C32 directs that an additional code should be reported for any nicotine dependence (F17-).

Procedure Codes

ØCBR8ZX **Excision of Epiglottis, Via Natural or Artificial Opening Endoscopic, Diagnostic[5]**

Ø7B23ZX **Excision of Left Neck Lymphatic, Percutaneous Approach, Diagnostic[6]**

ØWJ3XZZ **Inspection of Oral Cavity and Throat, External Approach[7]**

 KEY POINT

Tru-Cut needle biopsy.
Percutaneous approach by a notched needle in which a tissue specimen is cut, trapped, and withdrawn.

CODING AXIOM

Findings on pathology reports must be confirmed by the provider if they are to be reported for code assignment on inpatient encounters.

DEFINITIONS

Via natural or artificial opening endoscopic. ICD-10-PCS approach value 8. Entry of instrumentation through a natural or artificial external opening to reach and visualize the site of the procedure.

Rationale for Procedure Codes

In reviewing the operative note, it is clear portions of the epiglottis are excised via a laryngoscope and once this was removed, a separate incision was made to excise portions of the anterior neck mass/lymph node. Both procedures are performed as biopsies, and therefore a seventh character (qualifier) of X is appropriate to indicate that the procedures are diagnostic in nature. A code for the inspection of the oral cavity and tongue should be reported as well. The approach for the inspection is external, according to ICD-10-PCS coding guideline B5.3a.

MS-DRG

| 133 | Other Ear, Nose, Mouth and Throat O.R. Procedures with CC/MCC | RW 1.8573 |

If the secondary neoplasm of the lymph node is mistakenly coded as lymphadenopathy (per the preoperative diagnosis section of the operation report), the MS-DRG would group to lower-weighted 134 Other Ear, Nose, Mouth and Throat O.R. Procedures without CC/MCC (RW 1.0635).

OPERATIVE REPORT MDC 3—#2

Preoperative/postoperative diagnosis:
Right chronic mastoiditis, right mastoid cholesteatoma, right chronic otorrhea

Procedure performed:
Right tympanomastoidectomy with facial nerve monitoring

Procedure description:
After consent was obtained, the patient was taken to the operating suite and underwent general anesthesia with an endotracheal tube in supine position. The patient was rotated to 180 degrees. The nerve integrity monitor for the facial nerve was connected using surface electrodes. Then 1 percent Xylocaine with 1:100,000 epinephrine was injected into the postauricular incision site. The right ear was prepped and draped in the usual sterile fashion.

A #15 blade was used to create an incision that was carried up to the temporalis fascia. A temporalis fascial graft was obtained and set aside for routine drying procedure. Bovie suction cautery was used to create an incision along the linea temporalis, and a second incision was made inferiorly up to the inferior aspect of the bony external auditory canal. This periosteal flap was then elevated anteriorly with a Joseph elevator. This allowed access up to the junction of the cartilaginous and bony external auditory canal. A #15 blade was used to create an incision through the cartilaginous aspect of the external auditory canal parallel to the bony external auditory canal. This allowed visualization into the external auditory canal. The mastoid cortex was further visualized after periosteal elevation. A #5 cutting bur was used to perform a complete right mastoidectomy. The mastoid cavity was dissected anteriorly into the zygomatic root. The dissection was carried further posteriorly into the sinodural angle and inferiorly to the digastric insertion in the mastoid tip. Anteriorly, the dissection was performed medially to visualize the horizontal semicircular canal and fossa incudis. A #3 coarse diamond bur was used to further skeletonize posteriorly along the sigmoid sinus, superiorly along the tegmen tympani. A #.5 coarse diamond bur was used to dissect further into the zygomatic root and allow better access and visualization of the epitympanic region. Large amounts of cholesteatoma and granulation tissue were removed throughout the procedure. Upon adequate skeletonization and removal of cholesteatoma from the sinodural angle and epitympanum, attention was directed to the tympanic membrane. The tympanic membrane was very edematous. This was elevated from the annular groove anteriorly and dissected. Chorda tympani was visualized and preserved. Granulation tissue and polypoid masses were removed from the middle ear cavity. All tissue from the mastoid and middle ear cavity was sent to pathology for further evaluation. Further elevation of the tympanic membrane allowed visualization of the malleus and the incus.

The incudostapedial joint was seen, and careful dissection allowed visualization of the stapes capitulum. The malleus and incus complex was held anteriorly into the middle ear cavity for cholesteatoma removal.

Upon adequate removal of the cholesteatoma, irrigation was performed to ensure a good connection between the middle ear cavity and mastoid. The malleus and incus complex were then replaced to their original position. The incus was placed into the fossa incudis and the incudostapedial joint was rejoined. A small amount of fibrin glue was injected over the IS joint. Gelfilm cut in small circles was placed into the middle ear cavity, atop the promontory. Ciprodex-soaked Gelfoam was placed into the middle ear cavity. The temporalis fascia was placed underneath the original tympanic membrane anteriorly and brought out posteriorly along the bony external auditory canal. The Penrose drain and self-retaining retractors were removed. Under visualization with the microscope, the posterior cartilaginous external auditory canal and skin flap were replaced in their original position superficial to the temporalis fascia graft. Another layer of Ciprodex-soaked Gelfoam was placed lateral to the tympanic membrane and temporalis fascia graft.

The postauricular incision was closed in 3 layers with 3-0 Vicryl suture in an interrupted fashion. We started with the periosteal closure, then the dermal, and epidermal closure. The epidermis was closed with 5-0 fast gut suture in a running fashion. Antibiotic ointment was injected and a cotton ball inserted into the right external auditory canal. A Glasscock ear dressing was then placed.

The patient tolerated the procedure well. No complications. The patient was taken to postanesthesia care unit in satisfactory condition.

Code all relevant ICD-10-CM diagnosis and ICD-10-PCS procedure codes in accordance with official guidelines and coding conventions.

Diagnosis Codes:

_____

_____

Procedure Codes:

_____

_____

MS-DRG:

_____

_____

Answers and Rationale

Preoperative/postoperative diagnosis:

Right chronic mastoiditis,[1] right mastoid cholesteatoma,[2] right chronic otorrhea[3]

Procedure performed:

Right tympanomastoidectomy with facial nerve monitoring

Procedure description:

After consent was obtained, the patient was taken to the operating suite and underwent general anesthesia with an endotracheal tube in supine position. The patient was rotated to 180 degrees. The nerve integrity monitor for the facial nerve was connected using surface electrodes.[10] Then 1 percent Xylocaine with 1:100,000 epinephrine was injected into the postauricular incision site. The right ear was prepped and draped in the usual sterile fashion.

A #15 blade was used to create an incision that was carried up to the temporalis fascia. A temporalis fascial graft was obtained and set aside for routine drying procedure.[9] Bovie suction cautery was used to create an incision along the linea temporalis, and a second incision was made inferiorly up to the inferior aspect of the bony external auditory canal. This periosteal flap was then elevated anteriorly with a Joseph elevator. This allowed access up to the junction of the cartilaginous and bony external auditory canal. A #15 blade was used to create an incision through the cartilaginous aspect of the external auditory canal parallel to the bony external auditory canal. This allowed visualization into the external auditory canal.[4-9] The mastoid cortex was further visualized after periosteal elevation. A #5 cutting bur was used to perform a complete right mastoidectomy.[4] The mastoid cavity was dissected anteriorly into the zygomatic root. The dissection was carried further posteriorly into the sinodural angle and inferiorly to the digastric insertion in the mastoid tip. Anteriorly, the dissection was performed medially to visualize the horizontal semicircular canal and fossa incudis. A #3 coarse diamond bur was used to further skeletonize posteriorly along the sigmoid sinus, superiorly along the tegmen tympani. A #.5 coarse diamond bur was used to dissect further into the zygomatic root and allow better access and visualization of the epitympanic region. Large amounts of cholesteatoma and granulation tissue were removed throughout the procedure. Upon adequate skeletonization and removal of cholesteatoma from the sinodural angle and epitympanum, attention was directed to the tympanic membrane. The tympanic membrane was very edematous. This was elevated from the annular groove anteriorly and dissected.[5] Chorda tympani was visualized and preserved. Granulation tissue and polypoid masses were removed from the middle ear cavity.[7, 8] All tissue from the mastoid and middle ear cavity was sent to pathology for further evaluation. Further elevation of the tympanic membrane allowed visualization of the malleus and the incus.

The incudostapedial joint was seen, and careful dissection allowed visualization of the stapes capitulum. The malleus and incus complex was held anteriorly into the middle ear cavity for cholesteatoma removal.

Upon adequate removal of the cholesteatoma, irrigation was performed to ensure a good connection between the middle ear cavity and mastoid. The malleus and incus complex were then replaced to their original position. The incus was placed into the fossa incudis and the incudostapedial joint was rejoined. A small amount of fibrin glue was injected over the IS joint. Gelfilm cut in small circles was placed into the middle ear cavity, atop the promontory. Ciprodex-soaked Gelfoam was placed into the middle ear cavity. The temporalis fascia was placed underneath the original tympanic membrane anteriorly and brought out posteriorly along the bony external auditory canal.[6] The Penrose drain and self-retaining retractors were removed. Under visualization with the microscope, the posterior cartilaginous external auditory canal and skin flap were replaced in their original position superficial to the temporalis fascia graft. Another layer of Ciprodex-soaked Gelfoam was placed lateral to the tympanic membrane and temporalis fascia graft.

The postauricular incision was closed in 3 layers with 3-0 Vicryl suture in an interrupted fashion. We started with the periosteal closure, then the dermal, and epidermal closure. The epidermis was closed with 5-0 fast gut suture in a running fashion. Antibiotic ointment was injected and a cotton ball inserted into the right external auditory canal. A Glasscock ear dressing was then placed.

The patient tolerated the procedure well. No complications. The patient was taken to postanesthesia care unit in satisfactory condition.

Diagnosis Codes

H70.11	Chronic mastoiditis, right ear[1]
H71.21	Cholesteatoma of mastoid, right ear[2]
H92.11	Otorrhea, right ear[3]

Rationale for Diagnosis Codes

The pre- and postoperative diagnoses are the same. This makes the diagnosis code assignment straightforward. Be sure to choose the accurate diagnosis code based on the appropriate side of the body, in this case the right ear.

Procedure Codes

09TB0ZZ	Resection of Right Mastoid Sinus, Open Approach[4]
09R707Z	Replacement of Right Tympanic Membrane with Autologous Tissue Substitute, Open Approach[5,6]
09B50ZZ	Excision of Right Middle Ear, Open Approach[7]
09C50ZZ	Extirpation of Right Middle Ear, Open Approach[8]
0JB00ZZ	Excision of Scalp Subcutaneous Tissue and Fascia, Open Approach[9]
4A10X2Z	Monitoring of Central Nervous Conductivity, External Approach[10]

Rationale for Procedure Codes

Both a complete right mastoidectomy and tympanectomy are performed. Because these are described as being removed in their entirety, the appropriate root operation for these would be *Resection*. For the tympanectomy, however, the resection would not be reported separately, as a replacement (graft) procedure was done. The objective of a *Replacement* procedure is to put in a device that takes the place of some or all of a body part and includes taking out the body part.

In addition, granulation tissue and polypoid masses were removed from the middle ear, which is separately reportable as the middle ear is a different body part. The removal of granulation tissue would be reported as *Extirpation*, while the polypectomy portion of the procedure would be classified as an *Excision*. In *Extirpation* procedures, the objective is to remove solid material such as a foreign body, thrombus, or calculus from a body part.

The excision of the temporalis fascia for a graft is reported in addition to the grafting of the tympanic membrane (replacement), per *ICD-10-PCS Official Guidelines for Coding and Reporting* section B3.9. Lastly, the facial nerve monitoring was performed via external electrodes. According to the ICD-10-PCS classification, the facial nerve is considered part of the central nervous system.

MS-DRG

136	Sinus and Mastoid Procedures without CC/MCC	RW 1.1905

📖 **DEFINITIONS**

excision. Cutting out or off, without replacement, a portion of a body part.

extirpation. Taking or cutting out solid matter from a body part.

replacement. Putting in or on biological or synthetic material that physically takes the place and/or function of all or a portion of a body part (includes taking out the body part).

resection. Cutting out or off, without replacement, all of a body part.

OPERATIVE REPORT MDC 3—#3

Preoperative diagnosis:
Chronic obstructive adenotonsillitis with sleep apnea

Postoperative diagnosis:
Same

Procedure performed:
Tonsillectomy and adenoidectomy

Procedure description:
The patient was brought to the operating room, and general anesthesia was administered. The patient was prepped and draped in the usual sterile fashion. A Crowe-Davis mouth gag was placed in the mouth and a tongue depressor applied. The oropharynx was inspected.

The right tonsil was grasped and retracted out of its fossa and excised using electrocautery. This was repeated on the left tonsil. The patient was repositioned, and two #12-French red rubber Robinson catheters were placed within the nasal passage to provide soft palate retraction. The adenoids were then inspected using a laryngeal mirror. The hypertrophic adenoid pads were ablated via electrocautery. The oropharynx was irrigated and the red rubber catheters removed. Estimated blood loss was insignificant, and there were no complications. The patient left the operating room in good condition.

Code all relevant ICD-10-CM diagnosis and ICD-10-PCS procedure codes in accordance with official guidelines and coding conventions.

Diagnosis Codes:

_____

_____

Procedure Codes:

_____

_____

MS-DRG:

_____

_____

Answers and Rationale

Preoperative diagnosis:
Chronic[1] obstructive[2] adenotonsillitis[1] with sleep apnea[2]

Postoperative diagnosis:
Same

Procedure performed:
Tonsillectomy and adenoidectomy

Procedure description:
The patient was brought to the operating room, and general anesthesia was administered. The patient was prepped and draped in the usual sterile fashion. A Crowe-Davis mouth gag was placed in the mouth and a tongue depressor applied. The oropharynx was inspected.

The right tonsil was grasped and retracted out of its fossa and excised using electrocautery. This was repeated on the left tonsil.[3] The patient was repositioned, and two #12-French red rubber Robinson catheters were placed within the nasal passage to provide soft palate retraction. The adenoids were then inspected using a laryngeal mirror. The hypertrophic adenoid pads were ablated via electrocautery.[4] The oropharynx was irrigated and the red rubber catheters removed. Estimated blood loss was insignificant, and there were no complications. The patient left the operating room in good condition.

Diagnosis Codes

J35.Ø3   **Chronic tonsillitis and adenoiditis**[1]

G47.33   **Obstructive sleep apnea (adult) (pediatric)**[2]

Rationale for Diagnosis Codes

Chronic tonsillitis with adenoiditis is reported to J35.Ø3. Because is it associated with the *obstructive* adenotonsillitis, the sleep apnea is considered obstructive sleep apnea. Although there is a "code also" note under category G47, indicating that an additional code should be assigned for the underlying condition, this instructional note does not determine the sequencing of the two conditions. The reason for the procedure is the adenotonsillitis, making that the appropriate principal diagnosis.

Procedure Codes

ØCTPXZZ   **Resection of Tonsils, External Approach**[3]

ØC5QXZZ   **Destruction of Adenoids, External Approach**[4]

Rationale for Procedure Codes

It is important to note that the tonsils were removed and the adenoids were ablated. These are two distinct root operations in ICD-10-PCS. The appropriate root operation for the tonsils is *Resection*, or "cutting out or off, without replacement, all of a body part." Do not be misled by the term "excision" used in the operative note itself, as the entire tonsil on each side was removed, which would lead to the use of the root operation *Resection*. The procedure performed on the adenoids is considered *Destruction*, or "physical eradication of all or a portion of a body part by the direct use of energy, force, or a destructive agent." The approach value is *External* as there were no incisions or punctures needed to reach the operative site.

MS-DRG

134	Other Ear, Nose, Mouth and Throat O.R. Procedures without CC/MCC	RW 1.0635

CODING AXIOM

ICD-10-CM Official Guidelines for Coding and Reporting Section I.A.17:

A "code also" note instructs that two codes may be required to fully describe a condition, but this note does not provide sequencing direction.

CODING AXIOM

ICD-10-PCS Official Guidelines for Coding and Reporting Section B5.3a:

Procedures performed within an orifice on structures that are visible without the aid of any instrumentation are coded to the approach *External*.

OPERATIVE REPORT MDC 3—#4

Preoperative diagnosis:
Chronic sinusitis. Deviated nasal septum. Turbinate hypertrophy.

Postoperative diagnosis:
Same

Procedure performed:
Endoscopic sinus surgery with bilateral total ethmoidectomies, nasal polypectomy bilateral nasoantral windows, and partial excision of the middle turbinates

Procedure description:
The patient was identified, taken to the operating room, and placed in a neutral position. Smooth endotracheal anesthesia was induced. The patient was prepped and draped in the standard fashion. 1% lidocaine with 1:100,000 epinephrine was injected into the septum, uncinate process nasal polyps, and middle turbinates. Visualization with the sinus endoscope revealed a marked spur along the left septum impinging on the left inferior and the middle turbinate and a marked deviation of the superior septum to the right side precluding adequate visualization of the right middle turbinate. Therefore, a left hemitransfixation incision was performed, mucoperichondrial flaps elevated, 1.0 cm caudal and dorsal struts outlined and incised, and a portion of the perpendicular plate of the ethmoid, vomer, and quadrangular cartilage as well as a large maxillary crest spur were resected. The septum was shortened by approximately 1 mm to allow it to return to the midline, and the incision was closed with 4-0 chromic interrupted simple sutures.

Next, the left middle turbinate and middle meatus was identified, and a large polyp was seen to completely obstruct the middle meatus. The polyp was removed with power instrumentation and the insertion of the middle turbinate incised and the anterior two-thirds of the middle turbinate resected. The polyp was then further removed via the ethmoid sinus. The uncinate process was then infractured and sharply resected, gaining entrance to the maxillary sinus. A large polyp was then noted to almost completely fill the maxillary sinus on the left side, and this was removed with curved power instrumentation.

The ethmoid sinus was then entered again, and a marked polypoid and thickened mucosa was noted throughout. The fovea ethmoidalis and laminal papyracea were identified and used as landmarks for the procedure. The basal lamella was entered and the posterior cells also opened wider. Thicken mucosa was noted in the sinuses as well. The sinoethmoidal recess was evaluated and was seen to be free of polypoid tissue. The posterior insertion of the turbinate was cauterized with bipolar cautery as was the anterior insertion. The same procedure was performed on the opposite side with similar findings, except only a small polyp was noted in the right maxillary sinus. Splints coated in ointment were sutured to the nasal septum with 3-0 Prolene. The throat pack that was placed at the beginning of the case was removed, and the patient was extubated and transported to the recovery room in good and stable condition.

Code all relevant ICD-10-CM diagnosis and ICD-10-PCS procedure codes in accordance with official guidelines and coding conventions.

Diagnosis Codes:
_____

_____

Procedure Codes:
_____

_____

MS-DRG:
_____

_____

Answers and Rationale

Preoperative diagnosis:
Chronic sinusitis.[1] Deviated nasal septum.[2] Turbinate hypertrophy.[4]

Postoperative diagnosis:
Same

Procedure performed:
Endoscopic sinus surgery[5-8] with bilateral total ethmoidectomies,[5,6] nasal polypectomy[8,9] bilateral nasoantral windows, and partial excision of the middle turbinates[7]

Procedure description:
The patient was identified, taken to the operating room, and placed in a neutral position. Smooth endotracheal anesthesia was induced. The patient was prepped and draped in the standard fashion. 1% lidocaine with 1:100,000 epinephrine was injected into the septum, uncinate process nasal polyps, and middle turbinates. Visualization with the sinus endoscope revealed a marked spur along the left septum impinging on the left inferior and the middle turbinate and a marked deviation of the superior septum to the right side precluding adequate visualization of the right middle turbinate. Therefore, a left hemitransfixation incision was performed, mucoperichondrial flaps elevated, 1.0 cm caudal and dorsal struts outlined and incised, and a portion of the perpendicular plate of the ethmoid, vomer, and quadrangular cartilage as well as a large maxillary crest spur were resected. The septum was shortened by approximately 1 mm to allow it to return to the midline, and the incision was closed with 4-0 chromic interrupted simple sutures.[10]

Next, the left middle turbinate and middle meatus was identified, and a large polyp was seen to completely obstruct the middle meatus.[3-4] The polyp was removed with power instrumentation[9] and the insertion of the middle turbinate incised and the anterior two-thirds of the middle turbinate resected.[7] The polyp was then further removed entering via the ethmoid sinus. The uncinate process was then infractured and sharply resected, gaining entrance to the maxillary sinus. A large polyp was then noted to almost completely fill the maxillary sinus[4] on the left side, and this was removed with curved power instrumentation.[8]

The ethmoid sinus was then entered again, and a marked polypoid and thickened mucosa was noted throughout. The fovea ethmoidalis and laminal papyracea were identified and used as landmarks for the procedure. The basal lamella was entered and the posterior cells also opened wider.[5] Thicken mucosa was noted in the sinuses as well. The sinoethmoidal recess was evaluated and was seen to be free of polypoid tissue. The posterior insertion of the turbinate was cauterized with bipolar cautery as was the anterior insertion. The same procedure was performed on the opposite side with similar findings,[6] except only a small polyp was noted in the right maxillary sinus. Splints coated in ointment were sutured to the nasal septum with 3-0 Prolene. The throat pack that was placed at the beginning of the case was removed, and the patient was extubated and transported to the recovery room in good and stable condition.

Diagnosis Codes

J32.9	Chronic sinusitis, unspecified[1]
J34.2	Deviated nasal septum[2]
J33.8	Other polyp of sinus[3]
J34.3	Hypertrophy of nasal turbinates[4]

Rationale for Diagnosis Codes
The documentation of the chronic sinusitis and deviated nasal septum is fairly vague and nondescript. This means that there are no variables to consider when referring to the index, making coding straightforward. It is important to note that although the pre- and postoperative diagnoses do not mention polyps, the procedure description notes them multiple times throughout the sinuses. The polyps were treated via excision and therefore should be reported as additional diagnoses.

Procedure Codes

Ø9TV4ZZ	Resection of Left Ethmoid Sinus, Percutaneous Endoscopic Approach[5]
Ø9TU4ZZ	Resection of Right Ethmoid Sinus, Percutaneous Endoscopic Approach[6]
Ø9BL4ZZ	Excision of Nasal Turbinate, Percutaneous Endoscopic Approach[7]
Ø9BR4ZZ	Excision of Left Maxillary Sinus, Percutaneous Endoscopic Approach[8]

Ø9BN4ZZ   **Excision of Nasopharynx, Percutaneous Endoscopic Approach**[9]

Ø9SMØZZ   **Reposition Nasal Septum, Open Approach**[10]

Rationale for Procedure Codes

The only procedure that was not performed via the endoscope was the septal deviation repositioning. Although multiple procedures moved the septum, the objective was to place it into its correct anatomical position, which by ICD-10-PCS definition is the root operation *Reposition*. Polyps were encountered within the middle meatus, left maxillary sinus, and the ethmoid sinus. The one removed from the ethmoid sinus is included in the resection of the left ethmoid sinus; however, the other two should be reported as excisions of the anatomical site in which the polyp was removed. Note that, although the resection of the turbinate occurs multiple times, only one turbinate is resected and the procedure therefore is reported only once. Lastly, the bilateral ethmoidectomies should be reported as root operation *Resection* because the documentation indicates that the sinuses were removed in their entirety.

MS-DRG

136   **Sinus and Mastoid Procedures without CC/MCC**   **RW 1.1905**

MDC 4 Diseases and Disorders of the Respiratory System

OPERATIVE REPORT MDC 4—#1

Preoperative diagnosis:
Lung mass

Postoperative diagnosis:
Metastatic amelanotic melanoma

Indication:
A staging CT of the chest, abdomen, and pelvis reveals a single 4 cm lobulated mass lesion in the left lower lobe of the lung, confirmed to be amelanotic melanoma on biopsy. No further abnormalities are noted.

Procedure performed:
Thermal ablation of the lung tumor

Procedure description:
Grounding pads were placed on the patient, two on each thigh. After conscious sedation with Midazolam and Fentanyl and local anesthesia with intradermal and subcutaneous 1% lidocaine injection, a tiny incision was made into the skin. Under CT fluoroscopic guidance, a 10 cm long expandable 15-gauge StarBurst XL RF electrode was advanced into the lung mass. CT scan showed superomedial position of the electrode within the mass. A treatment algorithm with staged deployment was applied with the lesion ablated for 20 min at maximum deployment and target temperature of 90°C. Intermittent CT fluoroscopy was performed during the ablation cycle, and the electrode position was readjusted appropriately. The electrode was partially withdrawn at the end of the cycle and repositioned for further ablation. Repositioning and repeat ablation was performed two times to produce a thermal lesion that incorporates the tumor and nonmalignant lung parenchyma to create 1 cm wide surgical margin around the mass. Upon completion of the ablations, the needle was heated on withdrawal to minimize the risk of track ablation. Follow-up serial chest radiographs were performed, as per standard post-lung biopsy protocol, and were negative for a pneumothorax. The patient tolerated the procedure well and was discharged to recovery in satisfactory condition.

Code all relevant ICD-10-CM diagnosis and ICD-10-PCS procedure codes in accordance with official guidelines and coding conventions.

Diagnosis Codes:

_____

_____

Procedure Codes:

_____

_____

MS-DRG:

_____

_____

Answers and Rationale

Preoperative diagnosis:
Lung mass

Postoperative diagnosis:
Metastatic amelanotic melanoma[1,2]

Indication:
A staging[1,2] CT of the chest, abdomen, and pelvis reveals a single 4 cm lobulated mass lesion in the left lower lobe of the lung,[1,3] confirmed to be amelanotic melanoma on biopsy. No further abnormalities are noted.

Procedure performed:
Thermal ablation of the lung tumor[3]

Procedure description:
Grounding pads were placed on the patient, two on each thigh. After conscious sedation with Midazolam and Fentanyl and local anesthesia with intradermal and subcutaneous 1% lidocaine injection, a tiny incision was made into the skin. Under CT fluoroscopic guidance, a 10 cm long expandable 15-gauge StarBurst XL RF electrode was advanced into the lung mass.[3] CT scan showed superomedial position of the electrode within the mass. A treatment algorithm with staged deployment was applied with the lesion ablated for 20 min at maximum deployment and target temperature of 90°C. Intermittent CT fluoroscopy was performed during the ablation cycle, and the electrode position was readjusted appropriately. The electrode was partially withdrawn at the end of the cycle and repositioned for further ablation. Repositioning and repeat ablation was performed two times to produce a thermal lesion that incorporates the tumor and nonmalignant lung parenchyma to create 1 cm wide surgical margin around the mass.[3] Upon completion of the ablations, the needle was heated on withdrawal to minimize the risk of track ablation. Follow-up serial chest radiographs were performed, as per standard post-lung biopsy protocol, and were negative for a pneumothorax. The patient tolerated the procedure well and was discharged to recovery in satisfactory condition.

Diagnosis Codes

C78.02 **Secondary malignant neoplasm of left lung**[1]

C43.9 **Malignant melanoma of skin, unspecified**[2]

Rationale for Diagnosis Codes
The terms "Melanoma, Amelanotic" in the ICD-10-CM index instruct the coder to "*see* Melanoma, skin, by site." However, the lesion is documented as in the lung. Also, the Excludes2 note under C43 (Malignant melanoma of skin) indicates that, for sites other than skin, a malignant neoplasm of that site should be coded. The lung mass is also described as metastatic and was discovered on a staging CT. This makes it appropriate to identify the lung tumor as a secondary malignant neoplasm, with C78.02 correctly reporting the lung tumor. As staging was involved, the coder can assume that the melanoma of the skin is still under treatment. Therefore, a secondary code is assigned for the melanoma of the skin. The sequencing of the diagnoses is according to guidelines section I.C.2.b.

Procedure Codes

0B5J3ZZ **Destruction of Left Lower Lung Lobe, Percutaneous Approach**[3]

Rationale for Procedure Codes
The term "Ablation" in the ICD-10-PCS index directs the coder to the root operation *Destruction*. Even if the index is not consulted, the objective of destroying the tumor by thermal energy coincides with that of the same root operation. The approach is considered Percutaneous as only a small incision is used to place the probe under CT guidance.

MS-DRG

168 **Other Respiratory System O.R. Procedures without CC/MCC   RW 1.2950**

If the diagnoses are sequenced incorrectly, the result is a much higher-weighted and targeted MS-DRG 982 Extensive O.R. Procedure Unrelated to Principal Diagnosis with CC.

DEFINITIONS

staging. Determination of the course of a disease, as in the case of a malignancy, to determine whether the malignancy is confined to the primary tumor, has spread to one or more lymph nodes, or has metastasized.

CODING AXIOM

ICD-10-CM Official Guidelines for Coding and Reporting Section I.C.2.b:

Treatment of secondary site:

When a patient is admitted because of a primary neoplasm with metastasis and treatment is directed toward the secondary site only, the secondary neoplasm is designated as the principal diagnosis even though the primary malignancy is still present.

OPERATIVE REPORT MDC 4—#2

Preoperative diagnosis:
Multiple lung nodules

Postoperative diagnosis:
Small cell carcinoma of the upper lobe of right lung

Procedure performed:
Thoracoscopic segmental resection of lung nodules

Indications:
A 53-year-old female presents to the hospital for resection of multiple lung nodules of the upper lobe of the right lung identified by previous outpatient radiological examination. The patient has smoked for 35 years and is a current two-pack-per-day smoker. She also has a family history of lung cancer.

Procedure description:
Two small incisions were made in the chest wall and carried down into the chest cavity by blunt dissection. A trocar was inserted through a small intercostal incision in the right side of the chest wall. An endoscope was passed through the trocar and into the chest cavity. The right lung was partially collapsed by instilling air into the chest through a second trocar placed via a separate incision. The contents of the chest cavity were examined under direct visualization. Via an endoscope, images were obtained of the lesions, and the instruments were manipulated through the secondary sites, clamping blood vessels and bronchial tubes at the segments of the lung containing the nodules. With the clamps in place, the nodules were removed by dividing the vessel and bronchial tubes isolated by the clamps. The remaining lung tissue was repaired by suture and surgical clips. At the conclusion of the procedure, the endoscope and the trocar(s) were removed. A chest tube was inserted for drainage and re-expansion of the chest cavity. Surgical pathology examination is consistent with small cell carcinoma.

Code all relevant ICD-10-CM diagnosis and ICD-10-PCS procedure codes in accordance with official guidelines and coding conventions.

Diagnosis Codes:

_____

_____

Procedure Codes:

_____

_____

MS-DRG:

_____

_____

Answers and Rationale

Preoperative diagnosis:

Multiple lung nodules

Postoperative diagnosis:

Small cell carcinoma of the upper lobe of right lung[1]

Procedure performed:

Thoracoscopic segmental resection of lung nodules

Indications:

A 53-year-old female presents to the hospital for resection of multiple lung nodules of the upper lobe of the right lung identified by previous outpatient radiological examination. The patient has smoked for 35 years and is a current two pack per day smoker.[2] She also has a family history of lung cancer.[3]

Procedure description:

Two small incisions were made in the chest wall and carried down into the chest cavity by blunt dissection. A trocar was inserted through a small intercostal incision in the right side of the chest wall. An endoscope was passed through the trocar and into the chest cavity.[4] The right lung was partially collapsed by instilling air into the chest through a second trocar placed via a separate incision. The contents of the chest cavity were examined under direct visualization. Via an endoscope, images were obtained of the lesions, and the instruments were manipulated through the secondary sites, clamping blood vessels and bronchial tubes at the segments of the lung containing the nodules. With the clamps in place, the nodules were removed by dividing the vessel and bronchial tubes isolated by the clamps.[4] The remaining lung tissue was repaired by suture and surgical clips. At the conclusion of the procedure, the endoscope and the trocar(s) were removed. A chest tube was inserted for drainage and re-expansion of the chest cavity. Surgical pathology examination is consistent with small cell carcinoma.

Diagnosis Codes

C34.11	Malignant neoplasm of upper lobe, right bronchus or lung[1]
F17.210	Nicotine dependence, cigarettes, uncomplicated[2]
Z80.1	Family history of malignant neoplasm of trachea, bronchus, and lung[3]

Rationale for Diagnosis Codes

The small cell carcinoma is confirmed by pathology and documented by the surgeon as the postoperative diagnosis, making this the correct principal diagnosis. The documentation specifies that the patient has been smoking for 35 years, which is clearly nicotine dependence and warrants the assignment of a code from the F17 (nicotine dependence) category. It is also important to report the family history of the same condition for which the patient is being treated.

Procedure Codes

ØBBC4ZZ   Excision of Upper Right Lung Lobe, Percutaneous Endoscopic[4]

Rationale for Procedure Codes

Although specimens are routinely sent to pathology after the surgery, the procedure is not considered diagnostic (seventh character X) unless it is specified as being an intent of the procedure. The objective of this procedure is to remove the nodules, making the appropriate code a therapeutic code (seventh character Z).

MS-DRG

165	Major Chest Procedures without CC/MCC	RW 1.8148

If the procedure is mistakenly reported as a biopsy (ØBBC4ZX Excision of Upper Right Lung Lobe, Percutaneous Endoscopic, Diagnostic), the MS-DRG changes to the lower-weighted 168 Other Respiratory System O.R. Procedures without CC/MCC.

DEFINITIONS

atelectasis. Collapse of lung tissue affecting part or all of one lung, preventing normal oxygen absorption to healthy tissues.

thoracentesis. Surgical puncture of the chest cavity with a specialized needle or hollow tubing to aspirate fluid from within the pleural space for diagnostic or therapeutic reasons.

OPERATIVE REPORT MDC 4—#3

Preoperative diagnosis:
Atelectasis with pleural effusion

Postoperative diagnosis:
Same

Procedure performed:
Diagnostic thoracentesis

Procedure description:
A time-out was performed and the chest x-ray was reviewed, confirming the left side. The patient was prepped and draped in a sterile manner. The appropriate level was percussed and confirmed by ultrasound. 1% lidocaine was used for local anesthesia. A finder needle was introduced over the superior aspect of the rib to locate the pleural fluid. A 10-blade scalpel was used to nick the skin at the insertion site. The Safe-t-Centesis needle was then introduced through the skin incision into the pleural space. The thoracentesis catheter was then threaded without difficulty. Straw-colored transudate was aspirated. The catheter was then removed. No immediate complications were noted during the procedure. A post-procedure chest x-ray is pending at the time of this note. The fluid will be sent for studies.

Code all relevant ICD-10-CM diagnosis and ICD-10-PCS procedure codes in accordance with official guidelines and coding conventions.

Diagnosis Codes:

_____

_____

Procedure Codes:

_____

_____

MS-DRG:

_____

_____

Answers and Rationale

Preoperative diagnosis:
Atelectasis[2] with pleural effusion[1]

Postoperative diagnosis:
Same

Procedure performed:
Diagnostic thoracentesis[3]

Procedure description:
A time-out was performed and the chest x-ray was reviewed, confirming the left side.[3] The patient was prepped and draped in a sterile manner. The appropriate level was percussed and confirmed by ultrasound. 1% lidocaine was used to for local anesthesia. A finder needle was introduced over the superior aspect of the rib to locate the pleural fluid. A 10-blade scalpel was used to nick the skin at the insertion site. The Safe-t-Centesis needle was then introduced through the skin incision into the pleural space. The thoracentesis catheter was then threaded without difficulty. Straw-colored transudate was aspirated.[3] The catheter was then removed. No immediate complications were noted during the procedure. A post-procedure chest x-ray is pending at the time of this note. The fluid will be sent for studies.

Diagnosis Codes

J9Ø   **Pleural effusion, not elsewhere classified**[1]

J98.11   **Atelectasis**[2]

Rationale for Diagnosis Codes

Because there is no information about the type or cause of the atelectasis, the proper code assignment is the default code for atelectasis, J98.11.

Procedure Codes

ØW9B3ZX   **Drainage of Left Pleural Cavity, Percutaneous Approach, Diagnostic**[3]

Rationale for Procedure Codes

The thoracentesis was specified as diagnostic and was performed to drain the fluid from the pleural space to assist in obtaining an accurate diagnosis. The term "Thoracentesis" in the ICD-10-PCS index directs the coder to see the "Drainage, Anatomical Regions, General" table.

MS-DRG

187   **Pleural effusion with CC**   **RW 1.0835**

CODING AXIOM

ICD-10-PCS Official Guidelines for Coding and Reporting Section B3.4a:

Biopsy procedures are coded using the root operations Excision, Extraction or Drainage and the qualifier Diagnostic.

OPERATIVE REPORT MDC 4—#4

Preoperative diagnosis:
Hemoptysis

Postoperative diagnosis:
Same

Procedure performed:
Fiberoptic bronchoscopy with endobronchial and transbronchial biopsies

Procedure description:
The patient was brought to the endoscopy suite and was sedated using IV Versed. It should be noted that the patient has some tendency toward obstructive apnea while in the supine position. The fiberoptic scope was introduced via the right naris and passed into the hypopharynx. The vocal cords, false cords, arytenoid region, hypopharyngeal region, and the epiglottis were examined and found to be unremarkable. The trachea was inspected and found to be normal. The right bronchial tree was examined. The right upper lobe had three normal segments examined. The right middle lobe had two segments, the medial one was stenotic. A very small amount of increased mucus was present in this area. The right lower lobe was also inspected, revealing no abnormality. The left upper lobe and lower lobe were inspected to the subsegmental level, revealing no abnormalities.

Using fluoroscopy, a biopsy forceps was placed into the medial portion of the right middle lobe of the lung. Biopsies were taken from this region. Additional endobronchial biopsies were taken from the area near the stenotic orifice of the right middle lobe and its associated carina. The scope was removed, and fluoroscopy ensured that there was no pneumothorax. The patient tolerated the procedure well.

Code all relevant ICD-10-CM diagnosis and ICD-10-PCS procedure codes in accordance with official guidelines and coding conventions.

Diagnosis Codes:

_____

_____

Procedure Codes:

_____

_____

MS-DRG:

_____

_____

Answers and Rationale

Preoperative diagnosis:
Hemoptysis[1]

Postoperative diagnosis:
Same

Procedure performed:
Fiberoptic bronchoscopy with endobronchial and transbronchial biopsies

Procedure description:
The patient was brought to the endoscopy suite and was sedated using IV Versed. It should be noted that the patient has some tendency toward obstructive apnea while in the supine position. The fiberoptic scope was introduced via the right naris and passed into the hypopharynx. The vocal cords, false cords, arytenoid region, hypopharyngeal region, and the epiglottis were examined and found to be unremarkable. The trachea was inspected and found to be normal. The right bronchial tree was examined. The right upper lobe had three normal segments examined. The right middle lobe had two segments, the medial one was stenotic. A very small amount of increased mucus was present in this area. The right lower lobe was also inspected revealing no abnormality. The left upper lobe and lower lobe were inspected to the subsegmental level, revealing no abnormalities.

Using fluoroscopy, a biopsy forceps was placed into the medial portion of the right middle lobe of the lung. Biopsies were taken from this region.[2] Additional endobronchial biopsies were taken from the area near the stenotic orifice of the right middle lobe[4] and its associated carina.[3] The scope was removed, and fluoroscopy ensured that there was no pneumothorax. The patient tolerated the procedure well.

Diagnosis Codes

R04.2   Hemoptysis[1]

Rationale for Diagnosis Codes

The pre- and postoperative diagnosis is hemoptysis. Because no definitive diagnosis is documented, a code from the signs and symptoms chapter is used. While the physician documents the patient has "some tendency toward obstructive apnea while in the supine position," there is no documentation that obstructive apnea occurred during this procedure. Therefore, no code would be reported.

Procedure Codes

0BBD8ZX   **Excision of Right Middle Lung Lobe, Via Natural or Artificial Opening Endoscopic, Diagnostic[2]**

0BB28ZX   **Excision of Carina, Via Natural or Artificial Opening Endoscopic, Diagnostic[3]**

0BB58ZX   **Excision of Right Middle Lobe Bronchus, Via Natural or Artificial Opening Endoscopic, Diagnostic[4]**

Rationale for Procedure Codes

The tissue removed was from the right middle lung lobe and the endobronchial section of the right middle lobe and carina. As only a portion of the lung tissue was removed from these areas and not the entire lobe, the root operation is *Excision* for each site. Biopsies are often considered excisions under ICD-10-PCS. A procedure involving inserting an endoscope via a natural orifice is reported using the approach character value of 8. It is important to note that the qualifier character value (X) should indicate that a biopsy is considered a diagnostic procedure and that the inspection of the lungs (bronchoscopy) is not reported separately as it is included in the overall objective of the biopsy.

MS-DRG

168   **Other Respiratory System O.R. Procedures without CC/MCC**   **RW 1.2950**

 CODING AXIOM

ICD-10-PCS Official Guidelines for Coding and Reporting

Inspection procedures

Section B3.11a:

Inspection of a body part(s) performed in order to achieve the objective of a procedure is not coded separately.

Section B3.11b:

If multiple tubular body parts are inspected, the most distal body part (the body part furthest from the starting point of the inspection) is coded. If multiple non-tubular body parts in a region are inspected, the body part that specifies the entire area inspected is coded.

Section B3.11c:

When both an Inspection procedure and another procedure are performed on the same body part during the same episode, if the Inspection procedure is performed using a different approach than the other procedure, the Inspection procedure is coded separately.

OPERATIVE REPORT MDC 4—#5

Preoperative diagnosis:
Stab wound to the back

Postoperative diagnosis:
Stab wound to the back, arterial laceration; laceration lung

Procedure performed:
Emergency right thoracotomy; ligation of the intercostal artery at the 10th interspace; a partial right upper lobectomy; placement of right arterial femoral catheter.

Indications:
The patient is a 31-year-old male who is currently employed at a gas station. During an attempted robbery, the patient suffered a stab wound from a knife to the back at the right paraspinal region at the 10th interspace.

Procedure description:
The patient was brought to the operating room and placed on the operating table in a right-side-up lateral decubitus position. General anesthesia was administered via endotracheal tube. The patient became hemodynamically unstable during this positioning. The patient was prepped and draped quickly, and an emergency thoracotomy was performed to the right chest, at the fourth interspace. The chest was quickly opened and evacuated of approximately 1500 cc of blood. Bleeding at the 10th interspace was controlled with compression. Retractors were placed and continued pressure was maintained in this area.

An incision was made in the right groin for placement of a right arterial femoral catheter to gain arterial access for possible bypass as well as for blood pressure monitoring, blood draw access, and ABGs. The incision was carried down through the subcutaneous tissue, to the right femoral artery. An Angiocath was placed in the artery and secured to the skin.

Next, the pleura was dissected off the area of bleeding. The arterial intercostal space artery was acutely bleeding. The bleeding was controlled with 3-0 Prolene suture. A laceration of the lung was noted on the lower-most portion of the upper lobe posteriorly. The large GIA stapling device was placed over this laceration, and a portion of this lobe was resected. This was a very difficult dissection in a hard to get to area to control bleeding. It required multiple hemoclips. With adequate control of this bleeding and the laceration, the chest was irrigated with sterile saline and then antibiotic solution. Two chest tubes were placed and brought through inferior stab incisions, one right chest tube and one straight chest tube to the apex. These were secured with #0 silk sutures. Interrupted paracostal sutures were placed with #1 Polysorb sutures. The chest wall muscle was closed with #0 Vicryl layered sutures. The skin was closed with hemoclips. The groin incision was closed with interrupted 2-0 Vicryl and hemoclips. During the surgery the patient's blood loss was massive, He received 15 liters of crystalloid, 13 units of packed red blood cells, 1500cc of cell-saver blood, 2000 cc of chest tube salvaged blood, a 2 pack of platelets, and 3 units of fresh-frozen plasma via peripheral artery.

The patient was then taken to the intensive care unit in critical condition.

Code all relevant ICD-10-CM diagnosis and ICD-10-PCS procedure codes in accordance with official guidelines and coding conventions.

Diagnosis Codes:

_____

_____

Procedure Codes:

_____

_____

MS-DRG:

_____

_____

Answers and Rationale

Preoperative diagnosis:
Stab wound to the back

Postoperative diagnosis:
Stab wound to the back,[3] arterial laceration;[2] laceration lung[1]

Procedure performed:
Emergency right thoracotomy; ligation of the intercostal artery at the 10th interspace; a partial right upper lobectomy; placement of right arterial femoral catheter.

Indications:
The patient is a 31-year-old male who is currently employed at a gas station.[5,6] During an attempted robbery, the patient suffered a stab wound from a knife[4] to the back at the right paraspinal region at the 10th interspace.[1]

Procedure description:
The patient was brought to the operating room and placed on the operating table in a right-side-up lateral decubitus position. General anesthesia was administered via endotracheal tube. The patient became hemodynamically unstable during this positioning. The patient was prepped and draped quickly, and an emergency thoracotomy was performed to the right chest, at the fourth interspace. The chest was quickly opened and evacuated of approximately 1500 cc of blood. Bleeding at the 10th interspace was controlled with compression. Retractors were placed and continued pressure was maintained in this area.

An incision was made in the right groin for placement of a right arterial femoral catheter to gain arterial access for possible bypass as well as for blood pressure monitoring, blood draw access, and ABG's. The incision was carried down through the subcutaneous tissue, to the right femoral artery. An Angiocath was placed in the artery and secured to the skin.[9]

Next, the pleura was dissected off the area of bleeding. The arterial intercostal space artery was acutely bleeding.[2] The bleeding was controlled with 3-0 Prolene suture.[8] A laceration of the lung was noted on the lower-most portion of the upper lobe posteriorly. The large GIA stapling device was placed over this laceration, and a portion of this lobe was resected.[7] This was a very difficult dissection in a hard to get to area to control bleeding. It required multiple hemoclips. With adequate control of this bleeding and the laceration, the chest was irrigated with sterile saline and then antibiotic solution. Two chest tubes were placed and brought through inferior stab incisions, one right chest tube and one straight chest tube to the apex. These were secured with #0 silk sutures. Interrupted paracostal sutures were placed with #1 Polysorb sutures. The chest wall muscle was closed with #0 Vicryl layered sutures. The skin was closed with hemoclips. The groin incision was closed with interrupted 2-0 Vicryl and hemoclips.

During the surgery the patient's blood loss was massive. He received 15 liters of crystalloid, 13 units of packed red blood cells,[10] 1500 cc of cell-saver blood, 2000 cc of chest tube salvaged blood, a 2 pack of platelets,[11] and 3 units of fresh-frozen plasma[12] via peripheral artery.[10-12]

The patient was then taken to the intensive care unit in critical condition.

Diagnosis Codes

S27.331A   Laceration of lung, unilateral, initial encounter[1]

S25.511A   Laceration of intercostal blood vessels, right side, initial encounter[2]

S21.411A   Laceration without foreign body of right back wall of thorax with penetration into thoracic cavity[3]

X99.1XXA   Assault by knife, initial encounter[4]

Y92.524   Gas station as the place of occurrence of the external cause[5]

Y99.Ø   Civilian activity done for income or pay[6]

Rationale for Diagnosis Codes

The injuries are documented as a unilateral lung laceration and a laceration of the intercostal artery on the right side due to the stab injury. The lung injury should be sequenced first, according to *ICD-10-CM Official Guidelines for Coding and Reporting* section I.C.19.b.2. The indications section of the dictation states that the patient was stabbed, making the appropriate external cause code one that describes an assault with a knife. All four of these codes require a seventh character denoting the episode of care. In this case, this is the initial encounter, which is represented by an A. Two more codes are

---

🕯   **CODING AXIOM**

ICD-10-CM Official Guidelines for Coding and Reporting Section I.C.19.b.2:

When a primary injury results in minor damage to peripheral nerves or blood vessels, the primary injury is sequenced first with additional code(s) for injuries to nerves and spinal cord (such as category S04), and/or injury to blood vessels (such as category S15). When the primary injury is to the blood vessels or nerves, that injury should be sequenced first.

---

required to fully report this scenario. The first identifies the place of occurrence (gas station) and the second that the assault occurred while the patient was at work.

Procedure Codes

0BBC0ZZ	Excision of Right Upper Lung Lobe, Open Approach[7]
03QY0ZZ	Repair Upper Artery, Open Approach[8]
04HY02Z	Insertion of Monitoring Device into Lower Artery, Open Approach[9]
30253N1	Transfusion of Nonautologous Red Blood Cells into Peripheral Artery, Percutaneous Approach[10]
30253R1	Transfusion of Nonautologous Platelets into Peripheral Artery, Percutaneous Approach[11]
30253K1	Transfusion of Nonautologous Frozen Plasma into Peripheral Artery, Percutaneous Approach[12]

Rationale for Procedure Codes

The bleeding of the lung was controlled by resecting the injured part of the lung, which is identified as the lower portion of the upper right lobe. As only a portion of the lung was removed, the root operation for this part of the procedure is *Excision* of the right upper lobe via an *Open* approach. The intercostal artery was also repaired using a suture. Because no body part character value specifies the intercostal artery, the generic value Y, *Upper Artery* is used. It is also important to report the insertion of the Angiocath for monitoring and the transfusions. Each of the three separate types of blood transfusions administered—packed red blood cells, platelets, and fresh-frozen plasma—is coded.

MS-DRG

164	Major Chest Procedures with CC	RW 2.5822

MDC 5 Diseases and Disorders of the Circulatory System

OPERATIVE REPORT MDC 5—#1

Procedure description:
Insertion of a permanent ventricular demand pacemaker

Indications:
Tachy-brady syndrome

Technique:
Informed consent was obtained from the patient. He was transferred to the cardiac catheterization laboratory. His left infraclavicular region had been previously prepped and draped in the usual fashion and anesthetized with lidocaine. A pacemaker pocket was fashioned in the left infraclavicular subcutaneous tissue using a combination of sharp and blunt dissection. A single wire was inserted into the left subclavian vein using the Seldinger technique, following which an active fixation Medtronics lead, model #5076, was affixed to the region of the intraventricular septum. This was sutured in place using silk suture and the suture sleeve. Appropriate pacing parameters were obtained and were programmed to a KSR123 single-chamber, rate-responsive pacemaker. This was affixed to the fascia using single silk suture and the skin was closed in two layers and a sterile dressing was applied over the insertion site. The patient tolerated the procedure well and there were no complications.

Code all relevant ICD-10-CM diagnosis and ICD-10-PCS procedure codes in accordance with official guidelines and coding conventions.

Diagnosis Codes:

_____

_____

Procedure Codes:

_____

_____

MS-DRG:

_____

_____

Answers and Rationale

Procedure description:

Insertion of a permanent ventricular demand pacemaker[2,3]

Indications:

Tachy-brady syndrome[1]

Technique:

Informed consent was obtained from the patient. He was transferred to the cardiac catheterization laboratory. His left infraclavicular region had been previously prepped and draped in the usual fashion and anesthetized with lidocaine. A pacemaker pocket was fashioned in the left infraclavicular subcutaneous tissue using a combination of sharp and blunt dissection.[2] A single wire was inserted into the left subclavian vein using the Seldinger technique, following which an active fixation Medtronics lead, model #5076, was affixed to the region of the intraventricular septum. [3] This was sutured in place using silk suture and the suture sleeve. Appropriate pacing parameters were obtained and were programmed to a KSR123 single-chamber, rate-responsive pacemaker. [2] This was affixed to the fascia using single silk suture, and the skin was closed in two layers and a sterile dressing was applied over the insertion site. The patient tolerated the procedure well and there were no complications.

Diagnosis Codes

I49.5   **Sick sinus syndrome**[1]

Rationale for Diagnosis Codes

To find the appropriate code for tachy-brady syndrome, also known as tachycardia-bradycardia syndrome, the coder looks in the ICD-10-CM index under "syndrome," followed by "Tachycardia-bradycardia." The index leads to I49.5 Sick sinus syndrome, which has an includes note for "tachycardia-bradycardia syndrome." Note that tachy-brady syndrome cannot be reached via the index using the term "tachycardia." It can be located under "bradycardia," however.

Procedure Codes

ØJH6Ø5Z   **Insertion of Single Chamber Rate Responsive Pacemaker into Chest Subcutaneous Tissue and Fascia, Open Approach**[2]

Ø2HL3JZ   **Insertion of Pacemaker Lead into Left Ventricle, Percutaneous Approach**[3]

Rationale for Procedure Codes

The documentation in the operative note states that both a single-chamber rate responsive pacemaker and ventricular lead were inserted. This indicates that there should be two codes: one for the insertion of the generator and a second for the insertion of the lead. Both of these procedures are accurately represented by the ICD-10-PCS root operation *Insertion*. The insertion of the generator is specified as within the subcutaneous tissue of the chest and therefore the appropriate code can be found in the skin and subcutaneous tissue section. Since the lead was inserted in the left ventricle of the heart, the most accurate code is in the heart and great vessels section. It should be noted for the approach values that the verbiage "by sharp and blunt dissection" indicates an *Open* approach for the pacemaker generator. The single wire in the subclavian vein indicates a *Percutaneous* approach for the lead.

MS-DRG

244   **Permanent Cardiac Pacemaker Implant without CC/MCC**   **RW 2.1394**

It is important to note that both procedure codes are required to get to MS-DRG 244. If either of the procedure codes is reported without the other, the MS-DRG becomes 310 Cardiac Arrhythmia and Conduction Disorders without CC/MCC, which is nonsurgical and a carries a lower weight.

CODING AXIOM

ICD-10-CM Official Guidelines for Coding and Reporting Section I.B.15:

Syndromes:

Follow the Alphabetic Index guidance when coding syndromes. In the absence of Alphabetic Index guidance, assign codes for the documented manifestations of the syndrome.

OPERATIVE REPORT MDC 5—#2

Preoperative diagnoses:
Varicose veins on left lower extremity associated with prolonged pain, swelling, and night cramps

Postoperative diagnoses:
Same

History of Illness:
This 55-year-old female has used support stockings as a form of conservative treatment with some relief of symptoms, but presents now for surgical endovascular laser ablation. Physical examination reveals large (> 8mm) left upper and lower branch varices. Previously obtained duplex ultrasound (including color Doppler and pulsed wave Doppler interrogation) reveals incompetence of the saphenofemoral junction with left greater saphenous vein (GSV) reflux. The left GSV is enlarged (14.8 x 15.6 mm in diameter) in its entire course with multiple enlarged tributaries also demonstrating reflux.

Procedure description:
Ultrasound (US) mapping of the incompetent venous pathways was performed and the vein segment to be treated marked. The skin was sterilely cleaned and draped. The puncture site was anesthetized with 0.2% lidocaine. Using US guidance, the left greater saphenous vein was accessed and a sheath placed. A laser fiber was advanced through the sheath and positioned under US. Distal fiber tip location was confirmed with direct visualization of the red aiming beam through the skin. Perivenous tumescent anesthesia (0.2% lidocaine) was delivered along the entire length of the vein using US guidance. Fiber tip location was again confirmed with US and red aiming beam. An 810nm diode laser energy was delivered intraluminally using 14 watts in continuous mode for 184 seconds while withdrawing the laser fiber over a 34 cm long vein segment from the saphenofemoral junction to the knee. Manual compression was applied to the puncture site to obtain hemostasis. A small protective bandage was placed over the incision. A class II graduated support stocking was applied.

Code all relevant ICD-10-CM diagnosis and ICD-10-PCS procedure codes in accordance with official guidelines and coding conventions.

Diagnosis Codes:

_____

_____

Procedure Codes:

_____

_____

MS-DRG:

_____

_____

Answers and Rationale

Preoperative diagnoses:
Varicose veins on left lower extremity[1-4] associated with prolonged pain,[1] swelling,[2,3] and night cramps[2,4]

Postoperative diagnoses:
Same

History of Illness:
This 55-year-old female has used support stockings as a form of conservative treatment with some relief of symptoms, but presents now for surgical endovascular laser ablation.[5] Physical examination reveals large (> 8mm) left upper and lower branch varices. Previously obtained duplex ultrasound (including color Doppler and pulsed wave Doppler interrogation) reveals incompetence of the saphenofemoral junction with left greater saphenous vein (GSV) reflux. The left GSV is enlarged (14.8 x 15.6 mm in diameter) in its entire course with multiple enlarged tributaries also demonstrating reflux. [5]

Procedure description:
Ultrasound (US) mapping of the incompetent venous pathways was performed and the vein segment to be treated marked. The skin was sterilely cleaned and draped. The puncture site[5] was anesthetized with 0.2% lidocaine. Using US guidance, the left greater saphenous vein[5] was accessed and a sheath placed. A laser fiber was advanced through the sheath and positioned under US. Distal fiber tip location was confirmed with direct visualization of the red aiming beam through the skin. Perivenous tumescent anesthesia (0.2% lidocaine) was delivered along the entire length of the vein using US guidance. Fiber tip location was again confirmed with US and red aiming beam. An 810nm diode laser energy was delivered intraluminally using 14 watts in continuous mode for 184 seconds while withdrawing the laser fiber over a 34 cm long vein segment from the saphenofemoral junction to the knee. Manual compression was applied to the puncture site to obtain hemostasis. A small protective bandage was placed over the incision. A class II graduated support stocking was applied.

Diagnosis Codes

I83.812	Varicose veins of left lower extremities with pain[1]
I83.892	Varicose veins of left lower extremities with other complications[2]
M79.89	Other specified soft tissue disorders[3]
R25.2	Cramp and spasm[4]

Rationale for Diagnosis Codes
ICD-10-CM differentiates between varicose veins with complications and without. In this case, complications of pain, swelling, and cramps are listed. There is a specific code to account for the pain, but the swelling and cramps are classified under the "other complications" code. According to coding guidelines section I.B.9, "when the combination code lacks necessary specificity in describing the manifestation or complication, an additional code should be used as a secondary code." Therefore, additional codes for the swelling (M79.89) and cramps (R25.2) should also be reported.

Procedure Codes

Ø65Q3ZZ	Destruction of Left Greater Saphenous Vein, Percutaneous Approach[5]

Rationale for Procedure Codes
The term "Ablation" in the ICD-10-PCS index refers the coder to the root operation *Destruction*. As specified in the history and procedure sections of the operative note, the left greater saphenous vein is the vessel being treated. The laser is inserted through a puncture. No other instrumentation, such as an endoscope, was used during the procedure. This makes the approach, by ICD-10 definition, *Percutaneous*.

MS-DRG

263	Vein Ligation and Stripping	RW 2.0854

OPERATIVE REPORT MDC 5—#3

Preoperative diagnosis:
Atypical left hip and thigh pain

Postoperative diagnosis:
Thrombus causing chronic occlusion femoral-femoral bypass graft

Procedure performed:
Revision of femoral-femoral bypass graft

Indications:
This 70-year-old woman had a femoral-femoral bypass performed by me 12 years ago. In recent months she has developed some unusual left hip and thigh pain with just a few steps of walking. An arteriogram demonstrated an occluded femoral-femoral graft, wide open right iliac system and distal system, occluded left iliac, and a patent femoral bifurcation with pretty good runoff in the left lower extremity.

Procedure description:
The patient was placed in the supine position after spinal anesthesia. The abdomen, inguinal regions, and upper thighs were prepped and draped sterilely. A vertical incision was taken through the old left femoral scar. It was extended through subcutaneous tissue down to the left extent of the old femoral-femoral graft. This was dissected out and followed down to the femoral artery. The superficial femoral artery and profundus femoris arteries were identified and dissected free. The dissection was carried up on the lateral side of the femoral artery. The graft was transected, the artery was rotated out, and I was able to dissect out the medial aspect of the femoral artery.

The graft was excised from the artery. The patient was heparinized with 4000 units of heparin. Clamps were placed on the profundus femoris and superficial femoral arteries. The profundus femoris was quite a small artery, and I elected to extend the incision down onto the superficial femoral artery rather than onto the profundus femoris artery. The remaining old graft was inspected. Most of the graft was filled with serum. The preoperative arteriography showed that about the first 2 cm of the right side of the graft were open.

I passed a #5 Fogarty catheter over through to the right side of the graft and withdrew it and pulled back some old thrombus and I got back some bright red blood. I passed it once again through the anastomosis and then pulled it back and got a plug of thrombus with a meniscus and an excellent arterial flow. With the graft unoccluded, there was an excellent pulse suprapubically in the graft. The graft was filled with heparinized saline and then clamped with a graft clamp.

A length of 8 mm Dacron graft was brought to the table, and a portion of that was anastomosed end-to-end to the old graft with continuous 5-0 Prolene. The other end of this new graft was beveled and then anastomosed to the femoral artery with the toe extending onto the SFA. This anastomosis was completed with continuous 5-0 Prolene. Just prior to completion of the suture line, the vessels were back-flushed and clamped and the graft was flushed and clamped. The suture line was completed, and the knots were tied. Clamps were released, and there was noted to be an excellent pulse in the graft and also an excellent pulse in the outflow SFA and PFA. Hemostasis was obtained and the groin wound was closed. Dressings were applied and the patient was taken to the operating room in good condition.

Code all relevant ICD-10-CM diagnosis and ICD-10-PCS procedure codes in accordance with official guidelines and coding conventions.

Diagnosis Codes:
_____

_____

Procedure Codes:
_____

_____

MS-DRG:
_____

_____

Answers and Rationale

Preoperative diagnosis:
Atypical left hip and thigh pain

Postoperative diagnosis:
Thrombus causing chronic occlusion femoral-femoral bypass graft[1]

Procedure performed:
Revision of femoral-femoral bypass graft

Indications:
This 70-year-old woman had a femoral-femoral bypass performed by me 12 years ago. In recent months she has developed some unusual left hip and thigh pain with just a few steps of walking. An arteriogram demonstrated an occluded femoral-femoral graft, wide open right iliac system and distal system, occluded left iliac, [2] and a patent femoral bifurcation with pretty good runoff in the left lower extremity.

Procedure description:
The patient was placed in the supine position after spinal anesthesia. The abdomen, inguinal regions, and upper thighs were prepped and draped sterilely. A vertical incision was taken through the old left femoral[1,3] scar. It was extended through subcutaneous tissue down to the left extent of the old femoral-femoral graft. This was dissected out and followed down to the femoral artery. The superficial femoral artery and profundus femoris arteries were identified and dissected free. The dissection was carried up on the lateral side of the femoral artery. The graft was transected, the artery was rotated out, and I was able to dissect out the medial aspect of the femoral artery.

The graft was excised from the artery. The patient was heparinized with 4000 units of heparin. Clamps were placed on the profundus femoris and superficial femoral arteries. The profundus femoris was quite a small artery, and I elected to extend the incision down onto the superficial femoral artery rather than onto the profundus femoris artery. The remaining old graft was inspected. Most of the graft was filled with serum. The preoperative arteriography showed that about the first 2 cm of the right side of the graft were open. I passed a #5 Fogarty catheter over through to the right side of the graft and withdrew it and pulled back some old thrombus and I got back some bright red blood. I passed it once again through the anastomosis and then pulled it back and got a plug of thrombus with a meniscus and an excellent arterial flow.[3] With the graft unoccluded, there was an excellent pulse suprapubically in the graft. The graft was filled with heparinized saline and then clamped with a graft clamp.

A length of 8 mm Dacron graft was brought to the table, and a portion of that was anastomosed end-to-end to the old graft with continuous 5-0 Prolene.[3] The other end of this new graft was beveled and then anastomosed to the femoral artery with the toe extending onto the SFA. This anastomosis was completed with continuous 5-0 Prolene. Just prior to completion of the suture line, the vessels were back-flushed and clamped and the graft was flushed and clamped. The suture line was completed, and the knots were tied. Clamps were released, and there was noted to be an excellent pulse in the graft and also an excellent pulse in the outflow SFA and PFA. Hemostasis was obtained and the groin wound was closed. Dressings were applied and the patient was taken to the recovery room.

Diagnosis Codes

T82.868A   **Thrombosis of vascular prosthetic devices, implants and grafts, initial encounter**[1]

I74.5   **Embolism and thrombosis of iliac artery**[2]

Rationale for Diagnosis Codes
An occluded graft is considered a complication and should be coded as such. It is found in the index under thrombosis of an arterial graft. The iliac occlusion should also be reported as it demonstrates the severity of the occlusive disease in the left lower extremity.

Procedure Codes

Ø4WYØJZ   **Revision of Synthetic Substitute in Lower Artery, Open Approach**[3]

Rationale for Procedure Codes
The excision of the graft is considered part of the approach to the other procedures and is not reported. The thrombus is removed from the graft and seems to be described by the root operation *Extirpation*. However, the procedure is performed on the graft, which makes *Extirpation* not applicable as a root operation because when a procedure is performed on a device (in this case a graft), the root operation must include the device.

🕯️ **CODING AXIOM**

ICD-10-PCS Official Guidelines for Coding and Reporting Section B6.1c:

Procedures performed on a device only and not on a body part are specified in the root operations Change, Irrigation, Removal and Revision, and are coded to the procedure performed.

The objective of the procedure is to remove the occlusion and restore the function of the graft, which by ICD-10-PCS definition is the root operation *Revision*.

MS-DRG

253   **Other Vascular Procedures with CC**   **RW 2.6028**

OPERATIVE REPORT MDC 5—#4

Preoperative diagnosis:
Aortic valve stenosis

Postoperative diagnosis:
Aortic valve stenosis

Procedure performed:
Transcatheter aortic valve replacement (TAVR)

Indications:
A patient with severe aortic valve stenosis presents for TAVR. A diagnostic cardiac catheterization performed at a previous outpatient encounter was negative for significant coronary artery disease or other pathology and confirmed candidacy for endovascular replacement.

Procedure description:
The patient was prepped, draped, and transported to the operating suite with cardiopulmonary bypass on standby. Access was obtained through the femoral artery at the groin. The valve assembly was mounted on a specialized delivery catheter. A balloon tip catheter was advanced through the aorta to the aortic valve. A balloon valvuloplasty was performed with destruction of the native structure. The valvuloplasty catheter was removed, and the delivery catheter was advanced through the aorta to the valvuloplasty site. The bioprosthetic aortic valve was positioned and expanded in situ, attached to a stent frame across the native valve remnants. Once optimal placement was achieved, the prosthetic valve was tested and determined to be at optimal function. All instruments were removed. Hemostasis was obtained, and the patient was transported to the recovery room.

Code all relevant ICD-10-CM diagnosis and ICD-10-PCS procedure codes in accordance with official guidelines and coding conventions.

Diagnosis Codes:

_____

_____

Procedure Codes:

_____

_____

MS-DRG:

_____

_____

Answers and Rationale

Preoperative diagnosis:
Aortic valve stenosis

Postoperative diagnosis:
Aortic valve stenosis[1]

Procedure performed:
Transcatheter aortic valve replacement (TAVR)

Indications:
A patient with severe aortic valve stenosis presents for TAVR (transcatheter aortic valve replacement). A diagnostic cardiac catheterization performed at a previous outpatient encounter was negative for significant coronary artery disease or other pathology and confirmed candidacy for endovascular replacement.

Procedure description:
The patient was prepped, draped, and transported to the operating suite with cardiopulmonary bypass on standby. Access was obtained through the femoral artery at the groin.[2] The valve assembly was mounted on a specialized delivery catheter. A balloon tip catheter was advanced through the aorta to the aortic valve. A balloon valvuloplasty was performed with destruction of the native structure. The valvuloplasty catheter was removed, and the delivery catheter was advanced through the aorta to the valvuloplasty site. The bioprosthetic aortic valve was positioned and expanded in situ, attached to a stent frame across the native valve remnants. Once optimal placement was achieved, the prosthetic valve was tested and determined to be at optimal function.[2] All instruments were removed. Hemostasis was obtained and the patient was transported to the recovery room.

Diagnosis Codes

I35.0   **Nonrheumatic aortic (valve) stenosis**[1]

Rationale for Diagnosis Codes
Since the documentation does not give much specification with regard to the aortic stenosis, the default code I35.0 is used.

Procedure Codes

02RF38Z   **Replacement of Aortic Valve with Zooplastic Tissue, Percutaneous Approach**[2]

Rationale for Procedure Codes
The procedure's objective is to replace the aortic valve with a bioprosthetic valve. The diseased valve is destroyed via balloon valvuloplasty. However, this would not be coded in addition to the valve replacement as it is an inherent part of the procedure. This is specified in the *ICD-10-PCS Official Guidelines for Coding and Reporting* section B3.1b. It is important to note that a bioprosthetic valve is usually porcine, or "zooplastic," by ICD-10-PCS standards.

MS-DRG

221   **Cardiac Valve and Other Major Cardiothoracic Procedures   RW 4.5406 without Cardiac Catheterization without CC/MCC**

If right heart catheterization is performed for diagnostic purposes or further evaluation, it may be coded and reported, since a diagnostic catheterization is not inherent in the thoracic aortic valve repair (TAVR) procedure. Sampling and monitoring of intracardiac pressures, however, are inherent in the procedure and would not be coded separately.

Inappropriate reporting of diagnostic right heart catheterization is a focus of regulatory investigation. The higher-weighted, but incorrect, MS-DRG 218 Cardiac Valve and Other Major Cardiothoracic Procedures with Cardiac Catheterization without CC/MCC (RW 5.4815), would be at risk of denial.

🕯 **CODING AXIOM**

ICD-10-PCS Official Guidelines for Coding and Reporting Section B3.1b:

Components of a procedure specified in the root operation definition and explanation are not coded separately. Procedural steps necessary to reach the operative site and close the operative site, including anastomosis of a tubular body part, are also not coded separately.

OPERATIVE REPORT MDC 5—#5

Preoperative diagnosis:
Chest pain with fixed anterior defect on nuclear study

Postoperative diagnosis:
Unstable angina

Procedure performed:
Selective coronary angiography, right and left coronary arteries; contrast left ventriculography with left heart catheterization; PTCA with Taxus stent of the right coronary artery.

Indications:
The patient is a 53-year-old female with a markedly positive family history of coronary artery disease who presents with chest pain and a fixed anterior defect.

Procedure description:
The patient was brought to the catheterization suite where she was prepped and draped in the usual fashion and sedated using IV Versed and fentanyl. The skin and subcutaneous tissue overlying the right femoral artery was infiltrated with 1% lidocaine for local anesthesia. A 6-French sheath was placed in the right femoral artery. Diagnostic coronary angiography under fluoroscopy of the right and left coronary arteries using iso-osmolar contrast was performed with 6-French JL-4 and 6-French JR-4 diagnostic catheters, and a 6-French pigtail catheter was used to perform a left ventriculography, also under fluoroscopy with iso-osmolar contrast. It was determined that there was approximately 85-90% stenosis of the mid right coronary artery. A JR4 catheter was placed at the site of the stenosis, and the lesion was crossed with a guidewire. A 3.0 x 12 mm Taxus stent was deployed to a total of 14 atmospheres. Follow-up angiography demonstrated 0% residual stenosis. The catheter and sheath were removed and Angio-Seal plug was deployed. The patient was then transferred to the holding area in stable condition.

Findings:
There was 85-90% stenosis in the mid right coronary artery; percutaneous intervention was initiated. There is a 10% to 20% stenosis in the distal left main; this will be managed medically. There are no further significant obstructions in the coronary arteries. The left ventricular function is normal. There are no regional wall motion abnormalities. There is no mitral regurgitation.

Code all relevant ICD-10-CM diagnosis and ICD-10-PCS procedure codes in accordance with official guidelines and coding conventions.

Diagnosis Codes:
_____

_____

Procedure Codes:
_____

_____

MS-DRG:
_____

_____

Answers and Rationale

Preoperative diagnosis:
Chest pain with fixed anterior defect on nuclear study

Postoperative diagnosis:
Unstable angina[1]

Procedure performed:
Selective coronary angiography, right and left coronary arteries[5] contrast left ventriculography[6] with left heart catheterization; [4]PTCA with Taxus stent of the right coronary artery.[3]

Indications:
The patient is a 53-year-old female with a markedly positive family history of coronary artery disease[2] who presents with chest pain and a fixed anterior defect.

Procedure description:
The patient was brought to the catheterization suite where she was prepped and draped in the usual fashion and sedated using IV Versed and fentanyl. The skin and subcutaneous tissue overlying the right femoral artery was infiltrated with 1% lidocaine for local anesthesia. A 6-French sheath was placed in the right femoral artery. Diagnostic coronary angiography under fluoroscopy of the right and left coronary arteries using iso-osmolar contrast[5] was performed with 6-French JL-4 and 6-French JR-4 diagnostic catheters, and a 6-French pigtail catheter was used to perform a left ventriculography, also under fluoroscopy with iso-osmolar contrast.[6]

It was determined that there was approximately 85-90% stenosis of the mid right coronary artery.[1] A JR4 catheter was placed at the site of the stenosis, and the lesion was crossed with a guidewire. A 3.0 x 12 mm Taxus stent was deployed to a total of 14 atmospheres.[3] Follow-up angiography demonstrated 0% residual stenosis. The catheter and sheath were removed and Angio-Seal plug was deployed. The patient was then transferred to the holding area in stable condition.

Findings:
There was 85-90% stenosis in the mid right coronary artery; percutaneous intervention was initiated. There is a 10% to 20% stenosis in the distal left main,[1] this will be managed medically. There are no further significant obstructions in the coronary arteries. The left ventricular function is normal. There are no regional wall motion abnormalities. There is no mitral regurgitation.

Diagnosis Codes

I25.11Ø   **Atherosclerotic heart disease of native coronary artery with unstable angina pectoris[1]**

Z82.49   **Family history of ischemic heart disease and other diseases of the circulatory system[2]**

Rationale for Diagnosis Codes

The postoperative diagnosis is unstable angina. It is also noted that the patient has stenosis in the mid right coronary artery. The terms "Stenosis, Coronary Artery" in the index direct the coder to see "Disease, Heart, Ischemic, Atherosclerotic." Those terms provide an additional option of whether the stenosis is with angina pectoris. In this case it is, so there are further instructions to see "Arteriosclerosis, Coronary (artery)," leading to the selection of code I25.11Ø. The family history of coronary artery disease is also significant in a patient newly diagnosed with the disease.

Procedure Codes

Ø27Ø34Z   **Dilation of Coronary Artery, One Site with Drug-eluting Intraluminal Device, Percutaneous Approach[3]**

4AØ23N7   **Measurement of Cardiac Sampling and Pressure, Left Heart, Percutaneous Approach[4]**

B211YZZ   **Fluoroscopy of Multiple Coronary Arteries Using Other Contrast [5]**

B215YZZ   **Fluoroscopy of Left Heart Using Other Contrast[6]**

Rationale for Procedure Codes

The objective of a stent insertion is to open an abnormally closed blood vessel. This objective coincides with the ICD-10-PCS root operation *Dilation*. ICD-10-PCS does not supply body part character values for individual coronary arteries but rather gives the option of one, two, three, or four or more coronary artery *sites*. In this case, only one site

CODING AXIOM

ICD-10-CM Official Guidelines for Coding and Reporting Section I.C.9.b:

Atherosclerotic Coronary Artery Disease and Angina

ICD-10-CM has combination codes for atherosclerotic heart disease with angina pectoris. The subcategories for these codes are I25.11, Atherosclerotic heart disease of native coronary artery with angina pectoris and I25.7, Atherosclerosis of coronary artery bypass graft(s) and coronary artery of transplanted heart with angina pectoris.

When using one of these combination codes it is not necessary to use an additional code for angina pectoris. A causal relationship can be assumed in a patient with both atherosclerosis and angina pectoris, unless the documentation indicates the angina is due to something other than the atherosclerosis.

was expanded. The coder must know whether a Taxus stent is bare-metal or drug-eluting. Experienced coders of cardiac catheterization know that a Taxus stent is drug-eluting and would therefore be represented by the device character value of 4.

A diagnostic left heart catheterization was also performed, reported in the table "Measurement, Cardiac 4A02," as well as a diagnostic coronary arteriography of multiple coronary arteries and left ventriculography via fluoroscopy with "other" (iso-osmolar) contrast, in the table "Fluoroscopy, Heart, B21."

MS-DRG

**247   Percutaneous Cardiovascular Procedure with Drug-Eluting   RW 2.1307
            Stent without MCC**

The procedure code drives this MS-DRG. If the stent is reported incorrectly as a bare-metal stent (02703DZ), the resulting MS-DRG would be lower-weighted 249 Percutaneous Cardiovascular Procedure with Non Drug-Eluting Stent without MCC (RW 1.9140). Also interesting to note, I25.110 is one of the codes designated to serve as its own CC if reported as a principal diagnosis. Although this MS-DRG group (246 and 247) is divided only by MCC, it is important to note that in most circumstances, reporting I25.110 as principal diagnosis would result in an MS-DRG "with CC," even if the code is reported alone.

OPERATIVE REPORT MDC 5—#6

Preoperative diagnosis:
Coronary artery disease

Postoperative diagnosis:
Same

Procedure performed:
Coronary artery bypass graft

Indications:
The patient is a 57-year-old tobacco-dependent male who suffered a non-ST elevation myocardial infarction during a previous encounter three weeks ago. He was not stable enough at that time to endure an invasive procedure.

Procedure description:
The patient was brought to the operating suite, where he was placed under general anesthesia. Once adequate sedation was achieved, the patient was prepped and draped in the usual sterile fashion.

The left greater saphenous vein was removed. Hemostasis was achieved at the site with the use of silk clips and ligatures. The area was irrigated with saline and antibiotics and closed using 5-0 Prolene sutures. Attention was then turned to the chest, where a sternotomy was performed using the sternal saw, and the left internal mammary artery was located and harvested using clips. The patient was then placed on cardiopulmonary bypass for the remainder of the procedure. The right coronary artery was identified and grasped. An arteriotomy was performed in order to attach the saphenous vein graft using 7-0 Prolene. We then turned our attention to the left anterior descending artery. The left internal mammary was placed end-to-side, and anastomosis was performed using 7-0 Prolene here as well.

The blood flow was resumed to all grafts and the patient was removed from cardiopulmonary bypass without any complications. The heart began a normal rhythm spontaneously.

The sternum was repaired using sternal wires. The rest of the wound was closed in layers in the usual fashion, and sterile dressings were applied. The patient tolerated the procedure well and was escorted to the recovery room in stable condition.

Code all relevant ICD-10-CM diagnosis and ICD-10-PCS procedure codes in accordance with official guidelines and coding conventions.

Diagnosis Codes:

_____

_____

Procedure Codes:

_____

_____

MS-DRG:

_____

_____

Answers and Rationale

Preoperative diagnosis:
Coronary artery disease[1]

Postoperative diagnosis:
Same

Procedure performed:
Coronary artery bypass graft

Indications:
The patient is a 57-year-old tobacco-dependent[3] male who suffered a non-ST elevation myocardial infarction during a previous encounter three weeks ago.[2] He was not stable enough at that time to endure an invasive procedure.

Procedure description:
The patient was brought to the operating suite, where he was placed under general anesthesia. Once adequate sedation was achieved, the patient was prepped and draped in the usual sterile fashion.

The left greater saphenous vein was removed.[6] Hemostasis was achieved at the site with the use of silk clips and ligatures. The area was irrigated with saline and antibiotics and closed using 5-0 Prolene sutures. Attention was then turned to the chest, where a sternotomy was performed[4,5] using the sternal saw, and the left internal mammary artery was located and harvested using clips. The patient was then placed on cardiopulmonary bypass[7] for the remainder of the procedure. The right coronary artery was identified and grasped. An arteriotomy was performed in order to attach the saphenous vein graft using 7-0 Prolene.[4] We then turned our attention to the left anterior descending artery. The left internal mammary was placed end-to-side, and anastomosis was performed using 7-0 Prolene here as well.[5]

The blood flow was resumed to all grafts and the patient was removed from cardiopulmonary bypass without any complications. The heart began a normal rhythm spontaneously.

The sternum was repaired using sternal wires. The rest of the wound was closed in layers in the usual fashion, and sterile dressings were applied. The patient tolerated the procedure well and was escorted to the recovery room in stable condition.

Diagnosis Codes

I25.10	**Atherosclerotic heart disease of native coronary artery without angina pectoris**[1]
I21.4	**Non-ST elevation (NSTEMI) myocardial infarction**[2]
F17.200	**Nicotine dependence, unspecified, uncomplicated**[3]

Rationale for Diagnosis Codes
The procedure is being performed to correct the coronary artery disease. There is no mention of the disease occurring in conjunction with angina or a previous coronary artery bypass graft, so the default code of I25.10 is used. The report notes that the patient had and was treated for a non-ST elevated myocardial infarction three weeks ago. According to the *ICD-10-PCS Official Guidelines for Coding and Reporting,* a myocardial infarction that occurred within the past four weeks is coded as acute. Lastly, it is important to report the patient's tobacco dependence although the documentation does not specify in what form, such as cigarettes or chewing tobacco. Therefore, a more specific code cannot be assigned.

Procedure Codes

021009W	**Bypass Coronary Artery, One Site from Aorta with Autologous Venous Tissue, Open Approach**[4]
02100Z9	**Bypass Coronary Artery, One Site from Left Internal Mammary Artery, Open Approach**[5]
06BQ0ZZ	**Excision of Left Greater Saphenous Vein, Open Approach**[6]
5A1221Z	**Performance of Cardiac Output, Continuous**[7]

Rationale for Procedure Codes
Specific ICD-10-PCS guidelines address how to report coronary artery bypass grafts. The fourth-character body part identifies the body part bypassed "to" (coronary artery), including the number of sites (arteries) involved, and the seventh-character qualifier identifies the body part bypassed "from." Note that this is reversed for other types of

---

🕯 **CODING AXIOM**

ICD-10-CM Official Guidelines for Coding and Reporting Section I.C.9.e.1:

For encounters occurring while the myocardial infarction is equal to, or less than, four weeks old, including transfers to another acute setting or a postacute setting, and when the patient requires continued care for the myocardial infarction, codes from category I21 may continue to be reported. For encounters after the 4 week time frame and the patient is still receiving care related to the myocardial infarction, the appropriate aftercare code should be assigned, rather than a code from category I21. For old or healed myocardial infarctions not requiring further care, code I25.2 Old myocardial infarction, may be assigned.

ICD-10-PCS Official Guidelines for Coding and Reporting Section B3.6b:

Coronary arteries are classified by number of distinct sites treated, rather than number of coronary arteries or anatomic name of a coronary artery (e.g., left anterior descending). Coronary artery bypass procedures are coded differently from other bypass procedures as described in the previous guideline. Rather than identifying the body part bypassed from, the body part identifies the number of coronary artery sites bypassed to, and the qualifier specifies the vessel bypassed from.

Section B3.6c:

If multiple coronary artery sites are bypassed, a separate procedure is coded for each coronary artery site that uses a different device and/or qualifier.

bypasses. The sixth character, describing the device, identifies the material/tissue used to create either an excised graft (free) or indicates "no device" for a graft that remains attached at its origin. A separate procedure is reported for each type of graft that involves a different device or qualifier. In this case, there is one device of a free autologous vein (9) and no device for the internal mammary artery graft (Z), as it remains attached at its origin. The number of coronary arteries is one for each type of graft in this example. The qualifier for the vein graft is (from) aorta (W), and the second qualifier is (from) left internal mammary (9). The harvesting (excision) of the free graft is reported as an additional code, which must identify the vessel used. When the facility tracks and reports the cardiopulmonary bypass, add 5A1221Z.

MS-DRG

235	Coronary Bypass without Cardiac Catheterization with MCC	RW 5.8103

If the myocardial infarction is reported incorrectly as aftercare or history or not at all, the MS-DRG changes to 236 Coronary Bypass without Cardiac Catheterization without MCC (RW 3.8013).

DEFINITIONS

angina pectoris. Angina pectoris is chest pain due to myocardial ischemia, most often caused by atherosclerotic heart disease, but it may be due to coronary artery spasm, severe aortic stenosis or insufficiency, syphilitic aortitis, vasculitis, marked anemia, paroxysmal tachycardia with rapid ventricular rates, or any disease or disorder that markedly increases metabolic demands on the heart. Symptoms result from decreased oxygen supplied to the heart due to narrowed vessels, categorized as ischemia.

calcified coronary lesion. In the treatment of coronary atherosclerosis, calcified lesions present significant treatment challenges. Calcified coronary artery lesions are less amenable to angioplasty and stenting procedures due to the recalcitrant blockages caused by the hardened calcium deposits in the arteries.

OPERATIVE REPORT MDC 5—# 7

Preoperative diagnosis:
Coronary artery disease with calcified chronic total occlusion

Postoperative diagnosis:
Same

Procedure performed:
Coronary orbital atherectomy

Indications:
A 70-year-old male patient with hypertension, dyslipidemia, and coronary artery disease status post coronary artery bypass surgery (CABG) in 2005 is referred for cardiac catheterization. The patient complained of angina with an associated large area of inferolateral ischemia on stress imaging. A prior diagnostic cardiac catheterization was performed, which revealed a subtotal occlusion of the distal left main artery and patent left internal mammary artery (LIMA) to left anterior descending coronary artery (LAD) graft. The right coronary artery (RCA) was 95–100% chronically occluded with multiple calcified lesions.

Procedure description:
The patient was brought back for an elective intervention of the RCA secondary to his symptoms. Access was obtained using a 6-French with a hydrophilic Glidesheath in the right radial artery. An intra-arterial cocktail was injected to prevent radial artery spasm, and the hydrophilic sheath was then exchanged over a 35" J wire for a 7-Fr non-hydrophilic sheath. A 7 Fr guide was selectively engaged in the RCA. Due to a long area of very heavy calcification and severe angulation within the diseased segment, several different wires, and different tip shapes, failed to cross the lesions. Ultimately, a Fielder FC wire was able to pass through the lesion. The Fielder FC wire was exchanged for a 300 cm Viper wire. Under fluoroscopy, an orbital atherectomy system (Diamondback 360˚ coronary classic crown, CSI) was gently advanced over the Viper wire proximal to the lesion. Orbital atherectomy was performed in the entire proximal and mid severely calcified RCA with multiple passes with total atherectomy time of 7.5 minutes. Each pass (treatment time) was performed for 25–30 seconds with equal length resting periods after each pass. Initially five passes were executed at low revolution speed (80K rpm) with the final three passes performed at high revolution speed (120K rpm). Promus drug-eluting stents (3.5 x 38 mm and 3.5 x 18 mm) (Boston Scientific) were subsequently deployed over the Viper wire in overlapping fashion, covering the entire diseased segment. An excellent angiographic result was achieved with TIMI-3 flow .The sheath and catheters were removed, and the patient was transferred to the recovery room in stable condition.

Code all relevant ICD-10-CM diagnosis and ICD-10-PCS procedure codes in accordance with official guidelines and coding conventions.

Diagnosis Codes:

_____

_____

Procedure Codes:

_____

_____

MS-DRG:

_____

_____

Answers and Rationale

Preoperative Diagnosis:
Coronary artery disease with calcified chronic total occlusion [1,2,3]

Postoperative diagnosis:
Same

Procedure performed:
Coronary orbital atherectomy [7]

Indications:

A 70-year-old male patient with hypertension[4], dyslipidemia[5], and coronary artery disease[1] status post coronary artery bypass surgery (CABG) [6] in 2005 is referred for cardiac catheterization. The patient complained of angina[1] with an associated large area of inferolateral ischemia on stress imaging. A prior diagnostic cardiac catheterization was performed, which revealed a subtotal occlusion of the distal left main artery[1] and patent left internal mammary artery (LIMA) to left anterior descending coronary artery (LAD) graft. The right coronary artery (RCA) was 95–100% chronically occluded with multiple calcified lesions.[2,3]

Procedure description:

The patient was brought back for an elective intervention of the RCA secondary to his symptoms. Access was obtained using a 6-French with a hydrophilic Glidesheath in the right radial artery.[7,8] An intra-arterial cocktail was injected to prevent radial artery spasm and the hydrophilic sheath was then exchanged over a 35" J wire for a 7-Fr non-hydrophilic sheath. A 7 Fr guide was selectively engaged in the RCA. Due to a long area of very heavy calcification and severe angulation within the diseased segment, several different wires, and different tip shapes, failed to cross the lesions. Ultimately, a Fielder FC wire was able to pass through the lesion. The Fielder FC wire was exchanged for a 300 cm Viper wire. Under fluoroscopy, an orbital atherectomy system (Diamondback 360° coronary classic crown, CSI) was gently advanced over the Viper wire proximal to the lesion. Orbital atherectomy was performed in the entire proximal and mid severely calcified RCA artery[7] with multiple passes with total atherectomy time of 7.5 minutes. Each pass (treatment time) was performed for 25–30 seconds with equal length resting periods after each pass. Initially five passes were executed at low revolution speed (80K rpm) with the final three passes performed at high revolution speed (120K rpm). Promus drug-eluting stents (3.5 x 38 mm and 3.5 x 18 mm) (Boston Scientific) were subsequently deployed over the Viper wire in overlapping fashion, covering the entire diseased segment.[8] An excellent angiographic result was achieved with TIMI-3 flow. The sheath and catheters were removed, and the patient was transferred to the recovery room in stable condition.

Diagnosis Codes

I25.119	**Atherosclerotic heart disease of native coronary artery with unspecified angina pectoris**[1]
I25.82	**Chronic total occlusion of coronary artery**[2]
I25.84	**Coronary atherosclerosis due to calcified coronary lesion**[3]
I10	**Essential (primary) hypertension**[4]
E78.5	**Hyperlipidemia, unspecified**[5]
Z95.1	**Presence of aortocoronary bypass graft**[6]

Rationale for Diagnosis Codes

The indications state that the patient was experiencing angina with his coronary artery disease (CAD), which is captured with a combination code that describes both conditions. The chronic total occlusion of the right coronary artery (RCA) with a calcified lesion also must be coded separately to fully describe the condition being treated. The diagnosis codes further specify that a native artery was occluded rather than the previous bypass graft, which was found to be patent (unobstructed).

Procedure Codes

X2C0361	**Extirpation of Matter from Coronary Artery, One Site using Orbital Atherectomy Technology, Percutaneous Approach, New Technology Group 1**[7]
027034Z	**Dilation of Coronary Artery, one site, with drug- eluting intraluminal device, percutaneous approach**[8]

CODING AXIOM

ICD-10-PCS Official Guidelines for Coding and Reporting Section D1:

Section X codes are standalone codes. They are not supplemental codes. Section X codes fully represent the specific procedure described in the code title, and do not require any additional codes from other sections of ICD-10-PCS. When section X contains a code title which describes a specific new technology procedure, only that X code is reported for the procedure. There is no need to report a broader, nonspecific code in another section of ICD-10-PCS.

Rationale for Procedure Codes

The orbital atherectomy procedure is included in the new technology section (X) of ICD-10-PCS. This new section provides a place for codes that uniquely identify procedures that are not otherwise captured in PCS. Codes from this section can be used to capture data for new technology add-on payments or clinical trials. These codes are not meant to be permanently contained in this section but will be held there until further decisions are made affecting their use. The seventh character (qualifier) in this section indicates the year the code was created. For instance the seventh character this year (for fiscal 2016) will be 1, next year will be 2 and so on. The orbital atherectomy new technology code includes the root operation of *Extirpation*, which appropriately describes the intent of the procedure (defined as taking out solid matter from a body part).

As indicated by the new coding guideline D1, the new technology codes are standalone codes. This means that the new technology code would fully describe the entire procedure if only that procedure were performed. However, in this case when reading through the operative report, it mentions that two stents were deployed in the area where the atherectomy was performed. Since this stent deployment is considered a separate procedure, an additional code would be necessary to completely describe the technique performed. The objective of the stents is to keep the RCA expanded and patent, which would lead to the root operation of *Dilation* with the drug-eluting intraluminal device.

MS-DRG

247	Percutaneous Cardiovascular Procedure with Drug-eluting Stent w/o MCC	RW 2.1307

The placement of the stent drove the assignment of MS-DRG 247. The coronary atherectomy (new technology procedure) alone without stent placement would have resulted in a lower-weighted MS-DRG of 251 Percutaneous Cardiovascular Procedures without Coronary Artery Stent without MCC (RW 1.6863).

MDC 6 Diseases Disorders of the Digestive System

OPERATIVE REPORT MDC 6—#1

Preoperative diagnoses:
Chronic and severe abdominal pain occurring at the time of her menstrual cycle, alternating diarrhea and constipation, bloating, and occasional pain during urination (previous test for urinary tract infection came back negative)

Postoperative diagnoses:
Colon endometrioma

History of Illness:
There was no evidence of endometriosis when the patient underwent an oophorectomy two years earlier to remove a large ovarian cyst. An initial exam reveals a palpable fullness of approximately 4 cm at the right lower quadrant of the abdomen, and a subsequent transvaginal ultrasound shows a cystic mass approximately 4.5 cm by 5.0 cm.

Procedure description:
Following induction of endotracheal anesthesia, the patient is placed in the dorsolithotomy position and prepped and draped in the usual sterile fashion. An incision near the belly button is made and the abdomen is insufflated with CO_2 gas to raise the abdomen away from the internal organs. The laparoscope is inserted, and two more incisions are made for the insertion of additional surgical instruments during the procedure. The sigmoid colon is mobilized, revealing a lesion of the sigmoid, and a decision is made to perform an open segmental resection of the sigmoid colon. The dissection is carried down to the level of the rectum to fully mobilize the sigmoid colon. A segmental resection of the lesion is performed. The specimen is sent to pathology, and frozen section confirms the diagnosis of colon endometrioma. An end-to-end anastomosis is performed using a stapler technique. The staple holes are closed. The bowel is returned to the peritoneal cavity after completion of the anastomosis. The bowel is inspected using the laparoscope, and air is placed in the rectum to evaluate the anastomosis. The incisions are closed. There are no intraoperative or postoperative complications.

Code all relevant ICD-10-CM diagnosis and ICD-10-PCS procedure codes in accordance with official guidelines and coding conventions.

Diagnosis Codes:

_____

_____

Procedure Codes:

_____

_____

MS-DRG:

_____

_____

Answers and Rationale

Preoperative diagnoses:
Chronic and severe abdominal pain occurring at the time of her menstrual cycle, alternating diarrhea and constipation, bloating, and occasional pain during urination (previous test for urinary tract infection came back negative)

Postoperative diagnoses:
Colon endometrioma[1]

History of Illness:
There was no evidence of endometriosis when the patient underwent an oophorectomy two years earlier to remove a large ovarian cyst. An initial exam reveals a palpable fullness of approximately 4 cm at the right lower quadrant of the abdomen, and a subsequent transvaginal ultrasound shows a cystic mass approximately 4.5 cm by 5.0 cm.

Procedure description:
Following induction of endotracheal anesthesia, the patient is placed in the dorsolithotomy position and prepped and draped in the usual sterile fashion. An incision near the belly button is made and the abdomen is insufflated with CO2 gas to raise the abdomen away from the internal organs. The laparoscope is inserted[3] and two more incisions are made for the insertion of additional surgical instruments during the procedure. The sigmoid colon is mobilized, revealing a lesion of the sigmoid, and a decision is made to perform an open segmental resection of the sigmoid colon. The dissection is carried down to the level of the rectum to fully mobilize the sigmoid colon. A segmental resection of the lesion is performed. [2] The specimen is sent to pathology, and frozen section confirms the diagnosis of colon endometrioma. An end-to-end anastomosis is performed using a stapler technique. The staple holes are closed. The bowel is returned to the peritoneal cavity after completion of the anastomosis. The bowel is inspected using the laparoscope, and air is placed in the rectum to evaluate the anastomosis. The incisions are closed. There are no intraoperative or postoperative complications.

Diagnosis Codes

N80.5	**Endometriosis of intestine**[1]

Rationale for Diagnosis Codes
The term "Endometrioma" in the ICD-10-CM index refers to code N80.9 Endometriosis unspecified. However, the site of the endometrioma is specified and therefore a code specifying the site should be reported. According to *ICD-10-CM Official Guidelines for Coding and Reporting* section I.B.1, the Tabular List should always be consulted in addition to the Alphabetic Index to ensure the most appropriate and specific code is selected.

It would be inappropriate to report the symptoms listed under the preoperative diagnosis heading, as guidelines section I.B.4 states that codes for signs and symptoms should not be reported when there is a definitive associated diagnosis (endometrioma).

Procedure Codes

0DBN0ZZ	**Excision of Sigmoid Colon, Open Approach**[2]
0DJD4ZZ	**Inspection of Lower Intestinal Tract, Percutaneous Endoscopic Approach**[3]

Rationale for Procedure Codes
A diagnostic laparoscopy is performed at the beginning of the procedure. Once the surgeon decided to resect the sigmoid colon, the decision was made to convert to an *Open* approach. According to *ICD-10-PCS Official Guidelines for Coding and Reporting* section B3.2.d, if an endoscopic procedure is converted to open, report a percutaneous endoscopic inspection and a code for the open procedure. This is reiterated in guidelines section B3.11c, making it appropriate to report the laparoscopy in addition to the open segmental resection. It is important to note that a segmental resection by definition is an *Excision* in ICD-10-PCS. The anastomosis as closure of operative site is integral to the excision of a tubular body part; therefore, it is not reported separately according to guideline section B3.1b.

MS-DRG

331	**Major Small and Large Bowel Procedures without CC/MCC**	**RW 1.6491**

CODING AXIOM

ICD-10-PCS Official Guidelines for Coding and Reporting Section B3.1b:

Components of a procedure specified in the root operation definition and explanation are not coded separately. Procedural steps necessary to reach the operative site and close the operative site, including anastomosis of a tubular body part, are also not coded separately.

CODING AXIOM

ICD-10-PCS Official Guidelines for Coding and Reporting Section B3.2.d:

During the same operative episode, multiple procedures are coded if: The intended root operation is attempted using one approach, but is converted to a different approach.

OPERATIVE REPORT MDC 6—#2

Preoperative diagnosis:
Inguinal hernia

Postoperative diagnosis:
Same

Procedure performed:
Robot-assisted hernia repair

Procedure description:
A 55-year-old male patient with a right inguinal hernia was brought into the operating room, prepped, and anesthetized. The surgeon made three incisions in the abdominal wall, each 3 mm long, and then inserted trocars. The abdomen was inflated with air so the surgeon could visualize the operative space. A fiber optic camera was threaded into the patient's abdomen, and surgical instruments were inserted through the other trocars, then held by the arm of a robotic system. Sitting at the robotic operating console and using a headset, the surgeon began verbally directing the robot and manipulated these instruments inside the abdomen. A large inguinal hernia was located, and the surgeon directed the robotic arm to pull the hernia sac back into the abdominal cavity, exposing the abdominal wall defect. The repair was accomplished after extensive subcutaneous dissection, using a polypropylene mesh patch inserted through the operating port and placed inside the abdominal wall. The surgeon stapled the mesh to the pelvic bone and the abdominal muscles.

Code all relevant ICD-10-CM diagnosis and ICD-10-PCS procedure codes in accordance with official guidelines and coding conventions.

Diagnosis Codes:

_____

_____

Procedure Codes:

_____

_____

MS-DRG:

_____

_____

DEFINITIONS

inguinal hernia. Loop of intestine that protrudes through the abdominal peritoneum into the inguinal canal.

Answers and Rationale

Preoperative diagnosis:
Inguinal hernia[1]

Postoperative diagnosis:
Same

Procedure performed:
Robot-assisted[3] hernia repair

Procedure description:
A 55-year-old male patient with a right inguinal hernia[1-2] was brought into the operating room, prepped, and anesthetized. The surgeon made three incisions in the abdominal wall, each 3 mm long, and then inserted trocars. The abdomen was inflated with air so the surgeon could visualize the operative space. A fiber optic camera was threaded into patient's abdomen, and surgical instruments were inserted through the other trocars, then held by the arm of a robotic system.[2-3] Sitting at the robotic operating console and using a headset, the surgeon began verbally directing the robot and manipulated these instruments inside the abdomen. A large inguinal hernia was located, and the surgeon directed the robotic arm to pull the hernia sac back into the abdominal cavity, exposing the abdominal wall defect. The repair was accomplished after extensive subcutaneous dissection, using a polypropylene mesh patch inserted through the operating port and placed inside the abdominal wall.[2] The surgeon stapled the mesh to the pelvic bone and the abdominal muscles.

Diagnosis Codes

K40.90   **Unilateral inguinal hernia, without obstruction or gangrene, not specified as recurrent[1]**

Rationale for Diagnosis Codes
The hernia is specified as being on the right (unilateral) and in the inguinal region making the diagnosis coding straightforward.

Procedure Codes

0YU54JZ   **Supplement Right Inguinal Region with Synthetic Substitute, Percutaneous Endoscopic Approach[2]**

8E0W4CZ   **Robotic Assisted Procedure of Trunk Region, Percutaneous Endoscopic Approach[3]**

Rationale for Procedure Codes
The procedure's objective is to repair the bulge in the abdominal wall (hernia) in the inguinal region utilizing mesh. Under "Herniorrhaphy" in the index, whether or not a synthetic substitute, otherwise known as mesh, was used determines the root operation that correctly represents this procedure. In this case, because mesh is used, the table for "supplement" rather than "repair" should be consulted. The mesh is inserted to "supplement" the abdominal wall by ICD-10-PCS definitions. The fact that the procedure is being performed utilizing robotic assistance should also be reported. The appropriate table can be located in the ICD-10-PCS index under the terms "Robotic assisted procedure, Trunk region."

MS-DRG

352   **Inguinal and Femoral Hernia Procedures without CC/MCC**   **RW 0.9764**

OPERATIVE REPORT MDC 6—#3

Preoperative diagnosis:
Screening colonoscopy, rectal bleeding

Postoperative diagnosis:
Same, polyps

Procedure performed:
Colonoscopy with polypectomy

Indications:
A 65-year-old patient with a history of rectal bleeding presents to the hospital for a colonoscopy.

Procedure description:
The patient is given versed intravenously for conscious sedation. She is brought to the endoscopy suite and placed in a supine position and turned to a left lateral Sims' position. Perianal area is inspected, no palpable masses, no evidence of anal fissure and good sphincter tone is noted.

The colonoscope is inserted through the anus and advanced to the cecum without difficulty. The lumen of the colon is visualized. There is a 3 mm polyp on the mucosal folds of the descending colon which is snared. There is a 5 mm polyp in the rectum which is removed in its entirety with hot biopsy forceps. Internal hemorrhoids are present. No source of bleeding was identified. The colonoscope was withdrawn. The patient tolerated the procedure well.

Code all relevant ICD-10-CM diagnosis and ICD-10-PCS procedure codes in accordance with official guidelines and coding conventions.

Diagnosis Codes:

_____

_____

Procedure Codes:

_____

_____

MS-DRG:

_____

_____

Answers and Rationale

Preoperative diagnosis:
Screening colonoscopy for rectal bleeding[1]

Postoperative diagnosis:
Same, polyps[2,3]

Procedure performed:
Colonoscopy with polypectomy

Indications:
A 65-year-old patient with a history of rectal bleeding presents to the hospital for a colonoscopy.

Procedure description:
The patient is given Versed intravenously for conscious sedation. She is brought to the endoscopy suite and placed in a supine position and turned to a left lateral Sims' position. Perianal area is inspected, no palpable masses, no evidence of anal fissure and good sphincter tone is noted.

The colonoscope is inserted through the anus[5,6] and advanced to the cecum without difficulty. The lumen of the colon is visualized. There is a 3 mm polyp on the mucosal folds of the descending colon which is snared.[2,5] There is a 5 mm polyp in the rectum which is removed in its entirety with hot biopsy forceps.[3,6] Internal hemorrhoids are present.[4] No source of bleeding was identified.[1] The colonoscope was withdrawn. The patient tolerated the procedure well.

Diagnosis Codes

K62.5	Hemorrhage of anus and rectum[1]
D12.4	Benign neoplasm of descending colon[2]
K62.1	Rectal polyp[3]
K64.8	Other hemorrhoids[4]

Rationale for Diagnosis Codes

Although the physician described the colonoscopy as a screening, there was a problem being worked up via the colonoscopy; therefore, this cannot be considered a screening based on the definition of a screening colonoscopy. The reason for the procedure was rectal bleeding. Because there is no definitive diagnosis documented as being responsible for the bleeding, the principal diagnosis should be the rectal bleeding per *ICD-10-CM Official Guidelines for Coding and Reporting* section II.A: "Codes for symptoms, signs, and ill-defined conditions from chapter 18 are not to be used as principal diagnosis when a related definitive diagnosis has been established."

Procedure Codes

ØDBM8ZZ	Excision of Descending Colon, Via Natural or Artificial Opening Endoscopic[5]
ØDBP8ZZ	Excision of Rectum, Via Natural or Artificial Opening Endoscopic[6]

Rationale for Procedure Codes

The term "Polypectomy" in the index directs the coder to the table for *Excision* in the gastrointestinal section. This root operation coincides with the objective of the procedures, to remove the polyps.

MS-DRG

379	GI Hemorrhage without CC/MCC	RW 0.6712

Because the procedures are nonoperating room procedures, they are not considered in the grouping of this MS-DRG. Although any of the other three diagnoses sequenced as principal diagnosis would result in a higher-paying MS-DRG assignment (MS-DRG 394 Other Digestive System Diagnoses with CC), it would be inappropriate to report any of those based on the definition of principal diagnosis. Code K62.5 is considered a CC condition, so it would increase the MS-DRG assignment if reported in any position other than the principal diagnosis (which would be inappropriate in this case).

CODING AXIOM

ICD-10-CM Official Guidelines for Coding and Reporting Section I.C.21.c.5:

Screening is the testing for disease or disease precursors in seemingly well individuals so that early detection and treatment can be provided for those who test positive for the disease (e.g., screening mammogram).

The testing of a person to rule out or confirm a suspected diagnosis because the patient has some sign or symptom is a diagnostic examination, not a screening. In these cases, the sign or symptom is used to explain the reason for the test.

OPERATIVE REPORT MDC 6—#4

Preoperative diagnosis:
Crohn's disease and small bowel obstruction

Postoperative diagnosis:
Crohn's disease and small bowel obstruction

Procedure performed:
Resection of bowel obstruction of the small intestine

Indications:
A 45-year-old female was referred for severe abdominal pain in the lower right area and a change in bowel habits, mainly diarrhea. She has been treated for Crohn's disease since the age of 19 and maintained on drug therapy. Her x-ray showed small bowel obstruction, and she was taken to surgery.

Procedure description:
Once the patient was properly sedated and anesthesia administered, the physician made an abdominal incision. The surgeon resected a segment of jejunum and performed an anastomosis between the remaining bowel ends. The surgeon then identified a second section of small bowel. The selected segment of small bowel was isolated and divided proximally and distally; a partial excision of the terminal ileum was performed to release the obstruction. The remaining intestinal ends were reapproximated using staples. The incision was closed. The patient tolerated the procedure well.

Code all relevant ICD-10-CM diagnosis and ICD-10-PCS procedure codes in accordance with official guidelines and coding conventions.

Diagnosis Codes:

_____

_____

Procedure Codes:

_____

_____

MS-DRG:

_____

_____

Answers and Rationale

Preoperative diagnosis:
Crohn's disease and small bowel obstruction

Postoperative diagnosis:
Crohn's disease and small bowel obstruction[1]

Procedure performed:
Resection of bowel obstruction of the small intestine

Indications:
A 45-year-old female was referred for severe abdominal pain in the lower right area and a change in bowel habits, mainly diarrhea. She has been treated for Crohn's disease since the age of 19 and maintained on drug therapy. Her x-ray showed small bowel obstruction, and she was taken to surgery.

Procedure description:
Once the patient was properly sedated and anesthesia administered, the physician made an abdominal incision. The surgeon resected a segment of jejunum[2] and performed an anastomosis between the remaining bowel ends. The surgeon then identified a second section of small bowel. The selected segment of small bowel was isolated and divided proximally and distally; a partial excision of the terminal ileum was performed to release the obstruction. [3] The remaining intestinal ends were reapproximated using staples. The incision was closed. The patient tolerated the procedure well.

Diagnosis Codes

K50.012   Crohn's disease of small intestine with intestinal obstruction[1]

Rationale for Diagnosis Codes
The terms "Disease, Crohns" in the index refer the coder to "Enteritis, Regional." These terms further differentiate the diagnosis by multiple deciding factors. With the documentation provided in this case, the code assigned reflects the appropriate location (small intestine) and the complication (bowel obstruction).

Procedure Codes

0DBA0ZZ   Excision of Jejunum, Open Approach[2]

0DBB0ZZ   Excision of Ileum, Open Approach[3]

Rationale for Procedure Codes
Resection of a segment of intestine is reported by the root operation *Excision*. The approach was open, and the technique for closure of the operative site (intestine) was by anastomosis. Since the objective of the anastomosis is closure of the operative site, it is not reported and not considered a bypass, which is the alteration of the route of passage involving a tubular body part.

MS-DRG

348	Anal and Stomal Procedures with CC	RW 1.4486

Note that there is only one code yet the MS-DRG is categorized as with CC. This is because code K50.012 serves as a CC to itself. Meaning, if the combination code is reported as principal diagnosis there is automatically a CC for the encounter.

OPERATIVE REPORT MDC 6—#5

Preoperative diagnosis:
Hematemesis, history of esophageal ulcer, possible erosion

Postoperative diagnosis:
Esophageal ulcer with bleeding

Procedure performed:
EGD

Indications:
Patient with history of esophageal ulcer and possible erosion presented with hematemesis and acute blood loss anemia; also has a history of diabetes and hypertension

Procedure description:
Moderate sedation was achieved with IV Versed. Once it was determined that the patient was adequately anesthetized, the patient was prepped and draped in a usual sterile fashion. The scope was passed through the mouth and into the stomach. The esophagus was tortuous. Biopsy was taken from the ulcerated area near the esophagogastric junction using forceps and sent for pathology. There was a small amount of bleeding from the biopsy that did not present a problem. Endoscope removed, all supplies accounted for, and patient sent to recovery.

Code all relevant ICD-10-CM diagnosis and ICD-10-PCS procedure codes in accordance with official guidelines and coding conventions.

Diagnosis Codes:

_____

_____

Procedure Codes:

_____

_____

MS-DRG:

_____

_____

Answers and Rational

Preoperative diagnosis:
Hematemesis, history of esophageal ulcer, possible erosion

Postoperative diagnosis:
Esophageal ulcer with bleeding[1]

Procedure performed:
EGD

Indications:
Patient with history of esophageal ulcer and possible erosion presented with hematemesis and acute blood loss anemia;[2] also has a history of diabetes[3] and hypertension[4]

Procedure description:
Moderate sedation was achieved with IV Versed. Once it was determined that the patient was adequately anesthetized, the patient was prepped and draped in a usual sterile fashion. The scope was passed through the mouth and into the stomach.[5] The esophagus was tortuous. Biopsy was taken from the ulcerated area near the esophagogastric junction using forceps and sent for pathology.[5] There was a small amount of bleeding from the biopsy that did not present a problem. Endoscope removed, all supplies accounted for, and patient sent to recovery.

Diagnosis Codes

K22.11	Ulcer of esophagus with bleeding[1]
D62	Acute posthemorrhagic anemia[2]
E11.9	Type 2 diabetes mellitus without complications[3]
I10	Essential (primary) hypertension[4]

Rationale for Diagnosis Codes

Because the hematemesis is due to the bleeding esophageal ulcer, it is unnecessary and incorrect to report this diagnosis in conjunction with K22.11, which includes the ulcer and the bleeding. It is also important to report the codes for the acute blood loss anemia, unspecified diabetes, and hypertension that are documented in the "Indications" section.

Procedure Codes

0DB48ZX	Excision of Esophagogastric Junction, Via Natural or Artificial Opening Endoscopic Approach, Diagnostic[5]

Rationale for Procedure Codes

The procedure indicated by the title would be reported using the root operation *Inspection* if a biopsy were not performed in the full description of the procedure. The biopsy as documented is reported using the root operation *Excision*. Both the inspection and the excision would be reported if they were performed using different approaches, but since both were performed via natural opening with an endoscope, only the biopsy is reported. The qualifier X, meaning *Diagnostic*, is used as well to indicate that a biopsy was performed. The approach character value 8 indicates that the biopsy is performed via the esophagogastroduodenoscopy (EGD), via the oral cavity.

MS-DRG

381	Complicated Peptic Ulcer with CC	RW 1.0690

If the acute blood-loss anemia is reported incorrectly or omitted, the MS-DRG changes to the lower-weighted 382 Complicated Peptic Ulcer Without CC/MCC (RW 0.8238).

CODING AXIOM

ICD-10-PCS Official Guidelines for Coding and Reporting Section B3.11a:

When the root operation *Inspection* and another procedure are performed on the same body part during the same episode but the *Inspection* procedure is performed using a different approach, the *Inspection* procedure is coded separately.

☞ **KEY POINT**

It is recommended to assign codes after all documentation is available whenever possible. Await pathology findings to code to the highest level of specificity after the provider confirms those findings.

OPERATIVE REPORT MDC 6—#6

Preoperative diagnosis:
Rectal cancer

Postoperative diagnosis:
Same

Procedure performed:
Open pull-through resection of rectum

Indications:
An otherwise healthy and active 65-year-old male patient presented with cyclical symptoms of diarrhea, with which he experienced episodes of dyspnea associated with "flushing" of the skin. He had a history of diverticulosis coli and therefore had delayed seeking treatment by assuming his symptoms were attacks of his existing diverticular disease. Urinalysis results were positive for high levels of 5-HIAA. After localization of the tumor and biopsy on an outpatient basis, malignant carcinoma of the rectum was diagnosed. The patient then presented for surgical removal of malignant carcinoid tumor of the rectum and initiation of medical therapy for associated carcinoid syndrome.

Procedure description:
The patient was brought into the operating room, prepped, and anesthetized. The surgeon made an abdominal incision in preparation for an open pull-through resection of the rectum with an end-to-end anastomosis. The distal colon and rectum were mobilized within the abdomen to the level of the sphincter muscles. The colon was divided above the pelvic brim and the rectum at the level of the sphincter muscles and removed. The mucosa was stripped from the remaining distal colon. The sigmoid colon was pulled through the sphincter complex and approximated to the perianal tissue with sutures. The incision was closed.

Code all relevant ICD-10-CM diagnosis and ICD-10-PCS procedure codes in accordance with official guidelines and coding conventions.

Diagnosis Codes:

_____

_____

Procedure Codes:

_____

_____

MS-DRG:

_____

_____

Answers and Rationale

Preoperative diagnosis:
Rectal cancer

Postoperative diagnosis:
Same

Procedure performed:
Open pull-through resection of rectum

Indications:
An otherwise healthy and active 65-year-old male patient presented with cyclical symptoms of diarrhea, with which he experienced episodes of dyspnea associated with "flushing" of the skin. He has a history of diverticulosis coli[3] and therefore had delayed seeking treatment by assuming his symptoms were attacks of his existing diverticular disease. Urinalysis results were positive for high levels of 5-HIAA. After localization of the tumor and biopsy on an outpatient basis, malignant carcinoma of the rectum was diagnosed. The patient then presented for surgical removal of malignant carcinoid tumor of the rectum[1] and initiation of medical therapy for associated carcinoid syndrome.[2]

Procedure description:
The patient was brought into the operating room, prepped, and anesthetized. The surgeon made an abdominal incision in preparation for an open pull-through resection of the rectum with an end-to-end anastomosis. The distal colon and rectum were mobilized within the abdomen to the level of the sphincter muscles. The colon was divided above the pelvic brim and the rectum at the level of the sphincter muscles and removed. The mucosa was stripped from the remaining distal colon. The sigmoid colon was pulled through the sphincter complex and approximated to the perianal tissue with sutures.[4] The incision was closed.

Diagnosis Codes

C7A.026	Malignant carcinoid tumor of the rectum[1]
E34.0	Carcinoid syndrome[2]
Z87.19	Personal history of other diseases of the digestive system[3]

Rationale for Diagnosis Codes

The terms "Tumor, Carcinoid" in the ICD-10-CM index does *not* direct the coder to the Neoplasm Table but rather offers the choice between benign or malignant as a subterm, followed by the anatomical site. Therefore, coders referring to the Neoplasm Table first instead of the index would report an incorrect code for the malignancy. A "use additional code" note under category C7A instructs the coder to assign E34.0 if carcinoid syndrome (dyspnea and skin flushing) is also present. Lastly, diverticulosis coli is documented in the history, and there is no indication that it is symptomatic or that it is under treatment and the work-up ruled it out as the cause of the presenting symptom. Therefore, diverticulosis is coded as history only when it is not clinically significant to the encounter.

Procedure Codes

0DTP0ZZ	Resection of Rectum, Open Approach[4]

Rationale for Procedure Codes

The documentation provides enough information for the coder to know that the rectum was removed from above the pelvic brim to the anal sphincter, which includes the entire rectum. As the entire body part is removed, the root operation is *Resection*.

MS-DRG

333	Rectal Resection with CC	RW 2.4254

If the carcinoid syndrome is not reported, the MS-DRG changes to lower-weighted 334 Rectal Resection without CC/MCC (RW 1.6480).

⚓ **CODING AXIOM**

ICD-10-CM Official Guidelines for Coding and Reporting Section I.C.2:

The Neoplasm Table in the Alphabetic Index should be referenced first. However, if the histological term is documented, that term should be referenced first to determine which column in the Neoplasm Table is appropriate. For example, if the documentation indicates "adenoma," refer to that term in the Alphabetic Index, which instructs the coder to "see also neoplasm, by site, benign." The table provides the proper code based on the type of neoplasm and the site. It is important to select the proper column in the table that corresponds to the type of neoplasm. The Tabular List should then be referenced to verify that the correct code has been selected from the table and that a more specific site code does not exist.

OPERATIVE REPORT MDC 6—#7

Preoperative diagnoses:
Hematemesis

Postoperative diagnoses:
Grade 2 to 3 distal esophageal varices

Procedure performed:
Esophagogastroduodenoscopy with sclerotherapy of esophageal varices

Indication:
Hematemesis in the setting of alcohol abuse and dependence in a patient with known esophageal varices

Procedure description:
Informed consent was obtained. The patient was deemed to be ASA class II and therefore a candidate for conscious sedation. The patient was placed in the left lateral decubitus position. After conscious sedation was administered, endoscope was introduced in the mouth and passed under direct visualization without difficulty to the fourth portion of the duodenum. The endoscope was then slowly withdrawn and mucosal circumference was inspected. Examination of the duodenal mucosa and entire examined portions was unremarkable.

Examination of the gastric mucosa revealed erythema of the antrum. On retroflexion, there was no evidence of gastric varices. The GE junction was at 40 cm from the incisors. Between 36 and 40 cm from the incisors, there were varices distally in the esophagus that were grade 2 to 3 with a weal mark noticed. There was evidence of a slight bleed remaining in this area. The remainder of the esophageal examination was unremarkable. A 23-gauge needle was passed through the working channel of the endoscope, and ethanolamine oleate was injected in the para-variceal area. The endoscope was withdrawn. The patient tolerated the procedure well. There were no immediate complications.

Code all relevant ICD-10-CM diagnosis and ICD-10-PCS procedure codes in accordance with official guidelines and coding conventions.

Diagnosis Codes:

_____

_____

Procedure Codes:

_____

_____

MS-DRG:

_____

Answers and Rationale

Preoperative diagnoses:
Hematemesis[1]

Postoperative diagnoses:
Grade 2 to 3 distal esophageal varices[1]

Procedure performed:
Esophagogastroduodenoscopy with sclerotherapy[4] of esophageal varices

Indication:
Hematemesis in the setting of alcohol abuse and dependence[3] in a patient with known esophageal varices and acute blood loss anemia[2]

Procedure description:
Informed consent was obtained. The patient was deemed to be ASA class II and therefore a candidate for conscious sedation. The patient was placed in the left lateral decubitus position. After conscious sedation was administered, an endoscope was introduced in the mouth and passed under direct visualization without difficulty to the fourth portion of the duodenum. Endoscope was then slowly withdrawn and mucosal circumference was inspected. Examination of the duodenal mucosa and entire examined portions was unremarkable.

Examination of the gastric mucosa revealed minor erythema of the antrum. On retroflexion, there was no evidence of gastric varices. The GE junction was at 40 cm from the incisors. Between 36 and 40 cm from the incisors, there were varices distally in the esophagus that were grade 2 to 3 with a weal mark noticed. There was evidence of a slight bleed remaining in this area.[1] The remainder of the esophageal examination was unremarkable. A 23-gauge needle was passed through the working channel of the endoscope and ethanolamine oleate was injected in the para-variceal area.[4] The endoscope was withdrawn. The patient tolerated the procedure well. There were no immediate complications.

Diagnosis Codes

I85.01	Esophageal varices with bleeding[1]
D62	Acute posthemorrhagic anemia[2]
F10.20	Alcohol dependence, uncomplicated[3]

Rationale for Diagnosis Codes
The patient has evidence of bleeding in the area of the esophageal varices. This means that the appropriate code includes the bleeding and that the hematemesis would not be reported as this is a symptom of the underlying and definitive diagnosis. In the "Indications" section, the acute blood loss anemia is discussed. Lastly, the physician discusses alcohol abuse and dependence. It should be noted that there is an Excludes1 note under the alcohol abuse stating that the dependence should be reported instead of the abuse. Therefore, code F10.20 should be assigned.

Procedure Codes

3E0G8TZ	Introduction of Destructive Agent into Upper GI, Via Natural or Artificial Opening Endoscopic[4]

Rationale for Procedure Codes
The purpose of the procedure is to stop or control the bleeding of the varices using a destructive agent that does not destroy the vessels. The appropriate root operation could not be *Destruction* because the vessel is not eradicated. The root operation *Control* is not appropriate because this is not considered "postoperative" bleeding. Therefore, introduction of the sclerosing agent should be reported for the injection via the endoscope. This advice is consistent with AHA *Coding Clinic for ICD-10-CM and ICD-10-PCS*, first quarter 2013, page 27.

MS-DRG

369	Major Esophageal Disorders with CC	RW 1.0630

🕯 CODING AXIOM

ICD-10-PCS Official Guidelines for Coding and Reporting Section I.A.12.a:

Excludes 1:

A type 1 Excludes note is a pure excludes note. It means "NOT CODED HERE!" An Excludes1 note indicates that the code excluded should never be used at the same time as the code above the Excludes1 note. An Excludes1 is used when two conditions cannot occur together, such as a congenital form versus an acquired form of the same condition.

📖 DEFINITIONS

control. Stopping, or attempting to stop, postprocedural bleeding.

destruction. Ablation or eradication of a structure or tissue.

introduction. Putting in or on a therapeutic, diagnostic, nutritional, physiological, or prophylactic substance except blood or blood products.

MDC 7 Diseases and Disorders of the Hepatobiliary System and Pancreas

OPERATIVE REPORT MDC 7—#1

Preoperative Diagnosis:
Cholelithiasis, cholecystitis, umbilical hernia

Postoperative Diagnosis:
Same with acute and chronic cholecystitis

Procedure description:
The patient was taken to the operating room and following establishment of a satisfactory level of general anesthesia, the abdomen was prepped and draped in the usual sterile fashion. Next, an infraumbilical incision was made. The umbilical hernia sac was freed up. The sac was opened and the Origin trocar was inserted. The abdomen was insufflated and the laparoscope was introduced. Lateral and superior medial trocars were inserted under direct vision. The gallbladder showed signs of marked acute cholecystitis. There was also a very prominent lobe of the liver that folded over the gallbladder almost completely, obscuring the field of dissection. This made dissection extremely difficult in addition to the acute cholecystitis. There was at least an additional 30-45 minutes of operative time necessary due to the severe amount of inflammation and infection in the denuded bed. Ultimately, after a very tedious dissection, the triangle of Calot was cleared. The cystic duct and artery were identified. The cystic duct was doubly clipped at its junction with the gallbladder. The gallbladder was dissected away from the liver bed and removed through a port, after which all trocars were withdrawn, and wounds repaired, and the patient was taken to the recovery room in satisfactory condition.

Code all relevant ICD-10-CM diagnosis and ICD-10-PCS procedure codes in accordance with official guidelines and coding conventions.

Diagnosis Codes:

_____

_____

Procedure Codes:

_____

_____

MS-DRG:

_____

_____

Answers and Rationale

Preoperative Diagnosis:
Cholelithiasis, cholecystitis,[1] umbilical hernia[2]

Postoperative Diagnosis:
Same with acute and chronic cholecystitis[1]

Procedure description:
The patient was taken to the operating room and following establishment of a satisfactory level of general anesthesia, the abdomen was prepped and draped in the usual sterile fashion. Next, an infraumbilical incision was made. The umbilical hernia sac was freed up. The sac was opened[4] and the Origin trocar was inserted. The abdomen was insufflated and the laparoscope was introduced[3]. Lateral and superior medial trocars were inserted under direct vision. The gallbladder showed signs of marked acute cholecystitis. [1] There was also a very prominent lobe of the liver that folded over the gallbladder almost completely, obscuring the field of dissection. This made dissection extremely difficult in addition to the acute cholecystitis. [1] Ultimately, after a very tedious dissection, the triangle of Calot was cleared. The cystic duct and artery were identified. The gallbladder was dissected away from the liver bed and removed through a port[3], after which all trocars were withdrawn, and wounds repaired, and the patient was taken to the recovery room in satisfactory condition.

Diagnosis Codes

K80.12   **Calculus of gallbladder with acute and chronic cholecystitis without obstruction[1]**

K42.9   **Umbilical hernia without obstruction or gangrene[2]**

Rationale for Diagnosis Codes
The term "Cholecystitis" or "Cholelithiasis" in the ICD-10-CM index refer the coder to "Calculus, Gallbladder," which further distinguishes between acute, chronic, or acute on chronic and with or without obstruction. The documentation explicitly states "acute on chronic" but does not note whether there is obstruction. As there is no specific detail, the default is to code "without obstruction." The index and tabular listings for umbilical hernia are straightforward. There is no mention of obstruction or gangrene and therefore the classification system defaults to "without."

Procedure Codes

0FT44ZZ   **Resection of Gallbladder, Percutaneous Endoscopic Approach[3]**

0WQF0ZZ   **Repair Abdominal Wall, Open Approach[4]**

Rationale for Procedure Codes
Code 0FT44ZZ is assigned for the cholecystectomy. Category 0FT4 represents the resection or "cutting out or off, without replacement, all of a body part" of the gallbladder. The approach is *Laparoscopic*, described as percutaneous endoscopic in ICD-10-PCS. The physician also performed a herniorrhaphy of the umbilical hernia. Although the cholecystectomy was performed laparoscopically, the hernia repair was not. According to the operative report, an incision was made, the hernia was incised before the abdomen was insufflated and the laparoscope inserted, making the approach for the hernia repair *Open*, or a fifth character of 0.

MS-DRG

419   **Laparoscopic Cholecystectomy without C.D.E. without CC/MCC**   **RW 1.2540**

It is important to get the approach correct for the cholecystectomy as this is one of the factors driving the appropriate MS-DRG. If *Open* was selected rather than *Percutaneous Endoscopic*, the MS-DRG would be higher-weighted 416 Cholecystectomy Except by Laparoscope without C.D.E. without CC/MCC.

OPERATIVE REPORT MDC 7—#2

Preoperative diagnosis:
Pancreatic head mass

Postoperative diagnosis:
Pancreatic carcinoma

Procedure performed:
Stomach sparing pancreaticoduodenectomy Whipple procedure

Procedure description:
The patient was brought to the operating suite, and a general intubation anesthetic was administered. Foley catheter was placed for gravity drainage. The abdomen was prepped with Betadine and sterilely draped. With the patient in a supine position, a bilateral subcostal incision was made. The right colon was then taken off the duodenum and the anterior surface of the head of the pancreas. The gastrocolic ligament was taken down to reveal the body and tail of the pancreas. It was followed to the superior mesenteric vein to the under-surface of the pancreas. Attention was then directed to the superior border of the pancreas, where it was observed that the pancreatic mass had come to the extra-pancreatic tissue. A biopsy was taken at the junction of the first portion of the jejunum and this was positive for metastasis.

The area was dissected free from the hepatic artery and attention was directed to the gallbladder and the bile duct. The peritoneum of the gallbladder fundus was incised and the gallbladder removed. The common hepatic duct was transected, and the dissection was continued to the upper border of the head of the pancreas. The gastroduodenal artery and the hepatic artery were separated away from the superior border of the pancreas. A vessel loop was then passed around the neck of the pancreas, and the pancreas was then transected between the two rows of sutures. The duodenum and jejunal junction was transected, and the specimen (entire duodenum en bloc) was marked and sent to pathology.

The pancreas was elevated 4 cm off the splenic vein. A gastrotomy was made and 1 cm of the pancreas was invaginated into the stomach with the end of the jejunum closed over, and a pancreaticojejunostomy was made with interrupted 4-0 PDS suture attaching the pancreas to the jejunum. A gastroenterostomy was made to the greater curvature of the stomach in two layers, outer interrupted 3-0 silk and inner running 3-0 Monocryl sutures. The lumens were all checked, and the abdomen was well-irrigated. One drain was placed by the gastrojejunostomy and another drain by the pancreaticoenterostomy and brought out below the incision on the right and left and anchored to the skin with 3-0 nylon. After an accurate sponge, instrument, and needle count was conducted, the abdomen was closed with continuous 1-0 Panacryl. The skin was approximated with skin staples, dressings were placed, and the patient discharged to recovery in satisfactory condition.

Code all relevant ICD-10-CM diagnosis and ICD-10-PCS procedure codes in accordance with official guidelines and coding conventions.

Diagnosis Codes:

_____

_____

Procedure Codes:

_____

_____

MS-DRG:

_____

_____

Answers and Rationale

Preoperative diagnosis:
Pancreatic head[1] mass

Postoperative diagnosis:
Pancreatic carcinoma[1]

Procedure performed:
Stomach sparing pancreaticoduodenectomy Whipple procedure

Procedure description:
The patient was brought to the operating suite, and a general intubation anesthetic was administered. Foley catheter was placed for gravity drainage. The abdomen was prepped with Betadine and sterilely draped. With the patient in a supine position, a bilateral subcostal incision was made. The right colon was then taken off the duodenum and the anterior surface of the head of the pancreas. The gastrocolic ligament was taken down to reveal the body and tail of the pancreas. It was followed to the superior mesenteric vein to the under-surface of the pancreas. Attention was then directed to the superior border of the pancreas, where it was observed that the pancreatic mass had come to the extra-pancreatic tissue. A biopsy was taken at the junction of the first portion of the jejunum and this was positive for metastasis.[2,4]

The area was dissected free from the hepatic artery and attention was directed to the gallbladder and the bile duct. The peritoneum of the gallbladder fundus was incised and the gallbladder removed.[5] The common hepatic duct was transected, and the dissection was continued to the upper border of the head of the pancreas. The gastroduodenal artery and the hepatic artery were separated away from the superior border of the pancreas. A vessel loop was then passed around the neck of the pancreas, and the pancreas was then transected between the two rows of sutures.[3] The duodenum and jejunal junction was transected[6,7], and the specimen (entire duodenum en bloc) was marked and sent to pathology.

The pancreas was elevated 4 cm off the splenic vein. A gastrotomy was made and 1 cm of the pancreas was invaginated into the stomach with the end of the jejunum closed over, and a pancreaticojejunostomy was made with interrupted 4-0 PDS suture attaching the pancreas to the jejunum. A gastroenterostomy was made to the greater curvature of the stomach in two layers, outer interrupted 3-0 silk and inner running 3-0 Monocryl sutures. The lumens were all checked, and the abdomen was well-irrigated. One drain was placed by the gastrojejunostomy and another drain by the pancreaticoenterostomy and brought out below the incision on the right and left and anchored to the skin with 3-0 nylon. After an accurate sponge, instrument, and needle count was conducted, the abdomen was closed with continuous 1-0 Panacryl. The skin was approximated with skin staples, dressings were placed, and the patient discharged to recovery in satisfactory condition.

Diagnosis Codes

C25.0	**Malignant neoplasm of head of pancreas**[1]
C78.4	**Secondary malignant neoplasm of small intestine**[2]

Rationale for Diagnosis Codes

The preoperative diagnosis notes the specific site of the pancreatic cancer, allowing for the selection of a more detailed code. The body of the operative note discusses the metastasis to the jejunum.

Procedure Codes

0FBG0ZZ	**Excision of Pancreas, Open Approach**[3]
0DBA0ZX	**Excision of Jejunum, Open Approach, Diagnostic**[4]
0FT40ZZ	**Resection of Gallbladder, Open Approach**[5]
0DT90ZZ	**Resection of Duodenum, Open Approach**[6]
0DBA0ZZ	**Excision of Jejunum, Open Approach**[7]

Rationale for Procedure Codes

In this procedure, portions of the pancreas and jejunum were removed, making it appropriate to report two codes with the root operation *Excision*. The entire duodenum and gallbladder were removed, resulting in the root operation *Resection* for those removals. A biopsy of a jejunal lesion also was performed intraoperatively. A biopsy performed before an excision or resection should be reported, according to *ICD-10-PCS Official Guidelines for Coding and Reporting* section B3.4. The biopsy followed by the procedure are represented by two codes for the excision of the jejunum, one diagnostic

---

☼ CODING AXIOM

ICD-10-PCS Official Guidelines for Coding and Reporting Section B3.4b:

If a diagnostic Excision, Extraction, or Drainage procedure (biopsy) is followed by a more definitive procedure, such as Destruction, Excision or Resection at the same procedure site, both the biopsy and the more definitive treatment are coded.

---

and the other therapeutic. In a standard Whipple procedure, part of the stomach would be removed. In this stomach-sparing Whipple procedure, however, the stomach and pylorus were preserved, allowing for normal gastric function. According to *AHA Coding Clinic for ICD-10-CM and ICD-10-PCS*, third quarter, 2014, page 32, the anastomoses are inherent to the procedure and included in the code assignment.

MS-DRG

406	Pancreas, Liver and Shunt Procedures with CC	RW 2.8075

Without the code for the jejunal metastasis, the MS-DRG drops to the lower-weighted, sister MS-DRG 407 Pancreas, Liver and Shunt Procedures without CC/MCC.

OPERATIVE REPORT MDC 7—#3

Preoperative diagnosis:
Liver and splenic lacerations with hemoperitoneum, internal injuries without open wound

Postoperative diagnosis:
Same and gross peritonitis with early abscess formation

Procedure performed:
Diagnostic laparoscopy and drainage of gross hemoperitonitis and subdiaphragmatic abscess and pelvic abscess

Findings:
2.5 to 3 liters of fluid were aspirated from the peritoneal cavity, including a combination of foul-smelling old blood and bile. Interestingly, there was no gross purulence identified.

Indications:
This 26-year-old male patient was in a dirt bike accident last week in which he struck his abdomen against the handlebars. Subjectively, his abdomen has been tender but not painful. He did not seek medical attention until today when he became cold, clammy, and lethargic and his abdominal pain increased significantly. Work-up confirmed the above-mentioned injuries, and we proceeded to emergent surgery.

Procedure description:
After informed consent was obtained, the patient was brought to the operating room where the abdomen was prepped and draped in a normal standard fashion. Utilizing an infraumbilical Hasson technique, the peritoneal cavity was accessed. Once we gained access there was immediate drainage of foul-smelling old blood. There was no obvious purulence. We then suctioned through the umbilical post for 5-10 minutes and were able to remove one liter of this blood. Despite it being foul smelling, we did not identify any fecal or succus entericus.

We then placed the Hasson port in and started to take down the light adhesions. We placed two more 5mm ports in as capable and were able to take fluid collections. The right lower quadrant cecum was adherent to the anterior abdominal wall because of an old appendectomy. At that time we explored the entire abdomen, taking down and draining fluid collections from the right upper quadrant, left upper quadrant, and left gutter as well as left pelvis. The right upper quadrant fluid collections were more of old blood and fibrinous debris. The left upper quadrant next to where the fractured and ischemic liver lay was probably a collection of old bile and blood and because of the foul smell represented an early abscess formation. There was also green exudate throughout all the peritoneal tissues in this region. This also was continuous to the left gutter. Then there was also a new type of foul-smelling fluid collection within the pelvis of at least a liter. All these areas were aspirated laparoscopically, and the abdomen was irrigated with 10 liters of saline with the last 3 liters containing Kantrex solution. A 19 French Blake drain was then placed in the left upper quadrant, under the left lobe of the liver and exiting through the superior port.

We also explored some interloop areas and did not identify any undrained fluid collections. We could not identify every area of interloop bowel for fear of damaging any of the bowel. Therefore after irrigating, all the peritoneal surfaces appeared much cleaner. We placed a 19 French Blake drain deep in the pelvis, coming up the left gutter and out of the port site on the left.

We then removed ports under direct vision and closed the abdominal fascia with a combination of interrupted 0 figure-of-eight and 0 simple Vicryl sutures. The skin was closed with a combination of Dermabond and 4-0 Monocryl.

The patient did have an episode of hypotension near the end of the case, however. He responded with fluids. In addition, the peak pressure at the start of the case was 39 and at the end of the case was down to 23-24. However, because he may have aspirated at the beginning of the case and he had some oxygenation difficulties and this hemodynamic episode, we have elected to keep him intubated and move him to the ICU.

Code all relevant ICD-10-CM diagnosis and ICD-10-PCS procedure codes in accordance with official guidelines and coding conventions.

Diagnosis Codes:

_____

_____

Procedure Codes:

_____

_____

MS-DRG:

_____

_____

Answers and Rationale

Preoperative diagnosis:

Liver[1] and splenic[2] lacerations with hemoperitoneum, internal injuries without open wound

Postoperative diagnosis:

Same and gross peritonitis with early abscess formation[3]

Procedure performed:

Diagnostic laparoscopy and drainage of gross hemoperitonitis and subdiaphragmatic abscess and pelvic abscess

Findings:

2.5 to 3 liters of fluid were aspirated from the peritoneal cavity, including a combination of foul-smelling old blood and bile. Interestingly, no gross purulence was identified.

Indications:

This 26-year-old male patient was in a dirt bike accident in which he struck his abdomen against the handlebars.[6] Subjectively, his abdomen has been tender but not painful. He did not seek medical attention until today, when he became cold, clammy, and lethargic and his abdominal pain increased significantly. Work-up confirmed the above-mentioned injuries, and we proceeded to emergent surgery.

Procedure description:

After informed consent was obtained, the patient was brought to the operating room where the abdomen was prepped and draped in a normal standard fashion. Utilizing an infraumbilical Hasson technique, the peritoneal cavity was accessed. Once we gained access, there was immediate drainage of foul-smelling old blood. There was no obvious purulence. We then suctioned through the umbilical post for 5-10 minutes and were able to remove one liter of this blood.[8] Despite it being foul smelling, we did not identify any fecal or succus entericus.

We then placed the Hasson port in and started to take down the light adhesions. We placed two more 5mm ports in as capable and were able to take fluid collections. The right lower quadrant cecum was adherent to the anterior abdominal wall because of an old appendectomy. At that time we explored the entire abdomen, taking down and draining fluid collections from the right upper quadrant, left upper quadrant, and left gutter as well as left pelvis. The right upper quadrant fluid collections were more of old blood and fibrinous debris. The left upper quadrant next to where the fractured and ischemic liver lay was probably a collection of old bile and blood and because of the foul smell represented an early abscess formation. There was also green exudate throughout all the peritoneal tissues in this region. This also was continuous to the left gutter. Then there was also a new type of foul-smelling fluid collection within the pelvis of at least a liter. All these areas were aspirated laparoscopically,[7] and the abdomen was irrigated with 10 liters of saline[9] with the last 3 liters containing Kantrex solution.[10] A 19 French Blake drain was then placed in the left upper quadrant, under the left lobe of the liver and exiting through the superior port.

We also explored some interloop areas and did not identify any undrained fluid collections. We could not identify every area of interloop bowel for fear of damaging any of the bowel. Therefore after irrigating, all the peritoneal surfaces appeared much cleaner. We placed a 19 French Blake drain deep in the pelvis, coming up the left gutter and out of the port site on the left.

We then removed ports under direct vision and closed the abdominal fascia with a combination of interrupted 0 figure-of-eight and 0 simple Vicryl sutures. The skin was closed with a combination of Dermabond and 4-0 Monocryl.

The patient did have an episode of hypotension near the end of the case, however. He responded with fluids.[4,5] In addition, the peak pressure at the start of the case was 39 and at the end of the case was down to 23-24. However, because he may have aspirated at the beginning of the case and he had some oxygenation difficulties and this hemodynamic episode, we have elected to keep him intubated and move him to the ICU.

Diagnosis Codes

S36.113A	Laceration of liver, unspecified degree, initial encounter[1]
S36.039A	Unspecified laceration of spleen, initial encounter[2]
K65.1	Peritoneal abscess[3]

I97.791	Other intraoperative cardiac functional disturbances during other surgery[4]
I95.89	Other hypotension[5]
V86.59XA	Driver of other special all-terrain or other off-road motor vehicle injured in nontraffic accident, initial encounter[6]

Rationale for Diagnosis Codes

The spleen and liver lacerations caused the hemoperitoneum. The ICD-10-CM index categorizes hemoperitoneum to an unspecified injury of the intra-abdominal organs (S36.899-), which according to the documentation is incorrect as the spleen and liver are injured. Therefore the hemoperitoneum is included in the codes for the lacerations. The peritonitis and pelvic abscess are both included in code K65.1, according to the index. Lastly, the injury requires that an external cause of injury be reported. The documentation specifies that the patient was injured riding a dirt bike, which is listed in the includes note under V86.59-. The physician also mentions an intraoperative drop in the patient's blood pressure, which leads to treating the patient with IV fluids, keeping him on the ventilator, and transferring him to the ICU.

Procedure Codes

ØW9G4ZZ	Drainage of Peritoneal Cavity, Percutaneous Endoscopic Approach[7]
ØW9G3ZZ	Drainage of Peritoneal Cavity, Percutaneous Approach[8]
3E1M38Z	Irrigation of Peritoneal Cavity using Irrigating Substance, Percutaneous Approach[9]
3EØM329	Introduction of Other Anti-infective into Peritoneal Cavity, Percutaneous Approach[10]

Rationale for Procedure Codes

When the abdominal wall is pierced initially (percutaneous approach) to insert the laparoscope, fluid is expelled. Fluid and abscesses are further aspirated (root operation *Drainage* according to the ICD-10-PCS index) once the laparoscope is inserted (percutaneous endoscopic approach). This is followed by peritoneal lavage and then instillation of an antibiotic (only percutaneous approach is offered). All of these are reportable procedures.

MS-DRG

| 420 | Hepatobiliary Diagnostic Procedures with MCC | RW 3.6609 |

While both the spleen and liver lacerations caused the hemoperitoneum, according to the operative report, the abscess and peritonitis were a result of the fractured and ischemic liver. The splenic laceration was not addressed during the surgery. According to ICD-10-CM guideline I.C.19.b, "Coding of Injuries," the code for the most serious injury, as determined by the provider and the focus of treatment, is sequenced first. As the most serious injury, the liver laceration was selected as the principal diagnosis.

OPERATIVE REPORT MDC 7—#4

Preoperative diagnosis:
Malignant ascites with liver lesions on imaging

Postoperative diagnosis:
Confirmed hepatocellular carcinoma

Procedure performed:
Diagnostic laparoscopy and liver biopsy

Indications:
The patient is a 56-year-old male with a long-standing medical history that includes hepatitis C.

Procedure description:
The patient was brought to the operating room and placed in the supine position on the operating table. General anesthesia was induced. The abdomen was prepped and draped in the usual sterile manner. The patient was placed in Trendelenburg position. A 1 cm incision was made just below the umbilicus, and a catheter was inserted to drain the ascites. Approximately 150 ccs were removed. After the fluid was taken off, the abdomen was insufflated and a laparoscope and camera were introduced. The interior of the abdomen was examined. The liver had a pale pink granular appearance to it. There were fine nodules, whitish in appearance. Two biopsy specimens were obtained and sent to pathology. Hemostasis was achieved using electrocautery, and the laparoscope was removed. The skin incisions were closed using 3-0 Vicryl. Steri-strips and gauze were applied. The patient tolerated the procedure well and was taken to the post anesthesia care unit in good condition.

Code all relevant ICD-10-CM diagnosis and ICD-10-PCS procedure codes in accordance with official guidelines and coding conventions.

Diagnosis Codes:

_____

_____

Procedure Codes:

_____

_____

MS-DRG:

_____

_____

Answers and Rationale

Preoperative diagnosis:
Malignant ascites[2] with liver lesions on imaging

Postoperative diagnosis:
Confirmed hepatocellular carcinoma[1]

Procedure performed:
Diagnostic laparoscopy and liver biopsy

Indications:
The patient is a 56-year-old male with a long standing medical history that includes hepatitis C.[3]

Procedure description:
The patient was brought to the operating room and placed in the supine position on the operating table. General anesthesia was induced. The abdomen was prepped and draped in the usual sterile manner. The patient was placed in Trendelenburg position. A 1 cm incision was made just below the umbilicus, and a catheter was inserted to drain the ascites. Approximately 150 ccs were removed.[5] After the fluid was taken off, the abdomen was insufflated and a laparoscope and camera were introduced.[4] The interior of the abdomen was examined. The liver had a pale pink granular appearance to it. There were fine nodules, whitish in appearance. Two biopsy specimens were obtained and sent to pathology.[4] Hemostasis was achieved using electrocautery and the laparoscope was removed. The skin incisions were closed using 3-0 Vicryl. Steri-strips and gauze were applied. The patient tolerated the procedure well and was taken to the post anesthesia care unit in good condition.

Diagnosis Codes

C22.Ø   **Liver cell carcinoma**[1]

R18.Ø   **Malignant ascites**[2]

B18.2   **Chronic viral hepatitis C**[3]

Rationale for Diagnosis Codes
The postoperative diagnosis of confirmed hepatocellular carcinoma does not require that the coder locate "Liver" in the Neoplasm Table, The index terms "Carcinoma, Hepatocellular" refer to the complete code C22.Ø . It should be noted that under category C22 there is an instructional note to report a code for any hepatitis, if applicable, which in this case, is mentioned in the "Indications" section of the dictation. It can be noted that a "Long-term history" of hepatitis is synonymous with the term "chronic" and therefore the code for chronic hepatitis C would be reported. Lastly, the "Preoperative Diagnosis" section mentions the ascites, which is documented as due to the existing malignancy. The ascites is still present, as the first part of the procedure involved a drainage procedure for this condition.

Procedure Codes

ØFBØ4ZX   **Excision of Liver, Percutaneous Endoscopic Approach, Diagnostic**[4]

ØW9G3ZZ   **Drainage of Peritoneal Cavity, Percutaneous Approach**[5]

Rationale for Procedure Codes
The biopsy sites of the liver are not specified but generalized as "liver," which means that a more specific body part value cannot be applied and "Ø" Liver should be reported. The biopsies were performed via laparoscope which interprets to *Percutaneous Endoscopic* approach in ICD-10-CM. The qualifier in this scenario must reflect that the procedure is a biopsy, making the addition of "X" as the seventh character imperative to the correct code assignment. An additional code should be reported for the drainage of the ascites performed at the beginning of the procedure. Ascites is a build-up of fluid in the peritoneal cavity. Therefore, the drainage is of body part *Peritoneal Cavity*, character value G. As the laparoscope was inserted *after* the drainage, this procedure was performed percutaneously, not endoscopically. Also, this was a therapeutic drainage of fluid, not a diagnostic procedure.

MS-DRG

421   **Hepatobiliary Diagnostic Procedures with CC**   **RW 1.7451**

If the ascites is not reported, the MS-DRG changes to lower-weighted 422 Hepatobiliary Diagnostic Procedures without CC/MCC (RW 1.2941).

MDC 8 Diseases and Disorders of the Musculoskeletal System and Connective Tissue

OPERATIVE REPORT MDC 8—#1

Preoperative diagnoses:
L2 vertebral fracture

Postoperative diagnoses:
L2 vertebral fracture

Procedure performed:
Percutaneous vertebroplasty with fluoroscopic guidance

History of presenting illness:
This is a 56-year-old female with severe age-related osteoporosis and a spontaneous L2 vertebral fracture confirmed with x-ray. Having failed conservative management, she was brought to the operating room for percutaneous vertebroplasty.

Procedure description:
The patient was made comfortable in the prone position on padded rolls and was administered intravenous sedation. The lumbar region was prepped and draped in a standard fashion. Utilizing fluoroscopic control, the pedicles of L2 were identified bilaterally. On the left side, a spinal needle was used for determining the correct entry point into the vertebra after the skin had been infiltrated with 2 cc of 1% Xylocaine with Epinephrine. The needle was advanced down to the entry point, and more anesthesia was injected into the periosteal region. Then the cannula was introduced down through the same tract after a stab incision had been made in the skin with an 11 blade. The cannula was advanced into the vertebra with good fluoroscopic guidance in both the AP and lateral planes. In a similar fashion, the cannula on the right side was introduced down into the vertebral body.

The methyl methacrylate was mixed appropriately and injected down into the vertebra with good filling achieved on both the left and right sides. The cannulas were removed and the skin edges were reapproximated with Steri-Strips. The wound was dressed with dry gauze and Op-Site dressing. Counts were correct. Blood loss was negligible and the patient awoke from sedation and was transferred to recovery in stable condition.

Code all relevant ICD-10-CM diagnosis and ICD-10-PCS procedure codes in accordance with official guidelines and coding conventions.

Diagnosis Codes:

_____

_____

Procedure Codes:

_____

_____

MS-DRG:

_____

Answers and Rationale

Preoperative diagnoses:
L2 vertebral fracture

Postoperative diagnoses:
L2 vertebral fracture[1]

Procedure performed:
Percutaneous vertebroplasty[2] with fluoroscopic guidance

History of Presenting Illness:
This is a 56-year-old female who suffers from severe age-related osteoporosis and had a spontaneous L2 vertebral fracture[1] confirmed with x-ray. Having failed conservative management, she was brought to the operating room for percutaneous vertebroplasty.

Procedure description:
The patient was made comfortable in the prone position on padded rolls and was administered intravenous sedation. The lumbar region was prepped and draped in a standard fashion. Utilizing fluoroscopic control, the pedicles of L2 were identified bilaterally. On the left side, a spinal needle was used for determining the correct entry point into the vertebra after the skin had been infiltrated with 2 cc of 1% Xylocaine with Epinephrine. The needle was advanced down to the entry point, and more anesthesia was injected into the periosteal region. Then the cannula was introduced down through the same tract after a stab incision had been made in the skin with an 11 blade. The cannula was advanced into the vertebra with good fluoroscopic guidance[2] in both the AP and lateral planes. In a similar fashion, the cannula on the right side was introduced down into the vertebral body.

The methyl methacrylate was mixed appropriately and injected down into the vertebra with good filling achieved on both the left and right sides. [2] The cannulas were removed and the skin edges were reapproximated with Steri-Strips. The wound was dressed with dry gauze and Op-Site dressing. Counts were correct. Blood loss was negligible and the patient awoke from sedation and was transferred to recovery in stable condition.

Diagnosis Codes

M80.08XA   Age-related osteoporosis with current pathological fracture, vertebra(e), initial encounter for fracture[1]

Rationale for Diagnosis Codes
ICD-10-CM Official Guidelines for Coding and Reporting section I.C.13.d.2 dictates that if the patient has osteoporosis and suffers a spontaneous fracture or one due to a minor trauma, the fracture is assumed to be pathological in nature and a code from subcategory M80 should be reported rather than a traumatic fracture code. The seventh character of A for initial encounter is still applicable, even though the patient has been undergoing conservative treatment, because she is receiving active treatment for her condition. This is true regardless of whether the vertebroplasty was performed by a new physician or the same physician who treated her conservatively.

Procedure Codes

0QU03JZ   Supplement Lumbar Vertebra with Synthetic Substitute, Percutaneous Approach[2]

Rationale for Procedure Codes
The objective of the vertebroplasty is to reinforce the patient's vertebra(e) that have been damaged, in this case by injecting methyl methacrylate. This objective coincides with the root operation *Supplement* per ICD-10-PCS standards. The substance injected is a synthetic bone substitute. Lastly, the procedure is performed percutaneously as there is no incision, only a puncture and placement verified by fluoroscopy.

MS-DRG

517   Other Musculoskeletal System and Connective Tissue O.R.   RW 1.7716 Procedure without CC/MCC

CODING AXIOM

ICD-10-CM Official Guidelines for Coding and Reporting Section I.C.13.d.2:

A code from category M80, not a traumatic fracture code, should be used for any patient with known osteoporosis who suffers a fracture, even if the patient had a minor fall or trauma, if that fall or trauma would not usually break a normal, healthy bone.

CODING AXIOM

ICD-10-CM Official Guidelines for Coding and Reporting Section I.C.13.c:

7th character A is for use as long as the patient is receiving active treatment for the fracture. Examples of active treatment are: surgical treatment, emergency department encounter, evaluation and continuing treatment by the same or a different physician. While the patient may be seen by a new or different provider over the course of treatment for a pathological fracture, assignment of the 7th character is based on whether the patient is undergoing active treatment and not whether the provider is seeing the patient for the first time.

DEFINITIONS

comminuted. Fracture type in which the bone is splintered or crushed.

OPERATIVE REPORT MDC 8—#2

Preoperative diagnoses:
Gunshot wound to right lateral upper leg

Postoperative diagnoses:
GSW with open fracture of right femoral lateral condyle and patella

Procedures:
Extension, exploration, and debridement of gunshot wound, removal of bullet and bone fragments, ORIF femoral condyle fracture, internal fixation of the patellar fracture

Indication:
The patient is a 27-year-old male who was shot in the right upper lateral leg while cleaning his handgun at home. Review of x-rays revealed a foreign body and possible bone fragments of the knee. The patient also has a comminuted fracture of the right lateral femoral condyle. Plan to explore and debride the bullet track and remove the bullet and fragments in surgery. The fractures will be repaired and stabilized.

Procedure description:
Under general anesthesia a tourniquet was placed on the right upper thigh and the leg was exsanguinated with an Esmarch bandage. The right leg was prepped and draped in sterile fashion. The trajectory of the bullet was determined, and the wound was enlarged and extended. Debridement of particulate matter was completed and exploration of muscles, nerves, tendons, and vessels was completed. Hemostasis was obtained with Bovie cauterization. The wound was extended to visualize the fracture site. The bullet did not enter the joint capsule and it was intact. The bullet was removed and labeled. The lateral knee was explored and bone fragments were debrided. Kirschner wire was passed through the patella and fragment. A large fragment of the lateral femoral condyle was brought back into place and secured with two 3.5 mm lag screws. Follow-up x-rays confirmed placement. The tourniquet was deflated. The wound was irrigated with antibiotic solution. A drain was inserted. The incision was closed using 2-0 Vicryl and the skin was closed with 4-0 nylon suture. A sterile dressing of Xeroform, 4x4s, and sterile Webril with elastic bandage was applied. A knee immobilizer was placed. The patient was transferred to the recovery room in stable condition.

Code all relevant ICD-10-CM diagnosis and ICD-10-PCS procedure codes in accordance with official guidelines and coding conventions.

Diagnosis Codes:

_____

_____

Procedure Codes:

_____

_____

MS-DRG:

_____

_____

Answers and Rationale

Preoperative diagnoses:

Gunshot wound to right lateral upper leg

Postoperative diagnoses:

GSW[3] with open fractures of right femoral lateral condyle[2] and patella[1]

Procedures:

Extension, exploration, and debridement of gunshot wound,[7] removal of bullet and bone fragments,[8] ORIF femoral condyle fracture,[5] internal fixation of the patellar fracture[6]

Indication:

The patient is a 27-year-old male who was shot in the right upper lateral leg while cleaning his handgun at home.[3,4] Review of x-rays revealed a foreign body and possible bone fragments of the knee. The patient also has a comminuted fracture of the right lateral femoral condyle. Plan to explore and debride the bullet track and remove the bullet and fragments in surgery. The fractures will be repaired and stabilized.

Procedure description:

Under general anesthesia a tourniquet was placed on the right upper thigh and the leg was exsanguinated with an Esmarch bandage. The right leg was prepped and draped in sterile fashion. The trajectory of the bullet was determined, and the wound was enlarged and extended. Debridement of particulate matter was completed[7] and exploration of muscles, nerves, tendons, and vessels was completed. Hemostasis was obtained with Bovie cauterization. The wound was extended to visualize the fracture site. The bullet did not enter the joint capsule and it was intact. The bullet was removed and labeled.[8] The lateral knee was explored and bone fragments were debrided. [8] Kirschner wire was passed through the patella and fragment. [6] A large fragment of the lateral femoral condyle was brought back into place and secured with two 3.5 mm lag screws. [5] Follow-up x-rays confirmed placement. The tourniquet was deflated. The wound was irrigated with antibiotic solution. A drain was inserted. The incision was closed using 2-0 Vicryl and the skin was closed with 4-0 nylon suture. A sterile dressing of Xeroform, 4x4s, and sterile Webril with elastic bandage was applied. A knee immobilizer was placed. The patient was transferred to the recovery room in stable condition.

Diagnosis Codes

S72.421C **Displaced fracture of lateral condyle of right femur, initial encounter for open fracture type IIIA, IIIB, or IIIC[2]**

S82.001C **Unspecified fracture of right patella, initial encounter for open fracture type IIIA, IIIB, or IIIC[1]**

W34.00XA **Accidental discharge from unspecified firearms or gun, initial encounter[3]**

Y92.00 **Unspecified non-institutional (private) residence as the place of occurrence of the external cause[4]**

Rationale for Diagnosis Codes

In the "Indications" section, the femur fracture is specified as a comminuted fracture of the lateral condyle, making the appropriate code selection S72.42- as the location of the fracture does not include a specified type (comminuted) in ICD-10-CM. Conventions of ICD-10 state that if a fracture is not specified as nondisplaced, displaced is the default. The fractures are specified as open. They are considered type III, according to the Gustilo classification, because the wound has significant soft tissue injury. The fractures are sequenced based on guidelines section II.B.

Procedure Codes

0QSB04Z **Reposition Right Lower Femur with Internal Fixation Device, Open Approach[5]**

0QHD04Z **Insertion of Internal Fixation Device into Right Patella, Open Approach[6]**

0JCL0ZZ **Extirpation of Matter from Right Upper Leg Subcutaneous Tissue and Fascia, Open Approach[7]**

0QCB0ZZ **Extirpation of Matter from Right Lower Femur, Open Approach[8]**

 KEY POINT

Types of open fractures (Gustilo classification):

- Type I: The wound is less than 1 cm in length and clean.
- Type II: The wound is greater than 1 cm in length, clean, and there is minimal to no soft tissue injury.
- Type III: The wound is greater than 1 cm in length, and there is significant soft tissue injury. Type III fractures can be further classified as:
  - IIIA: There is enough local soft tissue to cover the wound and bone without the need for skin grafting.
  - IIIB: The injury to the soft tissue is significant enough that skin grafting is necessary to cover the bone
  - IIIC: The injury is associated with an arterial injury that requires repair

CODING AXIOM

ICD-10-PCS Official Guidelines for Coding and Reporting Section B3.15:

Reduction of a displaced fracture is coded to the root operation Reposition and the application of a cast or splint in conjunction with the Reposition procedure is not coded separately. Treatment of a nondisplaced fracture is coded to the procedure performed.

Rationale for Procedure Codes

Both of the fractures are treated with internal fixation, although only the femur fracture is noted to have been reduced. Therefore the fixation of the femur fracture is considered a reposition (with a device character of 4 to represent the internal fixation), and the patella treatment coincides with the root operation *Insertion* according to *ICD-10-PCS Official Guidelines for Coding and Reporting* section B3.15.

The knee exploration, removal of the bullet at the fracture site (foreign body), and debridement performed to remove the particulate matter are separately reportable per guideline B3.2.c, which states that "multiple procedures are coded if multiple root operations with distinct objectives are performed on the same body part." Although the soft tissue is not the exact body part, the debridement was performed to accomplish an objective other than approach the operative site. While it is described as a "debridement," this is reported with root operation *Extirpation* as the bullet, particulate matter, and right femoral condyle comminuted fracture bone fragments were loose within the wound tract.

MS-DRG:

481	Hip and Femur Procedures Except Major Joint with CC	RW 1.9790

According to guideline I. C.19.c.2, the principles of multiple coding of injuries should be followed in coding fractures. The guideline I. C.19.b states that the code for the most serious injury, as determined by the provider and the focus of treatment, is sequenced first. Guideline I. C.19.c.2 states that multiple fractures are sequenced in accordance with the severity of the fracture. The fracture of the lateral condyle of the femur was comminuted and required reduction and fixation and is thus both the most serious injury and the more severe fracture and should be assigned as the principal diagnosis. The patellar fracture acts as the CC.

If the patella was documented as the more severe fracture and sequenced as the principal diagnosis, the MS-DRG would change to higher-weighted MS-DRG 480 Hip and Femur Procedures Except Major Joint with MCC (the femur fracture acts as the MCC). The CC and MCC status of the femur and patella fractures is another indication of the difference in severity of the fractures.

If the debridement procedures were incorrectly coded as excisional, this would inappropriately group to either higher-weighted MS-DRG 464 Wound Debridement and Skin Graft Except Hand, for Musculo-Connective Tissue Disorders with CC (RW 3.0937), with femur fracture as the principal diagnosis, or MS-DRG 463 Wound Debridement and Skin Graft Except Hand, for Musculo-Connective Tissue Disorders with MCC (RW 5.1028), with patella fracture as the principal diagnosis.

OPERATIVE REPORT MDC 8—#3

Preoperative diagnoses:
Degenerative lumbar intravertebral disc disease

Postoperative diagnoses:
Degenerative lumbar intravertebral disc disease

Procedures:
Intradiscal electrothermal annuloplasty under fluoroscopic guidance

Indication:
Patient is a 55-year-old male with chronic back pain from years of construction work. MRI revealed degenerative disc disease at L4-L5 at the right posterior aspect. Preoperative discogram testing reproduced the patient's pain, and it was determined that intradiscal electrothermal annuloplasty would help to relieve his chronic pain.

Procedure description:
The patient was brought into the operating suite. After IV sedation by the anesthesiologist, the patient was placed face down and appropriately padded for the procedure. The lumbar back was prepped and draped for the procedure.

Under fluoroscopic guidance a catheter was inserted into the L4-L5 disc area on the right posterior aspect. The location of the catheter tip was verified and the electrothermal probe placed along the posterior portion of the disc. The probe was heated to 90 degrees Celsius and maintained for 17 minutes. After the probe cooled significantly, the electrothermal catheter was removed. The disc was injected with antibiotic and local anesthetic, and the catheter was removed.

The area is cleansed and a sterile dressing applied. The patient is placed in a low back brace, and follow-up instructions were given.

Code all relevant ICD-10-CM diagnosis and ICD-10-PCS procedure codes in accordance with official guidelines and coding conventions.

Diagnosis Codes:

_____

_____

Procedure Codes:

_____

_____

MS-DRG:

_____

_____

Answers and Rationale

Preoperative diagnoses:
Degenerative lumbar intravertebral disc disease[1,2]

Postoperative diagnoses:
Degenerative lumbar intravertebral disc disease[1,2]

Procedures:
Intradiscal electrothermal annuloplasty[2] under fluoroscopic guidance

Indication:
Patient is a 55-year-old male with chronic back pain from years of construction work. MRI revealed degenerative disc disease at L4-L5[1] at the right posterior aspect. Preoperative discogram testing reproduced the patient's pain, and it was determined that intradiscal electrothermal annuloplasty would help to relieve his chronic pain.

Procedure description:
The patient was brought into the operating suite. After IV sedation by the anesthesiologist, the patient was placed face down and appropriately padded for the procedure. The lumbar back was prepped and draped for the procedure.

Under fluoroscopic guidance a catheter was inserted into the L4-L5 disc area[2] on the right posterior aspect. The location of the catheter tip was verified and the electrothermal probe placed along the posterior portion of the disc. The probe was heated to 90 degrees Celsius and maintained for 17 minutes.[2] After the probe cooled significantly, the electrothermal catheter was removed. The disc was injected with antibiotic[4] and local anesthetic,[3] and the catheter was removed.

The area was cleansed and a sterile dressing applied. The patient was placed in a low back brace, and follow-up instructions were given.

Diagnosis Codes

M51.36   **Other intervertebral disc degeneration, lumbar region**[1]

Rationale for Diagnosis Codes
The terms "Degeneration, Intravertebral disc, Lumbar" in the index direct the coder to M51.36. The chronic back pain is not reported separately based on guidelines section I.C.6.b.1, which states that "a code from category G89 should not be assigned if the underlying (definitive) diagnosis is known, unless the reason for the encounter is pain control/ management and not management of the underlying condition."

Procedure Codes

0S523ZZ   **Destruction of Lumbar Vertebral Disc, Percutaneous Approach**[2]

3E0U3BZ   **Introduction of Local Anesthetic into Joints, Percutaneous Approach**[3]

3E0U329   **Introduction of Other Anti-infective into Joints, Percutaneous Approach**[4]

Rationale for Procedure Codes
Intradiscal electrothermal annuloplasty destroys part or all of the intravertebral disc, making the correct root operation *Destruction*. Both of the injections should also be reported since injecting the disc/disc space or intravertebral joint is invasive. Because the physician performs all of the procedures via a catheter under fluoroscopic guidance, the approach is considered *Percutaneous*.

MS-DRG

520	Back and Neck Procedures Except Spinal Fusion without CC/MCC	RW 1.1812

📖 **DEFINITIONS**

destruction. ICD-10-PCS root operation value 5. Physical eradication of all or a portion of a body part by the direct use of energy, force, or a destructive agent. None of the body part is physically taken out.

OPERATIVE REPORT MDC 8—#4

Preoperative diagnosis:
Torn lateral meniscus of the left knee

Postoperative diagnosis:
Torn lateral meniscus of the left knee and chondromalacia

Procedure description:
Arthroscopy, left knee, with meniscectomy and debridement of the articular flap medial femoral condyle

Indications:
A 68-year-old male patient complains of increasing pain to the left knee and was found to have a current torn lateral meniscus of the left knee.

Procedure performed:
The patient was placed supine on the operating room table. After general anesthesia was administered, the left lower extremity was prepped and draped in the usual sterile manner for arthroscopic surgery. The knee was arthroscoped through the standard medial and lateral portals, and the entire knee joint was evaluated. He was found to have chondromalacia of the medial femoral condyle, extensive tear of the lateral meniscus, and mild degenerative changes of the lateral compartment.

Using a combination of manual and power instrumentation, a lateral meniscectomy was performed. This was followed by removal of the unstable flap of cartilage of the medial femoral condyle. Next, an arthroscopic shaver and Stryker electrocautery at a very low setting were used to perform a chondroplasty and debridement of the articular cartilage in the involved areas of the medial femoral condyle.

After copious irrigation, all fragmented tissue was removed. The arthroscope was then removed. The skin portals were closed with a single 4-0 nylon stitch. The knee was injected with 20 cc of Marcaine and 1 cc of Kenalog 40. The patient was taken to the recovery room in stable condition. There were no complications. All sponge and instrument counts were correct.

Code all relevant ICD-10-CM diagnosis and ICD-10-PCS procedure codes in accordance with official guidelines and coding conventions.

Diagnosis Codes:

_____

_____

Procedure Codes:

_____

_____

MS-DRG:

_____

_____

Answers and Rationale

Preoperative diagnosis:
Torn lateral meniscus of the left knee

Postoperative diagnosis:
Torn lateral meniscus[1] of the left[1-4] knee and chondromalacia[2]

Procedure description:
Arthroscopy, left knee, with meniscectomy and debridement of the articular flap medial femoral condyle

Indications:
A 68-year-old male patient complains of increasing pain to the left knee and was found to have a current torn lateral meniscus of the left knee.

Procedure performed:
The patient was placed supine on the operating room table. After general anesthesia was administered, the left lower extremity was prepped and draped in the usual sterile manner for arthroscopic surgery. The knee was arthroscoped[3,4] through the standard medial and lateral portals, and the entire knee joint was evaluated. He was found to have chondromalacia of the medial femoral condyle, extensive tear of the lateral meniscus, and mild degenerative changes of the lateral compartment.

Using a combination of manual and power instrumentation, a lateral meniscectomy was performed.[3] This was followed by removal of the unstable flap of cartilage of the medial femoral condyle. Next, an arthroscopic shaver and Stryker electrocautery at a very low setting were used to perform a chondroplasty and debridement of the articular cartilage in the involved areas of the medial femoral condyle. [4]

After copious irrigation, all fragmented tissue was removed. The arthroscope was then removed. The skin portals were closed with a single 4-0 nylon stitch. The knee was injected with 20 cc of Marcaine and 1 cc of Kenalog 40. The patient was taken to the recovery room in stable condition. There were no complications. All sponge and instrument counts were correct.

Diagnosis Codes
S83.282A **Other tear of lateral meniscus, current injury, left knee, initial encounter[1]**

M94.262 **Chondromalacia, left knee[2]**

Rationale for Diagnosis Codes
The seventh character of "A" appended to S83.282 is appropriate because active treatment (i.e. surgical treatment) is considered an initial encounter.

Procedure Codes
0SBD4ZZ **Excision of Left Knee Joint, Percutaneous Endoscopic Approach[3]**

0SBD4ZZ **Excision of Left Knee Joint, Percutaneous Endoscopic Approach[4]**

Rationale for Procedure Codes
The easiest way to locate the appropriate root operation for a meniscectomy is to consult the ICD-10-PCS index, which refers the coder to the root operation of *Excision* or *Resection* of the lower joint. Because the entire joint is not being removed, *Excision* is the correct option for this procedure. The same procedure code is reported a second time for the chondroplasty or shaving/debridement of the articular cartilage flap. According to ICD-10-PCS guidelines, the same procedure can be reported more than once if the same root operation is performed on body parts represented by the same character.

MS-DRG
489 **Knee Procedures without Principal Diagnosis of Infection without CC/MCC** **RW 1.2991**

CODING AXIOM

ICD-10-CM Official Guidelines for Coding and Reporting Section I.C.19.a:

7th character "A," initial encounter is used while the patient is receiving active treatment for the condition. Examples of active treatment are: surgical treatment, emergency department encounter, and evaluation and continuing treatment by the same or a different physician.

CODING AXIOM

ICD-10-PCS Official Guidelines for Coding and Reporting Section B3.2.b:

During the same operative episode, multiple procedures are coded if: The same root operation is repeated in multiple body parts, and those body parts are separate and distinct body parts classified to a single ICD-10-PCS body part value.

OPERATIVE REPORT MDC 8—#5

Preoperative diagnosis:
Posttraumatic osteoarthropathy

Postoperative diagnosis:
Posttraumatic osteoarthropathy

Procedure performed:
Total hip arthroplasty

Indications:
This is a 67-year-old male who sustained a fracture of the right hip five years ago and subsequently developed osteoarthritis at the site. The patient presents for a total hip arthroplasty using a ceramic-on-ceramic prosthetic hip implant.

Procedure description:
After adequate anesthesia was achieved, the patient was prepped and draped in the usual sterile fashion. The patient was placed in a lateral decubitus position, an incision was made along the posterior aspect of the hip. The fascia lata was incised and the muscles around the hip joint were retracted to visualize the capsule. The capsule was incised, and the hip dislocated posteriorly. The femoral head and many osteophytes around the rim of the acetabulum were removed with an osteotome. The acetabulum was reamed out with a power reamer, exposing both subchondral and cancellous bone, and the acetabular component was inserted. The femoral canal was prepared using the power reamer. The stem was secured into the femoral shaft using bone cement. The femoral stem prosthesis was repositioned. The external rotator muscles were reattached. The hip was repositioned, and the external rotator muscles were reattached. The incision was repaired in layers with suction drains. The patient tolerated the procedure well and was transported to the recovery room in stable condition.

Code all relevant ICD-10-CM diagnosis and ICD-10-PCS procedure codes in accordance with official guidelines and coding conventions.

Diagnosis Codes:
_____

_____

Procedure Codes:
_____

_____

MS-DRG:
_____

_____

Answers and Rationale

Preoperative diagnosis:
Posttraumatic osteoarthropathy

Postoperative diagnosis:
Posttraumatic osteoarthropathy[1]

Procedure performed:
Total hip arthroplasty

Indications:
This is a 67-year-old male who sustained a fracture of the right hip five years ago and subsequently developed osteoarthritis at the site.[2] The patient presents for a total hip arthroplasty using a ceramic-on-ceramic prosthetic hip implant.[3]

Procedure description:
After adequate anesthesia was achieved, the patient was prepped and draped in the usual sterile fashion. The patient was placed in a lateral decubitus position, an incision was made along the posterior aspect of the hip. The fascia lata was incised and the muscles around the hip joint were retracted to visualize the capsule. The capsule was incised, and the hip dislocated posteriorly. The femoral head and many osteophytes around the rim of the acetabulum were removed with an osteotome. The acetabulum was reamed out with a power reamer,[3] exposing both subchondral and cancellous bone, and the acetabular component was inserted.[3] The femoral canal was prepared using the power reamer. The stem was secured into the femoral shaft using bone cement. The femoral stem prosthesis was repositioned.[3] The external rotator muscles were reattached. The hip was repositioned, and the external rotator muscles were reattached. The incision was repaired in layers with suction drains. The patient tolerated the procedure well and was transported to the recovery room in stable condition.

Diagnosis Codes

M16.51   **Unilateral post-traumatic osteoarthritis, right hip**[1]

S72.001S   **Fracture of unspecified part of neck of right femur, sequela**[2]

Rationale for Diagnosis Codes

"Osteoarthritis, Posttraumatic, Hip" in the ICD-10-CM index lists M16.5-. The documentation notes that the osteoarthritis was caused by a previous fracture, or is "sequela" of a hip fracture. Therefore, the code for the hip fracture, not otherwise specified, should be reported with a seventh character of "S" denoting that the osteoarthritis is a sequela of the fracture.

Procedure Codes

ØSR9Ø39   **Replacement of Right Hip Joint with Synthetic Substitute, Ceramic, Open Approach, Cemented**[3]

Rationale for Procedure Codes

Because the entire hip surface, both the acetabular and femoral, are replaced using ceramic prostheses, the root operation is *Replacement* and the body part is *Right Hip Joint*. The sixth character represents the device used—in this instance, the ceramic prosthesis. As the femoral end of the prosthetic was secured in place using a bone cement, the seventh character is qualifier "9," representing *Cemented*.

MS-DRG

470	Major Joint Replacement or Reattachment of Lower Extremity without MCC	RW 2.0816

OPERATIVE REPORT MDC 8—#6

Preoperative diagnosis:
Advanced degenerative changes at L3–4, L4–5

Postoperative diagnosis:
Advanced degenerative changes at L3–4, L4–5

Procedure performed:

1. Anterior lumbar discectomy with fusion, L3–4, L4–5 with bone grafting and Pro Osteen blocks

2. Placement of intervertebral interbody fusion device, that being a 14-mm, 12-degree Solitaire PEEK cage

3. Placement of intervertebral interbody fusion device, that being a 16-mm, 12-degree Solitaire PEEK cage

4. Segmental fixation, L3–L5, via screws passed through the cage into the vertebral bodies above and below L3–4, L4–5

Procedure description:
Through a left vertical paramedian retroperitoneal approach, the L3–4 and L4–5 disc spaces were approached, needles placed, and C-arm used for position confirmation. Starting at the L4–5 level, the disc was excised in toto with knife, grabbers, periosteal elevators, and curettes. Interspaces were then incised with the smooth Solitaire sizer and found to receive a 16-mm, 12-degree cage. The appropriate size rasp was used to prepare the endplates.

A 16 mm, 12 degree Solitaire cage intervertebral body fusion device was filled with Pro Osteon bone block and coated with autologous growth factor. The cage was impacted into the L4–5 disc space under C-arm control. Segmental fixation was then accomplished by placing two screws through the cage into the L4 vertebral body and one screw through the cage into the L5 vertebral body.

Attention was then directed to the L3–L4 level. The disc was excised in toto in a similar fashion followed by sizing with smooth sizers, and found to receive a 14 mm, 12 degree cage. An appropriate size rasp was used to prepare the endplate, and then a 14 mm, 12 degree Solitaire PEEK case was filled with Pro Osteon bone block, coated with autologous growth factor, and impacted into the L3–4 disc space under lateral C-arm control. Segmental fixation was accomplished by placing two screws through the cage into the L3 vertebral body and one screw through the cages into the L4 vertebral body. A morselized bone bank bone graft was placed anterior to the cage and coated with autologous growth factor.

Code all relevant ICD-10-CM diagnosis and ICD-10-PCS procedure codes in accordance with official guidelines and coding conventions.

Diagnosis Codes:

_____

_____

Procedure Codes:

_____

_____

MS-DRG:

_____

_____

CODING AXIOM

ICD-10-PCS Official Guidelines for Coding and Reporting

Fusion procedures of the spine

Section B3.10a:
The body part coded for a spinal vertebral joint(s) rendered immobile by a spinal fusion procedure is classified by the level of the spine (e.g. thoracic). There are distinct body part values for a single vertebral joint and for multiple vertebral joints at each spinal level.

Example: Body part values specify Lumbar Vertebral Joint, Lumbar Vertebral Joints, 2 or More, and Lumbosacral Vertebral Joint.

Section B3.10b:
If multiple vertebral joints are fused, a separate procedure is coded for each vertebral joint that uses a different device and/or qualifier.

Example: Fusion of lumbar vertebral joint, posterior approach, anterior column and fusion of lumbar vertebral joint, posterior approach, posterior column are coded separately.

Section B3.10c:
Combinations of devices and materials are often used on a vertebral joint to render the joint immobile. When combinations of devices are used on the same vertebral joint, the device value coded for the procedure is as follows:

- If an interbody fusion device is used to render the joint immobile (alone or containing other material like bone graft), the procedure is coded with the device value Interbody Fusion Device
- If bone graft is the only device used to render the joint immobile, the procedure is coded with the device value Nonautologous Tissue Substitute or Autologous Tissue Substitute
- If a mixture of autologous and nonautologous bone graft (with or without biological or synthetic extenders or binders) is used to render the joint immobile, code the procedure with the device value Autologous Tissue Substitute

Examples: Fusion of a vertebral joint using a cage style interbody fusion device containing morselized bone graft is coded to the device Interbody Fusion Device.

Fusion of a vertebral joint using a bone dowel interbody fusion device made of cadaver bone and packed with a mixture of local morselized bone and demineralized bone matrix is coded to the device Interbody Fusion Device.

Answers and Rationale

Preoperative diagnosis:
Advanced degenerative changes at L3–4, L4–5

Postoperative diagnosis:
Advanced degenerative changes at L3–4, L4–5[1]

Procedure performed:

1. Anterior lumbar discectomy with fusion,[3] L3–4, L4–5 with bone grafting and Pro Osteen blocks[2]

2. Placement of intervertebral interbody fusion device, that being a 14-mm, 12-degree Solitaire PEEK cage[2]

3. Placement of intervertebral interbody fusion device, that being a 16-mm, 12-degree Solitaire PEEK cage[2]

4. Segmental fixation, L3–L5, via screws passed through the cage into the vertebral bodies above and below L3–4, L4–5

Procedure description:
Through a left vertical paramedian retroperitoneal approach,[2] the L3–4 and L4–5 disc spaces were approached, needles placed, and C-arm used for position confirmation. Starting at the L4–5 level, the disc was excised in toto with knife, grabbers, periosteal elevators, and curettes.[3] Interspaces were then incised with the smooth Solitaire sizer and found to receive a 16-mm, 12-degree cage. The appropriate size rasp was used to prepare the endplates.

A 16 mm, 12 degree Solitaire cage intervertebral body fusion device was filled with Pro Osteon bone block and coated with autologous growth factor. The cage was impacted into the L4–5 disc space under C-arm control.[2] Segmental fixation was then accomplished by placing two screws through the cage into the L4 vertebral body and one screw through the cage into the L5 vertebral body.

Attention was then directed to the L3–L4 level. The disc was excised in toto in a similar fashion,[3] followed by sizing with smooth sizers, and found to receive a 14 mm, 12 degree cage. An appropriate size rasp was used to prepare the endplate, and then a 14 mm, 12 degree Solitaire PEEK case was filled with Pro Osteon bone block, coated with autologous growth factor, and impacted into the L3–4 disc space under lateral C-arm control.[2]

Segmental fixation was accomplished by placing two screws through the cage into the L3 vertebral body and one screw through the cages into the L4 vertebral body. A morselized bone bank bone graft was placed anterior to the cage and coated with autologous growth factor.

Diagnosis Codes

M47.816   Spondylosis without myelopathy or radiculopathy, lumbar region[1]

Rationale for Diagnosis Codes
The terms "Degenerative, Changes, Spine or Vertebra" directs the coder to the term "Spondylosis," which lists M47.816. Although the code appears complete, the ICD-10-CM coding guidelines section I.B.1 indicates that the tabular must also be consulted to ensure a seventh character is not required.

Procedure Codes

0SG1030   Fusion of 2 or more Lumbar Vertebral Joints with Interbody Fusion Device, Anterior Approach, Anterior Column, Open Approach[2]

0ST20ZZ   Resection of Lumbar Vertebral Disc, Open Approach[3]

Rationale for Procedure Codes
The ICD-10-PCS guidelines have a section dedicated to spinal fusions. These guidelines note that if the same device and the same approach are used on multiple vertebral joints in a single level (i.e., cervical, thoracic, lumbar) only one code is used. The guidelines further go on to state that if an interbody device (such as a PEEK cage) is used, whether or not bone is grafted, the appropriate device character is 3, *Interbody Fusion Device.*

It should be noted that if the same device is inserted via a different approach, two codes would be needed and would be differentiated by the seventh character value. The surgeon documented that the discs at L3-L4 and L4-L5 were removed "in toto." Therefore, the discectomy is coded as a resection. This is consistent with advice given in the *AHA Coding Clinic for ICD-10-CM and ICD-10-PCS*, second quarter 2014, pages 6–7.

MS-DRG

| 460 | Spinal Fusion Except Cervical without MCC | RW 3.9717 |

OPERATIVE REPORT MDC 8—#7

Preoperative diagnosis:
Subtalar joint degenerative joint disease

Postoperative diagnosis:
Same

Procedure performed:
Subtalar joint fusion with external fixation device

Procedure description:
The patient was brought in the operating room and placed in a supine position. General anesthesia was administered. Once adequate levels of anesthesia had been obtained, a time-out was called with the patient identification and the proposed procedure being agreed upon by the surgical team and operating room staff. The left foot was prepped and draped in the normal sterile fashion to include a pneumatic tourniquet placed about the left ankle.

Attention was directed to the lateral sinus tarsi region, where a 10 cm linear-type incision was made and deepened using blunt dissection. Bleeders were cauterized as necessary, and neurovascular structures were retracted medially and laterally as necessary. Dissection was carried out using blunt and sharp technique, revealing the subtalar joint. The capsule was incised, exposing the posterior and middle facets. Using an osteotome and mallet, the cartilage and subchondral plate was removed adequately to allow for eversion of the calcaneus, once fusion of the talus and calcaneus was achieved. The joint surfaces were prepared using a smaller osteotome for a shingling effect.

At this time, Trinity demineralized bone matrix was introduced into the joint space. An ICOS screw was introduced percutaneously through the dorsal aspect of the talar neck. This was placed through the neck and into the posterior aspect of the calcaneus. Under fluoroscopic guidance, it was noted that adequate compression of the subtalar joint was achieved. A MiniRail was then placed across the subtalar joint. Two pins were placed in the calcaneus, and two pins were placed in the body of the talus. Using the MiniRail compression system, it was noted that the joint was further reduced. Incision was closed deeply, taking care to reattach the capsular structures, followed by reapproximation of the peroneal tendon sheaths, using Vicryl suture. Subcutaneous tissues were reapproximated using simple interrupted Vicryl suturing. The skin was closed using a running locking Prolene suture. At this time, the surgical site was dressed with Xeroform, 4x4 gauze, Kling, Coban, and an Ace wrap.

The patient was taken to the postoperative care unit where vital signs were stable and intact. It was noted that neurovascular status of the left foot remained intact. Patient was discharged to home once he emerged successfully, without incident, from general anesthesia.

Code all relevant ICD-10-CM diagnosis and ICD-10-PCS procedure codes in accordance with official guidelines and coding conventions.

Diagnosis Codes:

_____

_____

Procedure Codes:

_____

_____

MS-DRG:

_____

_____

Answers and Rationale

Preoperative diagnosis:
Subtalar joint degenerative joint disease[1]

Postoperative diagnosis:
Same

Procedure performed:
Subtalar joint fusion with external fixation device[2]

Procedure description:
The patient was brought in the operating room and placed in a supine position. General anesthesia was administered. Once adequate levels of anesthesia had been obtained, a time-out was called with the patient identification and the proposed procedure being agreed upon by the surgical team and operating room staff. The left foot[1,2] was prepped and draped in the normal sterile fashion to include a pneumatic tourniquet placed about the left ankle.

Attention was directed to the lateral sinus tarsi region, where a 10 cm linear-type incision was made and deepened using blunt dissection. Bleeders were cauterized as necessary, and neurovascular structures were retracted medially and laterally as necessary. Dissection was carried out using blunt and sharp technique, revealing the subtalar joint.[2] The capsule was incised, exposing the posterior and middle facets. Using an osteotome and mallet, the cartilage and subchondral plate was removed adequately to allow for eversion of the calcaneus, once fusion of the talus and calcaneus was achieved. The joint surfaces were prepared using a smaller osteotome for a shingling effect.

At this time, Trinity demineralized bone matrix was introduced into the joint space. An ICOS screw was introduced percutaneously through the dorsal aspect of the talar neck. This was placed through the neck and into the posterior aspect of the calcaneus. Under fluoroscopic guidance, it was noted that adequate compression of the subtalar joint was achieved. A MiniRail was then placed across the subtalar joint.[2] Two pins were placed in the calcaneus, and two pins were placed in the body of the talus. Using the MiniRail compression system, it was noted that the joint was further reduced. Incision was closed deeply, taking care to reattach the capsular structures, followed by reapproximation of the peroneal tendon sheaths, using Vicryl suture. Subcutaneous tissues were reapproximated using simple interrupted Vicryl suturing. The skin was closed using a running locking Prolene suture. At this time, the surgical site was dressed with Xeroform, 4x4 gauze, Kling, Coban, and an Ace wrap.

The patient was taken to the postoperative care unit where vital signs were stable and intact. It was noted that neurovascular status of the left foot remained intact. Patient was discharged to home once he emerged successfully, without incident, from general anesthesia.

Diagnosis Codes

M19.072   Primary osteoarthritis, left ankle and foot[1]

Rationale for Diagnosis Codes

The terms "Degenerative, joint disease" in the index refer the coder to "Osteoarthritis," which is divided by primary and secondary, then by anatomical site. The documentation does not specify primary or secondary so the default is primary. The subtalar joint is in the foot.

Procedure Codes

0SGJ05Z   Fusion of Left Tarsal Joint with External Fixation Device, Open Approach[2]

Rationale for Procedure Codes

A subtalar fusion is reported using the root operation *Fusion*. Since the subtalar area is part of the tarsals (see Body Part Key), the *Lower Joints* section of ICD-10-PCS should be referenced to build the correct procedure code. It is noted that the procedure was performed via an *Open* approach. The procedure description in the op report above states that the fusion was performed using an external fixation device, represented by the character value 5 in the device section.

MS-DRG

505	Foot Procedures without CC/MCC	RW 1.2590

OPERATIVE REPORT MDC 8—#8

Pre and postoperative diagnosis:

Superior labrum anterior and posterior (SLAP) lesion and rotator cuff tear, right shoulder

Procedure performed:

- Arthroscopy with arthroscopic SLAP lesion repair.
- Subacromial decompression
- Rotator cuff repair

History and gross findings:

This is a 45-year-old Hispanic female suffering from increasing right shoulder pain for a few months. She had an injury to her right shoulder when she fell off of her neighbor's balcony at that time.

Procedure description:

The patient was placed supine upon the operative table after she was given interscalene and then general anesthesia by the anesthesia department. She was prepped and draped in the usual sterile manner. The portals were created. Attention was then turned to the SLAP lesion. The edges were debrided. We used the anterior portal to lift up the mechanism and created a superolateral portal through the rotator cuff and into the edge of the labrum. Further debridement was carried out here. A drill hole was made just on the articular surface superiorly for a knotless anchor. A pull-through suture of #2 fiber wire was utilized and pulled through. It was tied to the leader suture of the knotless anchor. This was pulled through, and one limb of the anchor loop was grabbed and the anchor impacted with a mallet. There was excellent fixation of the superior labrum. It was noted to be solid and intact. The anchor was placed safely in the bone. There was no room for further knotless or other anchors. After probing was carried out, hard copy Polaroid was obtained.

Attention was then turned to the articular side for the rotator cuff. It was debrided. Subchondral debridement was carried out to the tuberosity also. Care was taken to go to the subchondral region but not beyond. The bone was satisfactory. The arthroscope was then placed in the subacromial region. Gross bursectomy was carried out as well as in the gutters anterolaterally and posteriorly. Debridement was carried out further to the rotator cuff. A tendon-to-tendon repair was accomplished by placing a fiber wire across the tendon and suturing through the anterolateral portal. This was done with a sliding stitch and then two half stitches. There was excellent reduction of the tear.

Attention was then turned to the coracoacromial ligament. It was released along with periosteum and the undersurface of the anterior acromion. There was noted to be no evidence of significant spurring with only a mostly type-I acromion. Thus, it was not elected to perform subacromial decompression for bone with soft tissue only. An interrupted #4-0 nylon was utilized for portal closure. A 0.5% Marcaine was instilled subacromially. Adaptic, 4x4s, ABDs, and Elastoplast tape placed for dressing. The patient's arm was placed in an arm sling. She was transferred to PACU in apparent satisfactory condition. Expected surgical prognosis on this patient is good.

Code all relevant ICD-10-CM diagnosis and ICD-10-PCS procedure codes in accordance with official guidelines and coding conventions.

Diagnosis Codes:

_____

_____

Procedure Codes:

_____

_____

MS-DRG:

_____

_____

Answers and Rationale

Pre and postoperative diagnosis:

Superior labrum anterior and posterior (SLAP) lesion[1] and rotator cuff tear, right shoulder.[2]

Procedure performed:

- Arthroscopy with arthroscopic SLAP lesion repair
- Subacromial decompression
- Rotator cuff repair

History and gross findings:

This is a 45-year-old Hispanic female suffering from increasing right shoulder pain for a few months. She had an injury to her right shoulder when she fell off of her neighbor's balcony[3,4] at that time.

Procedure description:

The patient was placed supine upon the operative table after she was given interscalene and then general anesthesia by the anesthesia department. She was prepped and draped in the usual sterile manner. The portals were created. Attention was then turned to the SLAP lesion. The edges were debrided. We used the anterior portal to lift up the mechanism and created a superolateral portal through the rotator cuff and into the edge of the labrum. Further debridement was carried out here. A drill hole was made just on the articular surface superiorly for a knotless anchor. A pull-through suture of #2 fiber wire was utilized and pulled through. It was tied to the leader suture of the knotless anchor. This was pulled through, and one limb of the anchor loop was grabbed and the anchor impacted with a mallet. There was excellent fixation of the superior labrum. It was noted to be solid and intact. The anchor was placed safely in the bone.[6] There was no room for further knotless or other anchors. After probing was carried out, hard copy Polaroid was obtained.

Attention was then turned to the articular side for the rotator cuff. It was debrided. Subchondral debridement was carried out to the tuberosity also. Care was taken to go to the subchondral region but not beyond. The bone was satisfactory. The arthroscope was then placed in the subacromial region. Gross bursectomy was carried out as well as in the gutters anterolaterally and posteriorly. Debridement was carried out further to the rotator cuff. A tendon-to-tendon repair was accomplished by placing a fiber wire across the tendon and suturing through the anterolateral portal.[7] This was done with a sliding stitch and then two half stitches. There was excellent reduction of the tear.

Attention was then turned to the coracoacromial ligament. It was released along with periosteum and the undersurface of the anterior acromion.[5] There was noted to be no evidence of significant spurring with only a mostly type-I acromion. Thus, it was not elected to perform subacromial decompression for bone with soft tissue only. An interrupted #4-0 nylon was utilized for portal closure. A 0.5% Marcaine was instilled subacromially. Adaptic, 4x4s, ABDs, and Elastoplast tape placed for dressing. The patient's arm was placed in an arm sling. She was transferred to PACU in apparent satisfactory condition. Expected surgical prognosis on this patient is good.

Diagnosis Codes

S43.431A Superior glenoid labrum lesion of right shoulder, initial encounter[1]

S46.011A Strain of muscle(s) and tendon(s) of the rotator cuff of right shoulder, initial encounter[2]

W13.0XXA Fall from, out of or through balcony, initial encounter[3]

Y92.008 Other place in unspecified non-institutional (private) residence as the place of occurrence of the external cause[4]

Rationale for Diagnosis Codes

The ICD-10-CM code for the labral tear is straightforward if the term "Lesion, SLAP" is referenced in the index. The code for the rotator cuff tear is a little more difficult to discern as there is question as to whether the injury is traumatic or not. As the documentation specifies that this occurred secondary to a fall, the correct code would be the one specified as traumatic tear or sprain. The documentation of the fall from the balcony is also required to report the external cause and place of occurrence codes.

Procedure Codes

0MN14ZZ Release Right Shoulder Bursa and Ligament, Percutaneous Endoscopic Approach[5]

ØMM14ZZ Reattachment of Right Shoulder Bursa and Ligament, Percutaneous Endoscopic Approach[6]

ØLQ14ZZ Repair Right Shoulder Tendon, Percutaneous Endoscopic Approach[7]

Rationale for Procedure Codes

AHA's *Coding Clinic for ICD-10-CM and ICD-10-PCS*, third quarter 2013, pages 20–22 discuss the nature of a SLAP injury and that the correct body part character is from the shoulder bursa and ligaments section. It should also be noted that this same reference aids in identifying why the appropriate root operation is reattachment as that is ultimately the reason for the lesion repair. In addition to the SLAP repair, the rotator cuff repair, specified as tendon-to-tendon, must also be reported. Lastly, although the header states that a subacromial decompression was performed, the body of the operative report does not support this, and only a release of the coracoacromial ligament was performed due to "no evidence of significant spurring."

MS-DRG

502	Soft Tissue Procedures without CC/MCC	RW 1.1752

The MS-DRG surgical hierarchy uses the release of the coracoacromial ligament to drive the MS-DRG to 502. It is important to note that the *repair* of this ligament is included in a rotator cuff repair; however, the release especially after the rotator cuff repair, is not. If the release is not reported, the encounter groups to higher-weighted 512 Shoulder, Elbow or Forearm Procedure, Except Major Joint Procedure without CC/MCC (RW 1.3531).

OPERATIVE REPORT MDC 8—#9

Diagnosis:
Chondrosarcoma of the left fourth rib

Procedure performed:
Resection of the rib with chest wall reconstruction using a composite Marlex methyl methacrylate prosthesis

Procedure:
Patient was brought to the operating room, positioned supine. General anesthesia was induced. Patient was then placed into the lateral decubitus position with the left side up. An incision was made in oblique fashion overlying the 4th rib and taken down onto the chest wall. The musculature was divided with electrocautery. The costal cartilages were then divided giving adequate tumor clearance of 5 cm. The intercostal cartilages were divided with a sternal saw and care is taken to identify, ligate, and divide the intercostal vascular bundle. Approximately 7 cm of the 4th rib was resected. The defect in the anterior chest wall was assessed for a good clearance margin on all sides, and the prosthesis was sized. The Marlex mesh was folded and placed on the defect, then sewn as a pouch. The methyl methacrylate with gentamycin was stirred to a paste-like consistency, instilled, and uniformly spread inside the Marlex pouch. The pouch was molded to suit the contour of the anterior chest wall, then fixed to the defect with interrupted 0 Vicryl sutures to the costal cartilages of the 3rd and 5th ribs. The chest wall musculature was then closed in layers using Polysorb suture. The subcutaneous tissue was closed with a running 3-0 Polysorb and skin with a 4-0 Biosyn subcuticular stitch. The resected specimen was measured and sent for histological exam. The histology confirmed the diagnosis of a Grade I chondrosarcoma with complete excision margins. The patient had a satisfactory cosmetic and function outcome, and the prosthesis was found to be sitting well in a follow-up CT scan.

Code all relevant ICD-10-CM diagnosis and ICD-10-PCS procedure codes in accordance with official guidelines and coding conventions.

Diagnosis Codes:

_____

_____

Procedure Codes:

_____

_____

MS-DRG:

_____

Answers and Rationale

Diagnosis:
Chondrosarcoma of the left fourth rib[1]

Procedure performed:
Resection of the rib with chest wall reconstruction using a composite Marlex methyl methacrylate prosthesis

Procedure:
Patient was brought to the operating room, positioned supine. General anesthesia was induced. Patient was then placed into the lateral decubitus position with the left side up. An incision was made in oblique fashion overlying the 4th rib and taken down onto the chest wall.[2,3] The musculature was divided with electrocautery. The costal cartilages were then divided giving adequate tumor clearance of 5 cm. The intercostal cartilages were divided with a sternal saw and care was taken to identify, ligate, and divide the intercostal vascular bundle. Approximately 7 cm of the 4th rib was resected.[2] The defect in the anterior chest wall assessed for a good clearance margin on all sides and the prosthesis was sized. The Marlex mesh was folded and placed on the defect, then sewn as a pouch. The methyl methacrylate with gentamycin was stirred to a paste-like consistency, instilled, and uniformly spread inside the Marlex pouch. The pouch was molded to suit the contour of the anterior chest wall then fixed to the defect with interrupted 0 Vicryl sutures to the costal cartilages of the 3rd and 5th ribs.[3] The chest wall musculature was then closed in layers using Polysorb suture. The subcutaneous tissue was closed with a running 3-0 Polysorb and skin with a 4-0 Biosyn subcuticular stitch. The resected specimen was measured and sent for histological exam. The histology confirmed the diagnosis of a Grade I chondrosarcoma with complete excision margins. The patient had a satisfactory cosmetic and function outcome, and the prosthesis was found to be sitting well in a follow-up CT scan.

Diagnosis Codes

C41.3   **Malignant neoplasm of ribs, sternum and clavicle**[1]

Rationale for Diagnosis Codes
In the ICD-10-CM index, "Chondrosarcoma" leads the coder to the neoplasm table under "Malignant neoplasm, cartilage," which is reported using C41.3.

Procedure Codes

ØPB2ØZZ   **Excision of Left Rib, Open Approach**[2]

ØWU8ØJZ   **Supplement Chest Wall with Synthetic Substitute, Open Approach**[3]

Rationale for Procedure Codes
AHA *Coding Clinic for ICD-10-CM and ICD-10-PCS* fourth quarter 2012, pages 101–102, discuss a rib "resection" with chest wall reconstruction. It is most important to note that only a portion of the rib is removed, making the physician's documentation of a resection the incorrect root operation. The insertion of the Marlex mesh entails supplementing the chest wall rather than replacing it.

MS-DRG

517	**Other Musculoskeletal System and Connective Tissue O.R. Procedure without CC/MCC**	**RW 1.7716**

MDC 9 Diseases and Disorders of the Skin, Subcutaneous Tissue and Breast

OPERATIVE REPORT MDC 9—#1

Preoperative diagnosis:
Malignant melanoma of the left upper extremity

Postoperative diagnosis:
Same

Procedure performed:
Wide local excision of melanoma

Indications:
The patient is a 62-year-old white male who previously underwent an excisional biopsy of a malignant melanoma 1.6 cm in diameter near the posterolateral aspect of the left upper arm. Examination today shows a surgical scar. A margin of 1.8 cm was outlined in a radial fashion from the periphery of the scar. The patient also has a small keratotic lesion on the occipital scalp for which he requested excision.

Procedure description:
The patient was appropriately identified and placed in the supine position where general endotracheal anesthesia was induced and maintained. The left arm was positioned across the chest and supported. Betadine preparation was performed. Sterile drapes where applied.

Methylene blue was used to create an outline after measuring a 1.7 radius around the periphery of the scar. An incision was performed with a #15 blade. The full thickness of the skin and subcutaneous tissue was excised with Bovie electrocautery. Undermining was performed with the Bovie to create flaps. The subcutaneous tissue was then closed with interrupted, inverted sutures of #2-0 Vicryl. The skin was closed with multiple vertical mattress sutures of #3-0 nylon. Excellent closure without tension was obtained. A sterile dressing was applied.

All counts were reported as correct.

Attention was directed to the lesion on the occipital scalp. Again, Betadine prep was provided and a very small elliptical incision was fashioned and the lesion excised. The specimen was sent to pathology. Closure was provided with a single suture of #3-0 nylon, followed by Bacitracin ointment. The patient tolerated the procedure well and at its conclusion was transported to the postoperative recovery room in satisfactory condition.

It should be noted that the melanoma specimen from the arm was labeled with silk suture, the short suture marking the superior aspect and the long suture marking the posterolateral aspect. This material was sent to pathology.

Addendum:
The pathology report documents that the surgical margins around the upper extremity lesion were clear, with no further indications of malignant melanoma. The scalp lesion was found to be a benign actinic hyperkeratosis.

Code all relevant ICD-10-CM diagnosis and ICD-10-PCS procedure codes in accordance with official guidelines and coding conventions.

Diagnosis Codes:

_____

_____

Procedure Codes:

_____

_____

MS-DRG:

_____

_____

Answers and Rationale

Preoperative diagnosis:
Malignant melanoma of the left upper extremity[1]

Postoperative diagnosis:
Same

Procedure performed:
Wide local excision of melanoma

Indications:
The patient is a 62-year-old white male who previously underwent an excisional biopsy of a malignant melanoma 1.6 cm in diameter near the posterolateral aspect of the left upper arm. Examination today shows a surgical scar. A margin of 1.8 cm was outlined in a radial fashion from the periphery of the scar. The patient also has a small keratotic lesion on the occipital scalp for which he requested excision.

Procedure description:
The patient was appropriately identified and placed in the supine position where general endotracheal anesthesia was induced and maintained. The left arm was positioned across the chest and supported. Betadine preparation was performed. Sterile drapes where applied.

Methylene blue was used to create an outline after measuring a 1.7 radius around the periphery of the scar. An incision was performed with a #15 blade. The full thickness of the skin and subcutaneous tissue was excised with Bovie electrocautery.[3] Undermining was performed with the Bovie to create flaps. The subcutaneous tissue was then closed with interrupted, inverted sutures of #2-0 Vicryl. The skin was closed with multiple vertical mattress sutures of #3-0 nylon. Excellent closure without tension was obtained. A sterile dressing was applied.

All counts were reported as correct.

Attention was directed to the lesion on the occipital scalp. Again, Betadine prep was provided and a very small elliptical incision was fashioned and the lesion excised.[4] The specimen was sent to pathology. Closure was provided with a single suture of #3-0 nylon, followed by Bacitracin ointment. The patient tolerated the procedure well and at its conclusion was transported to the postoperative recovery room in satisfactory condition.

It should be noted that the melanoma specimen from the arm was labeled with silk suture, the short suture marking the superior aspect and the long suture marking the posterolateral aspect. This material was sent to pathology.

Addendum:
The pathology report documents that the surgical margins around the upper extremity lesion were clear, with no further indications of malignant melanoma. The scalp lesion was found to be a benign actinic hyperkeratosis.[2]

Diagnosis Codes

C43.62	Malignant melanoma of left upper limb, including shoulder[1]
L57.0	Actinic keratosis[2]

Rationale for Diagnosis Codes
Even though the malignant melanoma was completely excised on the previous episode of care, the treatment provided during this procedure (a wide excision) is still considered treatment for the initial malignancy. Code C43.62 is assigned as the first-listed diagnosis, reflecting the melanoma of the upper extremity. The final pathology report substantiates a benign actinic hyperkeratosis for the scalp lesion. When "Hyperkeratosis" is referenced in the ICD-10-CM index, the coder is directed to "*see also* Keratosis" or to use L85.9 Epidermal thickening, unspecified. "Keratosis" lists the subterm "Actinic," leading the coder to L57.0, a more specific code than L85.9.

Procedure Codes

0JBF0ZZ	Excision of Left Upper Arm Subcutaneous Tissue and Fascia, Open Approach[3]
0HB0XZZ	Excision of Scalp Skin, External Approach[4]

Rationale for Procedure Codes
The procedure codes are straightforward excisions of first the skin and subcutaneous tissue of the left upper arm and second of a small scalp (skin) lesion. Both of these

---

DEFINITIONS

actinic keratosis. Flat, scaly precancerous lesions appearing on dry, sun-aged, and overexposed skin, including the eyelids.

melanoma. Highly metastatic malignant neoplasm composed of melanocytes that occur most often on the skin from a preexisting mole or nevus but may also occur in the mouth, esophagus, anal canal, or vagina.

CODING AXIOM

ICD-10-PCS Official Guidelines for Coding and Reporting Section B3.5:

If the root operations *Excision, Repair, or Inspection* are performed on overlapping layers of the musculoskeletal system, the body part specifying the deepest layer is coded.

procedures can be found under the root operation *Excision* in their respective anatomical sections (skin and breast, subcutaneous tissue and fascia).

MS-DRG

572   Skin Debridement without CC/MCC   RW 1.0391

Although technically these are not considered "debridement," in the MS-DRG Grouper logic, a subcutaneous tissue and fascia open excision groups to the debridement MS-DRGs.

Operative Report MDC 9—#2

Preoperative diagnosis :
Perceived unacceptable cosmetic appearance

Postoperative diagnosis:
Same

Procedure performed:
Cosmetic rhinoplasty

Indications:
The 19-year-old female patient presented with dissatisfaction regarding the appearance of her nose. The visible dorsal hump and bony and cartilage irregularities the patient was concerned with were addressed. The nature of the operation was discussed with the patient as well as the risks, including bleeding, hematoma, infection, scarring, asymmetry, and airway difficulties. The patient expressed understanding and wished to proceed.

Procedure description:
After initiation of general anesthesia, the patient was prepped and draped in the routine fashion. After this was completed, the nose was irrigated with 1% lidocaine with epinephrine, and then a columellar chevron incision was performed resulting in bilateral rim incisions. The nasal skin was then retracted back. This allowed full exposure of the bony nasal structure. Approximately 1 mm thickness of the dorsal nasal bone was removed using a straight guarded osteotome. This was followed by medial osteotomies. The osteotome was switched to a 2 mm thickness, and lateral osteotomies were then carried out. The remaining irregular edges were smoothed with a rasp.

To narrow the nasal base, infracture of the nasal bones was performed with optimal results. Then, using a #15 blade, portions of the nasal cartilage were excised to straighten the dorsum. Once this was achieved, the cartilage was attached to the septum via interrupted 4-0 Prolene. Using the same suturing technique, the nasal tip was narrowed. Dissection was then carried down to the caudal septum, which protruded to the right of the medial crura. Approximately 3 mm of caudal septum was excised. Next, the anterior nasal spine was exposed, and the protruding sections were removed using a bone biter.

The skin was then draped over the bony structures and checked for symmetry and contour. Noting a defect in the nasal dorsum, the skin was retracted and a small piece of previously removed cartilage was crushed and placed over the defect. The skin was again redraped and the symmetry and contour were checked and found to be satisfactory. Hemostasis was confirmed. The incisions were closed using interrupted 6-0 Prolene. Nasal splints and Xeroform packs were placed. The procedure was well tolerated and the patient was awakened and discharged to the recovery room in stable condition.

Code all relevant ICD-10-CM diagnosis and ICD-10-PCS procedure codes in accordance with official guidelines and coding conventions.

Diagnosis Codes:
_____

_____

Procedure Codes:
_____

_____

MS-DRG:
_____

_____

Answers and Rationale

Preoperative diagnosis:
Perceived unacceptable cosmetic appearance[1]

Postoperative diagnosis:
Same

Procedure performed:
Cosmetic rhinoplasty[2]

Indications:
The 19-year-old female patient presented with dissatisfaction regarding the appearance of her nose. The visible dorsal hump and bony and cartilage irregularities the patient is concerned with were addressed.[1] The nature of the operation was discussed with the patient as well as the risks, including bleeding, hematoma, infection, scarring, asymmetry, and airway difficulties. The patient expressed understanding and wished to proceed.

Procedure description:
After initiation of general anesthesia, the patient was prepped and draped in the routine fashion. After this was completed, the nose was irrigated with 1% lidocaine with epinephrine, and then a columellar chevron incision was performed resulting in bilateral rim incisions. The nasal skin was then retracted back. This allowed full exposure of the bony nasal structure. Approximately 1 mm thickness of the dorsal nasal bone was removed using a straight guarded osteotome. This was followed by medial osteotomies. The osteotome was switched to a 2 mm thickness, and lateral osteotomies were then carried out. The remaining irregular edges were smoothed with a rasp.

To narrow the nasal base, infracture of the nasal bones was performed with optimal results. Then, using a #15 blade, portions of the nasal cartilage were excised to straighten the dorsum. Once this was achieved, the cartilage was attached to the septum via interrupted 4-0 Prolene. Using the same suturing technique, the nasal tip was narrowed. Dissection was then carried down to the caudal septum, which protruded to the right of the medial crura. Approximately 3 mm of caudal septum was excised. Next, the anterior nasal spine was exposed, and the protruding sections were removed using a bone biter.

The skin was then draped over the bony structures and checked for symmetry and contour. Noting a defect in the nasal dorsum, the skin was retracted and a small piece of previously removed cartilage was crushed and placed over the defect. The skin was again redraped and the symmetry and contour were checked and found to be satisfactory. Hemostasis was confirmed. The incisions were closed using interrupted 6-0 Prolene. Nasal splints and Xeroform packs were placed. The procedure was well tolerated and the patient was awakened and discharged to the recovery room in stable condition.

Diagnosis Codes

Z41.1 **Encounter for cosmetic surgery[1]**

Rationale for Diagnosis Codes
There is no physical ailment, disease, disorder, sign, or symptom to report for a patient that presents solely for an "unacceptable cosmetic appearance." Due to this, a Z code may be used to accurately represent the reason for the encounter, which in this case coincides with Z41.1.

Procedure Codes

Ø9ØKØ7Z **Alteration of Nose with Autologous Tissue Substitute, Open Approach[2]**

Rationale for Procedure Codes
The rhinoplasty is specified as a cosmetic procedure with documentation that this surgery is being performed to improve the patient's appearance. This would be reported with the root operation *Alteration*, which is defined as modifying the natural anatomic structure of a body part without affecting the function of the body part. The principal purpose is to improve appearance.

Alteration is coded for all procedures performed solely to improve appearance. All methods, approaches, and devices used for the objective of improving appearance are coded here.

If the procedure were being done for a medical condition, the appropriate root operations, such as *Excision, Supplement, Reposition*, etc., would be assigned

MS-DRG

581 **Other Skin, Subcutaneous Tissue and Breast Procedures without CC/MCC** **RW 1.1834**

OPERATIVE REPORT MDC 9—#3

Preoperative diagnosis:
Right breast masses on mammography

Postoperative diagnosis:
Breast masses pending pathology

Procedure performed:
Stereotactic core biopsies

Procedure description:
The procedure and risks were explained to the patient and consent was obtained.

The right breast was positioned, and images of the mass in the upper outer quadrant were obtained posteriorly. The breast was prepped for the procedure. The area was anesthetized with a local anesthetic, and a small incision was made in the breast. Using an 8 g Mammotome vacuum-assisted device, two passes were made through the area and two specimens were obtained. The specimen was marked as core #1. A micromarker was placed at the site of the core biopsy.

The patient's breast was then repositioned and images of the mass in the central region at the middle depth were obtained. The area was anesthetized with a local anesthetic, and a small incision was made in the breast. Using an 8 g Mammotome vacuum-assisted device, two passes were made through the area and two specimens were obtained from this site as well. The specimen was marked as core #2. A micromarker was placed at the site of the core biopsy. Postprocedure mammograms were performed to document placement of the clips.

There were no complications and the patient was taken to recovery in good condition.

Addendum:
The pathology report was reviewed by me (the surgeon). The upper outer quadrant mass is confirmed benign fibroadenoma. The central mass has been identified as fibrocystic disease. The patient has been informed of the pathology by my office staff.

Code all relevant ICD-10-CM diagnosis and ICD-10-PCS procedure codes in accordance with official guidelines and coding conventions.

Diagnosis Codes:

_____

_____

Procedure Codes:

_____

_____

MS-DRG:

_____

_____

Answers and Rationale

Preoperative diagnosis:
Right breast[1-3] masses on mammography

Postoperative diagnosis:
Breast masses pending pathology

Procedure performed:
Stereotactic core biopsies

Procedure description:
The procedure and risks were explained to the patient and consent was obtained.

The right breast was positioned and images of the mass in the upper outer quadrant were obtained posteriorly. The breast was prepped for the procedure. The area was anesthetized with a local anesthetic, and a small incision was made in the breast. Using an 8 g Mammotome vacuum-assisted device, two passes were made through the area and two specimens were obtained.[3] The specimen was marked as core #1. A micromarker was placed at the site of the core biopsy.

The patient's breast was then repositioned and images of the mass in the central region at the middle depth were obtained. The area was anesthetized with a local anesthetic, and a small incision was made in the breast. Using an 8 g Mammotome vacuum-assisted device, two passes were made through the area and two specimens were obtained from this site as well.[3] The specimen was marked as core #2. A micromarker was placed at the site of the core biopsy. Postprocedure mammograms were performed to document placement of the clips.

There were no complications and the patient was taken to recovery in good condition.

Addendum:
The pathology report was reviewed by me (the surgeon). The upper outer quadrant mass is confirmed benign fibroadenoma.[1] The central mass has been identified as fibrocystic disease.[2] The patient has been informed of the pathology by my office staff.

Diagnosis Codes

D24.1   **Benign neoplasm of right breast[1]**

N60.11   **Diffuse cystic mastopathy of right breast[2]**

Rationale for Diagnosis Codes
The physician confirms the diagnoses of fibroadenoma and fibrocystic disease in the addendum. The term "Fibroadenoma" in the ICD-10-CM index instructs the coder to go to "Neoplasm, Benign, by site."

Procedure Codes

ØHBT3ZX   **Excision of Right Breast, Percutaneous Approach, Diagnostic[3]**

Rationale for Procedure Codes
Because only a small portion of breast tissue is being removed, the root operation is *Excision*. The approach is *Percutaneous* as only a small incision was made to introduce the Mammotome. Since these procedures were performed as biopsies, the seventh character value should be X, *Diagnostic*. It is important to note that the *ICD-10-PCS Official Guidelines for Coding and Reporting* section B3.2.b clarifies that multiple procedures would not be coded since the biopsies were taken from the same breast classified to the same PCS body part value, and not from separate and distinct body parts within that PCS body part value.

MS-DRG

607   **Minor Skin Disorders without MCC**   **RW 0.7258**

In this case, as the breast biopsy isn't considered an operating room procedure under the current MS-DRG grouping methodology, the principal diagnosis is used for MS-DRG assignment.

📖 DEFINITIONS

fibroadenoma. Benign neoplasm of glandular epithelium frequently found in the breast.

🕯 CODING AXIOM

ICD-10-CM Official Guidelines for Coding and Reporting Section B3.2.b:

During the same operative episode, multiple procedures are coded if: The same root operation is repeated in multiple body parts, and those body parts are separate and distinct body parts classified to a single ICD-10-PCS body part value.

Example: Excision of the sartorius muscle and excision of the gracilis muscle are both included in the upper leg muscle body part value, and multiple procedures are coded.

OPERATIVE REPORT MDC 9—#4

Preoperative diagnosis:
Right breast mass

Postoperative diagnosis:
Right breast carcinoma

Procedure performed:
Attempted core needle biopsy right breast mass, Right breast excisional biopsy, sentinel node lymphadenectomy of the right axilla x 5 with preoperative lymphoscintigraphy, right breast partial mastectomy

Indications:
She had palpable breast mass, which was clinically suspicious by fine needle aspiration cytology, ultrasound, and clinical examination.

Procedure description:
The patient was prepped and draped in a routine sterile fashion. A core needle biopsy was attempted using a 16 gauge MD Tech biopsy gun, which was not successful at retrieving the core. An attempt was made to get negative margins; however, on grossing the specimen in this it abuts margins in the above-mentioned areas. Electrocautery was used for hemostasis, and a temporary dressing was applied while I took the specimen to pathology. When the frozen section returned as positive for adenocarcinoma, blue dye was injected into the base of the lumpectomy cavity towards the axilla for a total of 3 cc.

Transcutaneous mapping identified three areas of increased activity, one in the posterior Level 1 axilla, another in the lower Level 1 axilla, and another in Level 2 underneath the pectoralis musculature more medially. An incision was made within the clavipectoral fascia. Blue stain channels were identified; the first one obtained was the low Level 1 node. Afterward, efferent channels were individually clipped and removed. A similar procedure was then performed for the posterior Level 1 axilla cell node and the Level 2 sentinel node. Two intercostal brachial nerves were identified within this wound and were dissected and preserved. In scanning the bed, two further nodes were present within the midportion of Level 1 and were removed. No suspicious clinical adenopathy is clinically palpable. A temporary dressing is applied here as the first four nodes were sent for frozen section.

The partial mastectomy was accomplished by grasping the biopsy cavity anteriorly with Allis forceps. A cup was obtained about the entire periphery with the base of the wound being the pectoralis fascia off of the chest wall. Dense breast tissue was superior and medial with excrescences present. Suspicious palpable masses were also present within the rim of tissue. Essentially a quadrectomy was accomplished through this incision. Double clips were placed in four quadrants to mark the extent of the excision. Electrocautery was used for hemostasis. Closure was with interrupted 3-0 Vicryl for deep layer and a running 4-0 Monocryl for the skin. The sentinel nodes were returned as all benign. A 10 French round drain was brought out dependently and closure in likewise manner. Steri-Strips and Benzoin were applied and OPSITE is used to complete the dressing. Patient tolerated the procedure well.

Findings:
A dominant 3 cm mass was present within the lower outer quadrant of the right breast. Lymphatic mapping identified four nodes, and intraoperative mapping identified nodes that had been successfully removed, three of which were concordant with blue staining and the two others being localized by radioisotope alone.

Code all relevant ICD-10-CM diagnosis and ICD-10-PCS procedure codes in accordance with official guidelines and coding conventions.

Diagnosis Codes:

_____

_____

Procedure Codes:

_____

_____

MS-DRG:

_____

_____

Answers and Rationale

Preoperative diagnosis:
Right breast mass

Postoperative diagnosis:
Right breast carcinoma[1]

Procedure performed:
Attempted core needle biopsy right breast mass, Right breast excisional biopsy, sentinel node lymphadenectomy of the right axilla x 5 with preoperative lymphoscintigraphy, right breast partial mastectomy

Indications:
She had palpable breast mass, which was clinically suspicious by fine needle aspiration cytology, ultrasound, and clinical examination.

Procedure description:
The patient was prepped and draped in a routine sterile fashion. A core needle biopsy was attempted using a 16 gauge MD Tech biopsy gun, which was not successful at retrieving the core.[3] An excisional biopsy was then accomplished through a circumareolar incision.[4] An attempt was made to get negative margins; however, on grossing the specimen in this it abuts margins in the above-mentioned areas. Electrocautery was used for hemostasis, and a temporary dressing was applied while I took the specimen to pathology. When the frozen section returned as positive for adenocarcinoma[1], blue dye was injected into the base of the lumpectomy cavity towards the axilla for a total of 3 cc.

Transcutaneous mapping identified three areas of increased activity, one in the posterior Level 1 axilla, another in the lower Level 1 axilla, and another in Level 2 underneath the pectoralis musculature more medially. An incision was made within the clavipectoral fascia. Blue stain channels were identified; the first one obtained was the low Level 1 node. Afterward, efferent channels were individually clipped and removed. A similar procedure was then performed for the posterior Level 1 axilla cell node and the Level 2 sentinel node.[5] Two intercostal brachial nerves were identified within this wound and were dissected and preserved. In scanning the bed, two further nodes were present within the midportion of Level 1 and were removed. No suspicious clinical adenopathy is clinically palpable. A temporary dressing is applied here as the first four nodes were sent for frozen section.

The partial mastectomy was accomplished by grasping the biopsy cavity anteriorly with Allis forceps. A cup was obtained about the entire periphery with the base of the wound being the pectoralis fascia off of the chest wall. Dense breast tissue was superior and medial with excrescences present. Suspicious palpable masses were also present within the rim of tissue. Essentially a quadrectomy was accomplished through this incision.[2] Double clips were placed in four quadrants to mark the extent of the excision. Electrocautery was used for hemostasis. Closure was with interrupted 3-0 Vicryl for deep layer and a running 4-0 Monocryl for the skin. The sentinel nodes were returned as all benign. A 10 French round drain was brought out dependently and closure in likewise manner. Steri-Strips and Benzoin were applied and OPSITE is used to complete the dressing. Patient tolerated the procedure well.

Findings:
A dominant 3 cm mass was present within the lower outer quadrant of the right breast[1]. Lymphatic mapping identified four nodes, and intraoperative mapping identified nodes that had been successfully removed, three of which were concordant with blue staining and the two others being localized by radioisotope alone.

Diagnosis Codes

C50.511   Malignant neoplasm of lower-outer quadrant of right female breast[1]

Rationale for Diagnosis Codes
The final diagnosis is listed as breast carcinoma. Therefore the malignancy should be reported rather than the code for a breast mass.

Procedure Codes

0HBT0ZZ   Excision of Right Breast, Open Approach[2]

0HBT3ZX   Excision of Right Breast, Percutaneous Approach, Diagnostic[3]

0HBT0ZX   Excision of Right Breast, Open Approach, Diagnostic[4]

07B50ZX   Excision of Right Axillary Lymphatic, Open Approach, Diagnostic[5]

CODING AXIOM

ICD-10-PCS Official Guidelines for Coding and Reporting

Section B3.4b:
If a diagnostic Excision, Extraction, or Drainage procedure (biopsy) is followed by a more definitive procedure, such as Destruction, Excision or Resection at the same procedure site, both the biopsy and the more definitive treatment are coded.

Section B3.2d:
During the same operative episode, multiple procedures are coded if: The intended root operation is attempted using one approach, but is converted to a different approach.

Section B3.3:
If the intended procedure is discontinued, code the procedure to the root operation performed. If a procedure is discontinued before any other root operation is performed, code the root operation Inspection of the body part or anatomical region inspected.

Rationale for Procedure Codes

The biopsy is coded in addition to the more extensive procedure performed on the same site during the same session. Another very important guideline to consider is that when a procedure is converted to a different approach (*Percutaneous* to *Open*, for example) codes representing both approaches should be reported. With this in mind, four procedure codes should be assigned: the attempted needle core biopsy, the excisional biopsy, the removal of the lymph nodes, and the breast quadrectomy.

MS-DRG

583	**Mastectomy for Malignancy without CC/MCC**	RW 1.1856

OPERATIVE REPORT MDC 9—#5

Preoperative and postoperative diagnosis:
Complex open wound, left knee, 7x5 cm

Procedure performed:
Excisional preparation of wound with a split thickness skin graft, 7 x 5 cm, left thigh to left leg op wound

Indications:
This patient is a 57-year-old female who has rheumatoid arthritis. She now presents with an open wound of her left knee after sustaining a fall approximately seven weeks ago. Approximately one month following the injury, her wound appeared infected and was foul smelling with drainage. Debridement, meticulous dressing changes, and antibiotics have allowed this infected wound to progress to a nicely granulating wound without evidence of infection. On physical examination there is a large open wound that measures approximately 7x5 cm overlying the left knee as well as a small amount of undermining circumferentially, which has decreased considerably with wound care. She now presents for definitive wound closure.

Procedure description:
The patient was brought to the operating suite and general endotracheal anesthesia was induced. The patient was then prepped and draped in the usual sterile fashion. A 10 blade was used to excise the margin of the wound circumferentially. This was sent for permanent pathological analysis. A pulse lavage irrigation system was used to provide good irrigation of 2 liters of normal saline to this wound. Intraoperative cultures were then obtained. The back side of a Betadine scrub brush was utilized to sharply debride the granulation tissue. A 10 blade was also used for this purpose. Bovie cautery was used for hemostasis.

After the wound was thoroughly prepared by removing the granulation tissue as well as the margin of the wound, the wound edge was marsupialized with 4-0 chromic suture in a continuous running and interrupted fashion. This allowed for closure of the skin flaps, which were slightly undermined from the extensive pre-existing hematoma, and it allowed for better contour with the skin graft.

A skin graft was then harvested from the left anterior thigh with the Zimmer dermatome set at a thickness of 15/1,000 of an inch. The skin was then fashioned to fit the defect and tacked down with 4-0 chromic in a continuous running fashion.

A bolster was constructed with Xeroform, 3-0 silk pop-off sutures, mineral oil, cotton balls, and saline. Note that meticulous hemostasis was obtained prior to application of the bolster. Note also that a small amount of pie-crusting was performed to prevent a collection of blood under the graft itself.

A laparotomy pad soaked in dilute epinephrine solution, 1:1,000,000, was used for hemostasis of the left anterior thigh donor site. After hemostasis was achieved, a small area that had resulted in full-thickness skin removal was closed with 4-0 chromic in a continuous running fashion. Xeroform and Kerlix roll were then applied. Finally a long-leg posterior splint was constructed and applied.

There were no obvious complications. The patient tolerated the procedure well. She was taken to the recovery room in stable condition.

Code all relevant ICD-10-CM diagnosis and ICD-10-PCS procedure codes in accordance with official guidelines and coding conventions.

Diagnosis Codes:

_____

_____

Procedure Codes:

_____

_____

MS-DRG:

_____

_____

Answers and Rationale

Preoperative and postoperative diagnosis:
Complex open wound, left knee, 7x5 cm[1]

Procedure performed:
Excisional preparation of wound with a split thickness skin graft, 7 x 5 cm, left thigh to left leg op wound

Indications:
This patient is a 57-year-old female who has rheumatoid arthritis.[2] She now presents with an open wound of her left knee after sustaining a fall approximately seven weeks ago. Approximately one month following the injury, her wound appeared infected and was foul smelling with drainage. Debridement, meticulous dressing changes, and antibiotics have allowed this infected wound to progress to a nicely granulating wound without evidence of infection. On physical examination there is a large open wound that measures approximately 7x5 cm overlying the left knee as well as a small amount of undermining circumferentially, which has decreased considerably with wound care. She now presents for definitive wound closure.

Procedure description:
The patient was brought to the operating suite and general endotracheal anesthesia was induced. The patient was then prepped and draped in the usual sterile fashion. A 10 blade was used to excise the margin of the wound circumferentially. This was sent for permanent pathological analysis. A pulse lavage irrigation system was used to provide good irrigation of 2 liters of normal saline to this wound. Intraoperative cultures were then obtained. The back side of a Betadine scrub brush was utilized to sharply debride the granulation tissue. A 10 blade was also used for this purpose. Bovie cautery was used for hemostasis.

After the wound was thoroughly prepared by removing the granulation tissue as well as the margin of the wound, the wound edge was marsupialized with 4-0 chromic suture in a continuous running and interrupted fashion. This allowed for closure of the skin flaps, which were slightly undermined from the extensive pre-existing hematoma, and it allowed for better contour with the skin graft.

A skin graft was then harvested from the left anterior thigh with the Zimmer dermatome set at a thickness of 15/1,000 of an inch.[4] The skin was then fashioned to fit the defect and tacked down with 4-0 chromic in a continuous running fashion.[3]

A bolster was constructed with Xeroform, 3-0 silk pop-off sutures, mineral oil, cotton balls, and saline. Note that meticulous hemostasis was obtained prior to application of the bolster. Note also that a small amount of pie-crusting was performed to prevent a collection of blood under the graft itself.

A laparotomy pad soaked in dilute epinephrine solution, 1:1,000,000, was used for hemostasis of the left anterior thigh donor site. After hemostasis was achieved, a small area that had resulted in full-thickness skin removal was closed with 4-0 chromic in a continuous running fashion. Xeroform and Kerlix roll were then applied. Finally a long-leg posterior splint was constructed and applied.

There were no obvious complications. The patient tolerated the procedure well. She was taken to the recovery room in stable condition.

Diagnosis Codes
S81.002A Unspecified open wound, left knee, initial encounter[1]

M06.9 Rheumatoid arthritis, unspecified[2]

Rationale for Diagnosis Codes
The documentation does not specify what type of wound is on the left knee, only that it is an open wound. This is reported using a code from category S81.0, according to the ICD-10-CM index. The seventh character should still represent an initial encounter although the patient has been seen more than once. This is because the wound is still under active treatment and the seventh-character extension for a subsequent encounter is for use when the injury is no longer under active treatment. The rheumatoid arthritis should be reported as a secondary diagnosis as it is a chronic condition.

Procedure Codes
0HRLX74 Replacement of Left Lower Leg Skin with Autologous Tissue Substitute, Partial Thickness, External Approach[3]

0HBJXZZ Excision of Left Upper Leg Skin, External Approach[4]

CODING AXIOM

ICD-10-CM Official Guidelines for Coding and Reporting Section I.C.19.a:

7th character "A," initial encounter is used while the patient is receiving active treatment for the condition. Examples of active treatment are: surgical treatment, emergency department encounter, and evaluation and continuing treatment by the same or a different physician.

7th character "D" subsequent encounter is used for encounters after the patient has received active treatment of the condition and is receiving routine care for the condition during the healing or recovery phase. Examples of subsequent care are: cast change or removal, an x-ray to check healing status of fracture, removal of external or internal fixation device, medication adjustment, other aftercare and follow up visits following treatment of the injury or condition.

CODING AXIOM

ICD-10-PCS Official Guidelines for Coding and Reporting Section B3.9:

If an autograft is obtained from a different body part in order to complete the objective of the procedure, a separate procedure is coded.

Rationale for Procedure Codes

The objective of the procedure is to replace the skin of the left knee. This coincides with the root operation *Replacement*. To build the correct skin graft ICD-10-PCS code, the coder must note that the graft was done with autologous tissue and was split or partial thickness. The excision of the graft tissue from the left anterior thigh should be reported separately, according to *ICD-10-PCS Official Guidelines for Coding and Reporting* section B3.9. The wound exploration and preparation would not be reported in addition to the graft procedure as these were performed to ready the site for the skin graft.

MS-DRG

| 578 | Skin Graft Except for Skin Ulcer or Cellulitis without CC/MCC | RW 1.3812 |

If the seventh-character extension on the diagnosis code for the open wound of the knee is reported mistakenly as "D" Subsequent Encounter, the MS-DRG changes to 941 O.R. Procedure with Diagnoses of Other Contact with Health Services without CC/MCC (RW 1.3589).

MDC 10 Endocrine, Nutritional and Metabolic Diseases and Disorders

OPERATIVE REPORT MDC 10—#1

Preoperative diagnosis:
Left thyroid mass

Postoperative diagnosis:
Carcinoma of the left thyroid lobe, possible Hürthle cell, possible papillary.

Indications:
The patient noted a large lump in the left side of the neck. On evaluation by the primary physician, it was felt this was a solid lesion. It was cold on thyroid scanning. The patient was euthyroid. It was felt the patient needed surgical excision of this large mass by thyroid lobectomy, followed by subtotal or total thyroidectomy if carcinoma was identified.

Procedure description:
With the patient under satisfactory general anesthesia, the neck was prepped and draped in a sterile fashion.

A curvilinear incision was made along the skin lines above the sternal notch. The skin, subcutaneous tissue, and platysma were incised. Large subplatysmal flaps were created superiorly to the level of the thyroid notch and inferiorly to the level of the sternal notch. The strap muscles were split along the midline and retracted laterally. The large left thyroid lobe was dissected from its loose attachments laterally. The superior pole was taken down with ligatures of 2-0 silk and Hemoclips as needed. Mobilizing the lobe inferiorly similarly, the inferior pedicles were taken down with ligatures as well. Rotating the gland medially allowed visualization of the course of the recurrent laryngeal nerve. Hemoclips were used for hemostasis and control of any small tributaries. Following retraction of the entire gland off the trachea, the isthmus was divided with hemostatic ligatures of 2-0 silk. The isthmus was sent for pathologic examination. The pathologist identified carcinoma in the gland with features suggestive of Hürthle cell carcinoma or papillary. With this information, it was elected to proceed with a total thyroidectomy.

A similar dissection was carried out on the right side with the superior pedicle being controlled first with ligatures of 2-0 silk and Hemoclips. Laterally and inferiorly, the loose attachments were taken down. The inferior pedicle was subsequently divided in a similar manner as the superior pedicle. Rotating the gland medially and identifying the course of the recurrent laryngeal nerve, a superior parathyroid gland was found, dissected off the thyroid gland, and left intact. Hemostasis was again achieved with Hemoclips. A small tributary that was entered in the gland during the dissection was kept on top of the thyroid gland all the way through. Again, the peritracheal attachments were taken down with ligatures of 2-0 silk. The isthmus was also removed separately.

Both sides of the neck were checked for hemostasis, thoroughly lavaged, and pressure reevaluated. No evidence of bleeding or oozing was noted. The wound was closed with the strap muscles, then closed with 3-0 Vicryl. The platysmal flaps were closed with 3-0 Vicryl as well. The skin was closed with 4-0 Prolene subcuticular suture.

The patient tolerated the procedure well. The patient was taken to the recovery room in satisfactory condition. The patient had good vocal cord function in the recovery room.

Code all relevant ICD-10-CM diagnosis and ICD-10-PCS procedure codes in accordance with official guidelines and coding conventions.

Diagnosis Codes:

_____

_____

Procedure Codes:

_____

_____

MS-DRG:

_____

_____

Answers and Rationale

Preoperative diagnosis:
Left thyroid mass

Postoperative diagnosis:
Carcinoma of the left thyroid lobe, possible Hürthle cell, possible papillary.[1]

Indications:
The patient noted a large lump in the left side of the neck. On evaluation by the primary physician, it was felt this was a solid lesion. It was cold on thyroid scanning. The patient was euthyroid. It was felt the patient needed surgical excision of this large mass by thyroid lobectomy, followed by subtotal or total thyroidectomy if carcinoma was identified.[2]

Procedure description:
With the patient under satisfactory general anesthesia, the neck was prepped and draped in a sterile fashion.

A curvilinear incision was made along the skin lines above the sternal notch. The skin, subcutaneous tissue, and platysma were incised. Large subplatysmal flaps were created superiorly to the level of the thyroid notch and inferiorly to the level of the sternal notch. The strap muscles were split along the midline and retracted laterally. The large left thyroid lobe was dissected from its loose attachments laterally.[2] The superior pole was taken down with ligatures of 2-0 silk and Hemoclips as needed. Mobilizing the lobe inferiorly similarly, the inferior pedicles were taken down with ligatures as well. Rotating the gland medially allowed visualization of the course of the recurrent laryngeal nerve. Hemoclips were used for hemostasis and control of any small tributaries. Following retraction of the entire gland off the trachea, the isthmus was divided with hemostatic ligatures of 2-0 silk. The isthmus was sent for pathologic examination. The pathologist identified carcinoma in the gland[1] with features suggestive of Hürthle cell carcinoma or papillary. With this information, it was elected to proceed with a total thyroidectomy.[2]

A similar dissection was carried out on the right side[2] with the superior pedicle being controlled first with ligatures of 2-0 silk and Hemoclips. Laterally and inferiorly, the loose attachments were taken down. The inferior pedicle was subsequently divided in a similar manner as the superior pedicle. Rotating the gland medially and identifying the course of the recurrent laryngeal nerve, a superior parathyroid gland was found, dissected off the thyroid gland, and left intact. Hemostasis was again achieved with Hemoclips. A small tributary that was entered in the gland during the dissection was kept on top of the thyroid gland all the way through. Again, the peritracheal attachments were taken down with ligatures of 2-0 silk. The isthmus was also removed separately.

Both sides of the neck were checked for hemostasis, thoroughly lavaged, and pressure reevaluated. No evidence of bleeding or oozing was noted. The wound was closed with the strap muscles, then closed with 3-0 Vicryl. The platysmal flaps were closed with 3-0 Vicryl as well. The skin was closed with 4-0 Prolene subcuticular suture.

The patient tolerated the procedure well. The patient was taken to the recovery room in satisfactory condition. The patient had good vocal cord function in the recovery room.

Diagnosis Codes

C73   **Malignant neoplasm of thyroid gland**[1]

Rationale for Diagnosis Codes
Although the specific type of carcinoma is not known, it is still specified that the tumor on the thyroid is malignant and therefore the first column (Malignant Primary) of the Neoplasm Table in ICD-10-CM should be used to report the thyroid carcinoma. If documented, add a secondary code to identify any dysfunction such as hypo or hyperthyroidism.

Procedure Codes

ØGTKØZZ   **Resection of Thyroid Gland, Open Approach**[2]

Rationale for Procedure Codes
Initially only the left lobe of the thyroid was excised. Following confirmation of a malignant diagnosis, the right lobe was then resected during the same operative episode. Reporting codes for the right lobe and the left lobe would be inappropriate as there is a body part character to represent the entire thyroid. Each lobe would be reported separately only if the lobes were removed during different operative sessions.

MS-DRG

627   **Thyroid, Parathyroid and Thyroglossal Procedures**   **RW 0.9108**
        without CC/MCC

☼ CODING AXIOM

ICD-10-PCS Official Guidelines for Coding and Reporting Section B3.8:

PCS contains specific body parts for anatomical subdivisions of a body part, such as lobes of the lungs or liver and regions of the intestine. Resection of the specific body part is coded whenever all of the body part is cut out or off, rather than coding Excision of a less specific body part.

OPERATIVE REPORT MDC 10—#2

Preoperative diagnosis:
Recalcitrant exogenous obesity

Postoperative diagnosis:
Recalcitrant exogenous obesity

Procedure performed:
Laparoscopic vertical sleeve gastrectomy

Indications:
A 38-year-old female with a BMI of 41.1 presents for laparoscopic vertical sleeve gastrectomy as treatment for morbid obesity.

Procedure description:
The patient was transported to the operative suite, prepped, and draped for surgery. Following appropriate anesthesia, a trocar was placed though an incision above the umbilicus, insufflating the abdominal cavity. The laparoscope and additional trocars were placed through small portal incisions in the abdomen. The stomach was visualized and divided through the greater curvature, from the left crus of the diaphragm to a point distal to the pylorus. The short gastric vessels were coagulated, and gastric staplers were used. A gastric tube was formed and the remaining 80 percent of the stomach was excised without incident. The instruments were removed and the incisions were closed.

Code all relevant ICD-10-CM diagnosis and ICD-10-PCS procedure codes in accordance with official guidelines and coding conventions.

Diagnosis Codes:
_____

_____

Procedure Codes:
_____

_____

MS-DRG:
_____

_____

Answers and Rationale

Preoperative diagnosis:
Recalcitrant exogenous obesity[1]

Postoperative diagnosis:
Recalcitrant exogenous obesity

Procedure performed:
Laparoscopic vertical sleeve gastrectomy[3]

Indications:
A 38-year-old female with a BMI of 41.1[2] presents for laparoscopic vertical sleeve gastrectomy as treatment for morbid obesity.[1]

Procedure description:
The patient was transported to the operative suite, prepped and draped for surgery. Following appropriate anesthesia, a trocar was placed though an incision above the umbilicus, insufflating the abdominal cavity. The laparoscope and additional trocars were placed through small portal incisions in the abdomen.[3] The stomach was visualized and divided through the greater curvature, from the left crus of the diaphragm to a point distal to the pylorus. The short gastric vessels were coagulated, and gastric staplers were used. A gastric tube was formed and the remaining 80 percent of the stomach was excised[3] without incident. The instruments were removed and the incisions were closed.

Diagnosis Codes

E66.01   Morbid (severe) obesity due to excess calories[1]

Z68.41   Body mass index (BMI) 40.0-44.9, adult[2]

Rationale for Diagnosis Codes

The patient's obesity is described as morbid in the indications section of the operative note. Neither the term recalcitrant nor exogenous provides enough detail or information that would clarify which obesity code is correct. The default code for morbid obesity is E66.01. There is a code also note for this category that instructs the user to include a code for the body mass index (BMI) if known. In this case, the BMI is documented as 41.1.

Procedure Codes

0DB64Z3   Excision of Stomach, Percutaneous Endoscopic Approach, Vertical[3]

Rationale for Procedure Codes

The procedure is pretty straightforward in that the laparoscope is inserted and 80 percent of the stomach is removed to form a tube or sleeve. Note that the seventh-character value 3 is used as the physician states that this was a "vertical sleeve gastrectomy."

MS-DRG

621   O.R. Procedures for Obesity without CC/MCC   RW 1.5484

It is important to note that while normally code Z68.41 Body mass index (BMI) 40.0-44.9, adult, is a CC, this code is excluded as a CC with a principal diagnosis of E66.01 Morbid (severe) obesity due to excess calories.

 DEFINITIONS

BMI. Body mass index. Tool for calculating weight appropriateness in adults. The Centers for Disease Control and Prevention places adult BMIs in the following categories: below 18.5, underweight; 18.5-24.9, normal; 25.0-29.9 overweight; 30.0 and above, obese. BMI may be a factor in determining medical necessity for bariatric procedures.

morbid obesity. Accumulation of excess fat in the subcutaneous connective tissue with increased weight beyond the limits of skeletal requirements, defined as 125 percent or more over the ideal body weight. It is often associated with serious conditions that can become life threatening, such as diabetes, hypertension, and arteriosclerosis.

OPERATIVE REPORT MDC 10—#3

Preoperative diagnosis:
Pheochromocytoma

Postoperative diagnosis:
Adrenal cortical carcinoma

Procedure performed:
Adrenalectomy

Indications:
The patient is a 71-year-old gentleman who presented with poorly controlled hypertension and a large right adrenal mass with presumptive diagnosis of pheochromocytoma, who now presents for resection.

Procedure description:
The patient was brought to the operating room and intubated without difficulty. After adequate positioning, the patient was prepped and draped in standard fashion. Incision was then made in the midclavicular line and approximately 6 cm inferior to the subcostal margin. Veress needle was inserted in the abdominal cavity and pneumoinsufflation was obtained to a partial pressure of 15 mmHg. Under direct visualization an 11 mm trocar and port was placed in the right anterior axillary line as well as several other trocars placed along the subcostal margin approximately 4 cm inferior. The right lobe of the liver was retracted anteriorly, and the triangular ligament from the origin of the adrenal gland to up toward the diaphragm was taken down. Visualization was somewhat difficult as this was a larger tumor. The tumor was not able to be retracted using the grasper therefore the procedure was converted to a GelPort technique.

A large incision was then made between the subcostal margin and the anterior superior iliac spine, carried down to the subcutaneous tissue, after which GelPort was deployed. Then the gland was retracted laterally by hand. Mobilization was continued until the adrenal vein was encountered and divided. Mobilization was continued inferiorly. Unexpectedly it appeared that the adrenal gland was densely adherent to the lateral wall of the vena cava. At this point it became prudent to convert to an open procedure given the probability that this was eroding into the vena cava. Therefore, an incision was made along the line of the trocars sharply with 10 blade, carried down to subcutaneous tissue and the musculature with the electrocautery device. The superior gland was then mobilized. The plane was extremely difficult; therefore, dissection had to begin laterally. The peritoneum and then subsequently the lateral attachments were taken down with harmonic shears. Mobilization was continued inferiorly until the superior renal artery was encountered. Unfortunately, this was included with the tumor and therefore was taken down with a clamp, cut and tie technique using 3-0 Vicryl ties. Mobilization then continued towards the inferior aspect and subsequently the medial aspect. The renal artery, or at least a portion of the renal artery, was draped up very close to this tumor but was able to be dissected away sharply. There was a small side branch encountered directly off the cava that did have some bleeding that was controlled with a 5-0 Prolene suture ligature. Posterior dissection was then started. This was tedious at times and there were multiple vessels present. These were controlled with a clamp, cut and tie technique using 3-0 Vicryl ties. The gland was rocked directly up onto the cava. At this point the lateral aspect of the vena cava was completely isolated, and there was simply no plane between the tumor and the cava. Therefore, a side-biting Satinsky clamp was selected. A portion of the lateral aspect of the vena cava was then occluded, after which a resection of the vena cava with Metzenbaum scissors was performed. This was then sent for frozen section. A venorrhaphy was performed with a running 5-0 Prolene suture. The vena cava was inspected. The staple line was noted to be hemostatic. Copious irrigation ensued without active bleeding. The internal oblique and transversalis fascia was then closed with a #1 PDS in running fashion. External oblique was closed with #1 skin staples. A sterile dressing was applied. The patient tolerated the procedure well. There were no complications. Sponge and needle counts were correct x2. Estimated blood loss was less than 50 ml. The patient was extubated in the operating room and transferred to the post anesthesia care unit in stable condition.

Code all relevant ICD-10-CM diagnosis and ICD-10-PCS procedure codes in accordance with official guidelines and coding conventions.

Diagnosis Codes:

_____

_____

Procedure Codes:

_____

_____

MS-DRG:

_____

_____

Answers and Rationale

Preoperative diagnosis:
Pheochromocytoma

Postoperative diagnosis:
Adrenal cortical carcinoma[1]

Procedure performed:
Adrenalectomy

Indications:
The patient is a 71-year-old gentleman who presented with poorly controlled hypertension[2] and a large right adrenal mass[1,3,4] with presumptive diagnosis of pheochromocytoma, who now presents for resection.

Procedure description:
The patient was brought to the operating room and intubated without difficulty. After adequate positioning, the patient was prepped and draped in standard fashion. Incision was then made in the midclavicular line and approximately 6 cm inferior to the subcostal margin. Veress needle was inserted in the abdominal cavity and pneumoinsufflation was obtained to a partial pressure of 15 mmHg. Under direct visualization an 11 mm trocar and port was placed in the right anterior axillary line as well as several other trocars placed along the subcostal margin approximately 4 cm inferior. The right lobe of the liver was retracted anteriorly, and the triangular ligament from the origin of the adrenal gland to up toward the diaphragm was taken down. Visualization was somewhat difficult as this was a larger tumor. The tumor was not able to be retracted using the grasper therefore the procedure was converted to a GelPort technique.

A large incision was then made between the subcostal margin and the anterior superior iliac spine, carried down to the subcutaneous tissue, after which GelPort was deployed. Then the gland was retracted laterally by hand. Mobilization was continued until the adrenal vein was encountered and divided. Mobilization was continued inferiorly. Unexpectedly it appeared that the adrenal gland was densely adherent to the lateral wall of the vena cava.[4] At this point it became prudent to convert to an open procedure given the probability that this was eroding into the vena cava. Therefore, an incision was made along the line of the trocars sharply with 10 blade, carried down to subcutaneous tissue and the musculature with the electrocautery device.[3,5] The superior gland was then mobilized. The plane was extremely difficult; therefore, dissection had to begin laterally. The peritoneum and then subsequently the lateral attachments were taken down with harmonic shears. Mobilization was continued inferiorly until the superior renal artery was encountered. Unfortunately, this was included with the tumor and therefore was taken down with a clamp, cut and tie technique using 3-0 Vicryl ties. Mobilization then continued towards the inferior aspect and subsequently the medial aspect. The renal artery, or at least a portion of the renal artery, was draped up very close to this tumor but was able to be dissected away sharply. There was a small side branch encountered directly off the cava that did have some bleeding that was controlled with a 5-0 Prolene suture ligature. Posterior dissection was then started. This was tedious at times and there were multiple vessels present. These were controlled with a clamp, cut and tie technique using 3-0 Vicryl ties. The gland was rocked directly up onto the cava. At this point the lateral aspect of the vena cava was completely isolated, and there was simply no plane between the tumor and the cava. Therefore, a side-biting Satinsky clamp was selected. A portion of the lateral aspect of the vena cava was then occluded, after which a resection of the vena cava with Metzenbaum scissors was performed.[3,5] This was then sent for frozen section. A venorrhaphy was performed with a running 5-0 Prolene suture. The vena cava was inspected. The staple line was noted to be hemostatic. Copious irrigation ensued without active bleeding. The internal oblique and transversalis fascia was then closed with a #1 PDS in running fashion. External oblique was closed with #1 skin staples. A sterile dressing was applied. The patient tolerated the procedure well. There were no complications. Sponge and needle counts were correct x2. Estimated blood loss was less than 50 ml. The patient was extubated in the operating room and transferred to the post anesthesia care unit in stable condition.

Diagnosis Codes

C74.Ø1	Malignant neoplasm of cortex of right adrenal gland[1]
I1Ø	Essential (primary) hypertension[2]

Rationale for Diagnosis Codes

The terms "Carcinoma, Cortical Adrenal" in the ICD-10-CM index list code C74.0-. The tabular indicates that the fifth character should be 1 to indicate that the carcinoma is of the right adrenal gland.

Procedure Codes

0GT30ZZ   **Resection of Right Adrenal Gland, Open Approach**[3]

0GN34ZZ   **Release Right Adrenal Gland, Percutaneous Endoscopic Approach**[4]

06B00ZZ   **Excision of Inferior Vena Cava, Open Approach**[5]

Rationale for Procedure Codes

The procedure started as a laparoscopic procedure and was converted to an open procedure. According to *ICD-10-PCS Official Guidelines for Coding and Reporting* sections B3.2.d and B3.3, if a procedure is converted from one approach to another two codes are required, one for the discontinued procedure and one for the final procedure. During the laparoscopic portion of the procedure, the right adrenal gland was mobilized, which coincides with the root operation *Release*. The resection of the gland was completed during the open phase of the procedure. Also it should be noted that in this case, an additional procedure was performed because the tumor has infiltrated the vena cava. Therefore, a portion of that organ also needed to be removed, which should be reported.

MS-DRG

615	Adrenal and Pituitary Procedures without CC/MCC	RW 1.4254

CODING AXIOM

ICD-10-PCS Official Guidelines for Coding and Reporting

Section B3.2.d:

During the same operative episode, multiple procedures are coded if: The intended root operation is attempted using one approach, but is converted to a different approach.

Section B3.3:

If the intended procedure is discontinued, code the procedure to the root operation performed. If a procedure is discontinued before any other root operation is performed, code the root operation Inspection of the body part or anatomical region inspected.

DEFINITIONS

BKA. Below-the-knee amputation.

OPERATIVE REPORT MDC 10—#4

Preoperative diagnosis:
Nonhealing diabetic right foot ulcer

Postoperative diagnosis:
Same

Procedure performed:
BKA

Indications:
The patient is a 68-year-old male a long-standing history of type I diabetes mellitus. He has nonhealing ulcers of bilateral feet and has been seeing wound care for many years for debridement and whirlpool treatments. The patient failed conservation attempts and was admitted for amputation of the right foot for worsening diabetic foot ulcers and bone necrosis.

Procedure description:
The patient was taken to the operating room and placed on the operating room table in the right lateral decubitus position. Spinal anesthesia was induced. The patient was placed supine and the right leg was prepped and draped in the usual sterile fashion. It should be noted that a tourniquet was applied but was not necessary during surgery. A transmetatarsal incision with a 10-blade scalpel was made around the foot. There was no bleeding or viable tissue at this site so at this point a midfoot amputation was aborted and a below-the-knee amputation was opted for. Attention was turned to the mid-tibia area and a circumferential incision was made here, leaving more posterior skin for ample closure. The incision was then carried down further into the soft tissue, fascia, muscles, and tendons, clamping blood vessels as needed. The peroneal and tibial nerves were located and divided proximally. The peroneal and tibial arteries were identified and tied off. An oscillating hand saw was used to cut the tibia approximately 3 cm proximal to the skin incision and the fibula 2 cm above this. The ends of both bones were rasped to smooth the surface and edges. Hemostasis was obtained and the wound was closed in layers. Sterile dressings were placed. There were no complications. The patient was transported to the post-anesthesia recovery unit in fair condition.

Code all relevant ICD-10-CM diagnosis and ICD-10-PCS procedure codes in accordance with official guidelines and coding conventions.

Diagnosis Codes:

_____

_____

Procedure Codes:

_____

_____

MS-DRG:

_____

_____

Answers and Rationale

Preoperative diagnosis:
Nonhealing diabetic right foot ulcer[1]

Postoperative diagnosis:
Same

Procedure performed:
BKA[3]

Indications:
The patient is a 68-year-old male a long-standing history of type I diabetes mellitus.[1] He has nonhealing ulcers of bilateral feet and has been seeing wound care for many years for debridement and whirlpool treatments. The patient failed conservation attempts and was admitted for amputation[4] of the right foot for worsening diabetic foot ulcers[1] and bone necrosis.[2]

Procedure description:
The patient was taken to the operating room and placed on the operating room table in the right lateral decubitus position. Spinal anesthesia was induced. The patient was placed supine and the right leg was prepped and draped in the usual sterile fashion. It should be noted that a tourniquet was applied but was not necessary during surgery. A transmetatarsal incision with a 10-blade scalpel was made around the foot. There was no bleeding or viable tissue at this site so at this point a midfoot amputation was aborted and a below-the-knee amputation was opted for. Attention was turned to the mid-tibia area and a circumferential incision was made here, leaving more posterior skin for ample closure. The incision was then carried down further into the soft tissue, fascia, muscles, and tendons, clamping blood vessels as needed. The peroneal and tibial nerves were located and divided proximally. The peroneal and tibial arteries were identified and tied off. An oscillating hand saw was used to cut the tibia approximately 3 cm proximal to the skin incision and the fibula 2 cm above this.[3] The ends of both bones were rasped to smooth the surface and edges. Hemostasis was obtained and the wound was closed in layers. Sterile dressings were placed. There were no complications. The patient was transported to the post-anesthesia recovery unit in fair condition.

Diagnosis Codes

E10.621 **Type 1 diabetes mellitus with foot ulcer**[1]

L97.514 **Non-pressure chronic ulcer of other part of right foot with necrosis of bone**[2]

Rationale for Diagnosis Codes
Diabetic foot ulcers require two codes to fully report the condition. This is noted in the instructional notes under category E10.621, which instruct the coder to use an additional code to specify the site of the ulcer, and those under category L97, which direct the coder to code first any associated underlying condition of the ulcer. The preoperative diagnosis section of the operative report links the type I diabetes to the foot ulcer, making it necessary to report the code for the diabetic foot ulcer first. The report further details that the ulcer includes bone necrosis; this is included in the ulcer code and does not require an additional code. It is important to note that if the ulcer were specified as the heel or midfoot, the code from L97 would describe a complication/comorbidity (CC). However, the code supported by the documentation (unspecified site of foot) provided does not describe a CC.

Procedure Codes

0Y6H0Z2 **Detachment at Right Lower Leg, Mid, Open Approach**[3]

Rationale for Procedure Codes
The term "Amputation" in the ICD-10-PCS index references the root operation "Detachment." In this case it is documented as a below-the-knee amputation at the mid-tibial level, leading to the lower extremity section. The body part character H specifies right lower leg, and the qualifier character value 2 indicates that the amputation occurred at the mid-lower leg. No code is needed for the first incision, and the multiple-procedure guideline (*ICD-10-PCS Official Guidelines for Coding and Reporting*, section B3.3) does not apply since the intended procedure was not discontinued; instead, it was performed with the same intent and approach but just at a higher anatomical site.

☼ CODING AXIOM

ICD-10-CM Official Guidelines for Coding and Reporting Section I.A.13:

Certain conditions have both an underlying etiology and multiple body system manifestations due to the underlying etiology. For such conditions, the ICD-10-CM has a coding convention that requires the underlying condition be sequenced first followed by the manifestation. Wherever such a combination exists, there is a "use additional code" note at the etiology code, and a "code first" note at the manifestation code. These instructional notes indicate the proper sequencing order of the codes, etiology followed by manifestation.

☼ CODING AXIOM

ICD-10-PCS Official Guidelines for Coding and Reporting Section B3.3:

If the intended procedure is discontinued, code the procedure to the root operation performed. If a procedure is discontinued before any other root operation is performed, code the root operation Inspection of the body part or anatomical region inspected.

MS-DRG

618   **Amputation of Lower Limb for Endocrine, Nutritional,**   RW 1.1804
        and Metabolic Disorders without CC/MCC

If the site of the foot ulcer were documented as midfoot or heel rather than not specified, the MS-DRG would change to 617 Amputation of Lower Limb for Endocrine, Nutritional, and Metabolic Disorders with CC (RW 2.0064).

MDC 11 Diseases and Disorders of the Kidney and Urinary Tract

OPERATIVE REPORT MDC 11—#1

Preoperative diagnoses:
Left ureteral stricture

Postoperative diagnoses:
Left ureteral stricture

Procedure description:
The patient presented with a previously identified stricture of the distal left ureter. The patient was placed prone on the imaging table, and the area over the left flank was prepped and draped in typical sterile fashion. Using ultrasound guidance, the needle was advanced into the distal portion of the collecting system of the left kidney. A glidewire was advanced through the needle and under fluoroscopic guidance was directed down the ureter. The tract was then serially dilated and an 8 French sheath was placed into the collecting system. Contrast was injected, demonstrating a dilated renal pelvis and the area of stricture in the distal ureter. The glidewire was then inserted and guided through the stricture into the bladder. A double J 8 French ureteral catheter was then guided through the area of stricture and advanced into the bladder. Contrast was injected through the sheath and demonstrated satisfactory placement of the stent with good flow through the catheter. The glidewire was withdrawn, looping the proximal end of the ureteral stent in the renal pelvis. A separate nephrostomy drainage catheter was then placed in the renal pelvis and left to external drainage. The catheter was secured to the skin and a sterile bandage applied over the site. There were no complications and the patient left the department in satisfactory condition.

Code all relevant ICD-10-CM diagnosis and ICD-10-PCS procedure codes in accordance with official guidelines and coding conventions.

Diagnosis Codes:

_____

_____

Procedure Codes:

_____

_____

MS-DRG:

_____

_____

Answers and Rationale

Preoperative diagnoses:
Left ureteral stricture

Postoperative diagnoses:
Left ureteral stricture[1]

Procedure description:
The patient presented with a previously identified stricture of the distal left ureter. The patient was placed prone on the imaging table, and the area over the left flank was prepped and draped in typical sterile fashion. Using ultrasound guidance, the needle was advanced into the distal portion of the collecting system of the left kidney.[2,3] A glidewire was advanced through the needle and under fluoroscopic guidance was directed down the ureter. The tract was then serially dilated[3] and an 8 French sheath was placed into the collecting system. Contrast was injected, demonstrating a dilated renal pelvis and the area of stricture in the distal ureter. The glidewire was then inserted and guided through the stricture into the bladder. A double J 8 French ureteral catheter was then guided through the area of stricture and advanced into the bladder. Contrast was injected through the sheath and demonstrated satisfactory placement of the stent with good flow through the catheter. The glidewire was withdrawn, looping the proximal end of the ureteral stent in the renal pelvis.[3] A separate nephrostomy drainage catheter was then placed in the renal pelvis and left to external drainage.[2] The catheter was secured to the skin and a sterile bandage applied over the site. There were no complications and the patient left the department in satisfactory condition.

Diagnosis Codes

N13.5   **Crossing vessel and stricture of ureter without hydronephrosis[1]**

Rationale for Diagnosis Codes

The term "Stricture, Ureter" in the ICD-10-CM index lists multiple selections for ureteral stricture based on documentation. Because there is no mention of hydronephrosis, infection, or pyelonephritis accompanying the stricture, code N13.5 is the appropriate selection.

Procedure Codes

ØT913ØZ   **Drainage of Left Kidney with Drainage Device, Percutaneous[2]**

ØT773DZ   **Dilation of Left Ureter with Intraluminal Device, Percutaneous[3]**

Rationale for Procedure Codes

The procedures were performed percutaneously, since the patient was placed in a prone position and the needle was inserted over the flank into the renal collecting system. There is no endoscope described in this operative note. A nephrostomy catheter is inserted for external drainage. According to the *ICD-10-PCS Official Guidelines for Coding and Reporting* section B6.2, "a separate procedure to put in a drainage device is coded to the root operation *Drainage* with the device value *Drainage Device.*" Dilation of the ureter occurs as well as a stent insertion into the left ureter. As the stent is placed for dilation, it is included in the dilation procedure code as the sixth character D Intraluminal device.

MS-DRG

661   **Kidney and Ureter Procedures for Non-neoplasm**   **RW 1.3981**
            without CC/MCC

DEFINITIONS

stricture. Narrowing of an anatomical structure.

OPERATIVE REPORT MDC 11—#2

Preoperative diagnosis:
ESRD

Postoperative diagnosis:
ESRD

Procedure performed:
Renal transplant

Indications:
This 45-year-old male with a history of type I diabetic end stage renal disease presented for kidney transplant. Induction therapy of 500 mg of Solu-Medrol and 20 mg Simulect was given intravenously prior to arrival in the operating room. The donor is the patient's cousin. Dr. Smith will be performing a right donor nephrectomy in the adjoining surgical suite.

Procedure description:
The patient was intubated and general anesthesia was induced. The patient's right groin area was prepped and draped in sterile fashion. A curvilinear incision in the right groin was made and dissection was carried down through the subcutaneous tissue and external oblique muscle. The peritoneum was accessed via an incision through the transverse abdominus muscle. The muscles were pulled back and held in place using a retractor. The inferior epigastric and round ligaments were ligated. The right external iliac artery and vein were exposed. The lymphatics anterior to the artery were clamped. The donor kidney with one artery and one vein was received after having been prepped in the adjoining operating suite. The donor ureter was cleaned off and the artery and vein were separated. Dopamine was started. Vascular clamps were placed on both the vein and the artery. A 4 mm coronary punch was used to make an arteriotomy in the right renal artery. An end-to-side anastomosis with the right external iliac vein was performed utilizing 5-0 Prolene running sutures. This same procedure was performed on the right renal vein, and again anastomosis to the right external iliac vein was performed. 80 mg of Lasix and 12 mg of Mannitol were given intravenously. The vascular clamps were released. The kidney had satisfactory color and was perfusing properly. The kidney was then irrigated with warm saline, and urine was made on the table signifying proper kidney function. The retractors were repositioned for better access to the bladder. The ureter was cut short and an extravesical bladder anastomosis was made with a running 5-0 Prolene suture. A JP drain was inserted. The fascia and muscular layers were closed as in a layered fashion using #1 PDS suture. 3-0 Vicryl were used to close the subcutaneous tissue and staples for the skin. The patient was extubated and taken to the recovery room in satisfactory condition.

Code all relevant ICD-10-CM diagnosis and ICD-10-PCS procedure codes in accordance with official guidelines and coding conventions.

Diagnosis Codes:

_____

_____

Procedure Codes:

_____

_____

MS-DRG:

_____

_____

☼ **CODING AXIOM**

ICD-10-CM Official Guidelines for Coding and Reporting Section I.B.7:

"Use additional code" notes are found in the Tabular List at codes that are not part of an etiology/manifestation pair where a secondary code is useful to fully describe a condition. The sequencing rule is the same as the etiology/manifestation pair, "use additional code" indicates that a secondary code should be added.

Answers and Rationale

Preoperative diagnosis:
ESRD

Postoperative diagnosis:
ESRD

Procedure performed:
Renal transplant

Indications:
This 45-year-old male with a history of type I diabetic end stage renal disease[1,2] presented for kidney transplant. Induction therapy of 500 mg of Solu-Medrol and 20 mg Simulect was given intravenously prior to arrival in the operating room. The donor is the patient's cousin.[3] Dr. Smith will be performing a right donor nephrectomy in the adjoining surgical suite.

Procedure description:
The patient was intubated and general anesthesia was induced. The patient's right groin area was prepped and draped in sterile fashion. A curvilinear incision in the right groin was made and dissection was carried down through the subcutaneous tissue and external oblique muscle. The peritoneum was accessed via an incision through the transverse abdominus muscle.[3] The muscles were pulled back and held in place using a retractor. The inferior epigastric and round ligaments were ligated. The right external iliac artery and vein were exposed. The lymphatics anterior to the artery were clamped. The donor kidney with one artery and one vein was received after having been prepped in the adjoining operating suite.[3] The donor ureter was cleaned off and the artery and vein were separated. Dopamine was started. Vascular clamps were placed on both the vein and the artery. A 4 mm coronary punch was used to make an arteriotomy in the right renal artery. An end-to-side anastomosis with the right external iliac vein was performed utilizing 5-0 Prolene running sutures. This same procedure was performed on the right renal vein, and again anastomosis to the right external iliac vein was performed. 80 mg of Lasix and 12 mg of Mannitol were given intravenously. The vascular clamps were released. The kidney had satisfactory color and was perfusing properly. The kidney was then irrigated with warm saline, and urine was made on the table signifying proper kidney function.[3] The retractors were repositioned for better access to the bladder. The ureter was cut short and an extravesical bladder anastomosis was made with a running 5-0 Prolene suture. A JP drain was inserted. The fascia and muscular layers were closed as in a layered fashion using #1 PDS suture. 3-0 Vicryl were used to close the subcutaneous tissue and staples for the skin. The patient was extubated and taken to the recovery room in satisfactory condition.

Diagnosis Codes

E10.22   Type 1 diabetes mellitus with diabetic chronic kidney disease[1]

N18.6   End-stage renal disease[2]

Rationale for Diagnosis Codes
End-stage renal disease is the final stage of chronic kidney disease. In the indications section of the operative note, the physician states that the ESRD is the result of type I diabetes. Therefore, according to the conventions in the ICD-10-CM Tabular List, the code for diabetes with diabetic chronic kidney disease should be reported first followed by a code identifying the ESRD. Although there is a "use additional code" note under N18.6 that instructs the coder to report dialysis status, there is no documentation of dialysis in this instance. Therefore reporting Z99.2 Dependence on renal dialysis, would be incorrect.

Procedure Codes

0TY00Z0   Transplantation of Right Kidney, Allogeneic, Open Approach[3]

Rationale for Procedure Codes
A transplant entails receiving all or a portion of a body part from another individual (or animal) to replace that body part that is dysfunctioning. In this case, the donor was the patient's cousin, making the qualifier (character value 7) *Allogenic*. The donor nephrectomy would not be reported here as it involves a different patient with a different encounter.

MS-DRG

652   Kidney Transplant   RW 3.1540

OPERATIVE REPORT MDC 11—#3

Preoperative diagnosis:
Left renal calculus

Postoperative diagnosis:
Left renal calculus

Procedure performed:
ESWL

Indications:
A stone measuring 4 mm located in the left upper calyx was visualized on imaging.

Procedure description:
A scout film was taken in the AP projection and the approximate position of the stone was marked on the patient's abdomen. The patient was then positioned over the plenum and coupled with mineral oil and water bag. X-ray exposures were then made in the oblique projection.

Stone position was determined and marked on exposed film. IV contrast was used for stone localization.

The targeted stone was then brought into the F2 focus using table coordinates generated by the computer digitizing process. Following position confirmation, treatment was begun. A total of 2000 shocks were administered at a power setting of 24 KV using EKG override. A total of 12 IRIS images and film were taken during the procedure to confirm stone targeting and to assess stone disintegration.

Post-treatment films showed indeterminate results.

The patient tolerated the procedure well and left the lithotripsy room in good condition. Antibiotics were not administered. Foley catheter was not used.

Code all relevant ICD-10-CM diagnosis and ICD-10-PCS procedure codes in accordance with official guidelines and coding conventions.

Diagnosis Codes:

_____

_____

Procedure Codes:

_____

_____

MS-DRG:

_____

_____

DEFINITIONS

ESWL. Extracorporeal shockwave lithotripsy. Destruction of calcified substances in the gallbladder or urinary system by means of directing shock waves at the calculus through a liquid medium to smash the concretion into small particles that can then be passed out of the body.

DEFINITIONS

external. ICD-10-PCS approach value X. Procedures performed directly on the skin or mucous membrane and procedures performed indirectly by the application of external force through the skin or mucous membrane.

fragmentation. ICD-10-PCS root operation value F. Breaking solid matter in a body part into pieces. Physical force (e.g., manual, ultrasonic) applied directly or indirectly is used to break the solid matter into pieces. The solid matter may be an abnormal byproduct of a biological function or a foreign body. The pieces of solid matter are not taken out.

Answers and Rationale

Preoperative diagnosis:
Left renal calculus

Postoperative diagnosis:
Left renal calculus[1]

Procedure performed:
ESWL

Indications:
A stone measuring 4 mm located in the left upper calyx was visualized on imaging.

Procedure description:
A scout film was taken in the AP projection and the approximate position of the stone was marked on the patient's abdomen. The patient was then positioned over the plenum and coupled with mineral oil and water bag. X-ray exposures were then made in the oblique projection.

Stone position was determined and marked on exposed film. IV contrast was used for stone localization.

The targeted stone was then brought into the F2 focus using table coordinates generated by the computer digitizing process. Following position confirmation, treatment was begun. A total of 2000 shocks were administered at a power setting of 24 KV using EKG override. A total of 12 IRIS images and film were taken during the procedure to confirm stone targeting and to assess stone disintegration.[2]

Post-treatment films showed indeterminate results.

The patient tolerated the procedure well and left the lithotripsy room in good condition. Antibiotics were not administered. Foley catheter was not used.

Diagnosis Codes

N20.0   **Calculus of kidney[1]**

Rationale for Diagnosis Codes
Coding a renal calculus (also known as a kidney stone) is straightforward when the ICD-10-CM index is referenced.

Procedure Codes

0TF4XZZ   **Fragmentation in Left Kidney Pelvis, External Approach[2]**

Rationale for Procedure Codes
Extracorporeal shockwave lithotripsy (ESWL) is performed to break a calculus into small pieces that can pass naturally and less painfully through the urinary tract. The objective of this procedure coincides with the ICD-10-PCS definition of *Fragmentation*. ESWL is performed externally by exposing the stone to shockwaves from outside the body. Therefore the approach value is X *External*.

Note: Based on *AHA Coding Clinic for ICD-10-CM and ICD-10-PCS*, second quarter 2015, page 7, if fragmentation (lithotripsy) is performed and the stone fragments are removed from the body, then *Extirpation* (removal of solid matter from a body part) would be coded instead of *Fragmentation*. *Extirpation* includes any previous fragmentation of the solid matter prior to removal.

MS-DRG

692   **Urinary Stones with ESW Lithotripsy without CC/MCC**   RW 1.2566

OPERATIVE REPORT MDC 11—#4

Preoperative diagnosis:
Transitional cell carcinoma of the bladder

Postoperative diagnosis:
Transitional cell carcinoma of the bladder

Procedure performed:
Cystoscopy with fulguration of greater than 5 cm of bladder tumor

Indications:
This is an 46-year-old male with a long history of transitional cell carcinoma with multiple recurrences and multiple resections. The patient's last procedure was 10 weeks ago when early in the resection his bladder was perforated and the procedure was terminated without completion of tumor resection. The patient presents now for complete resection.

Procedure description:
The patient was taken to the operating room where he received spinal anesthesia. However, as we were setting up the patient it was obvious that the spinal anesthesia had failed and at that time a general anesthetic with LMA was administered. The patient was then placed in the dorsal lithotomy position and prepped and draped in the usual sterile fashion.

A 21-French cystoscope was then inserted with the finding of a soft bulbar stricture, which was easily passed with the scope. Prostatic urethra was opened. Upon entering the bladder, there was a fairly large area of tumor evident on the posterior aspect extending up onto the dome and some at the anterior and right lateral bladder neck. This all appeared fairly superficial. We then switched to the resectoscope with the roller bar electrode through the resectoscope. We then proceeded to fulgurate all areas of evident tumor.

The patient tolerated this well. At the end of the case, a 16-French Foley catheter was inserted and the patient's urine was draining light pink. Drains consist only of a 16-French Foley catheter. There were no complications. The patient was extubated and taken to the post-anesthesia care unit in stable condition and then transferred to the floor for observation.

Code all relevant ICD-10-CM diagnosis and ICD-10-PCS procedure codes in accordance with official guidelines and coding conventions.

Diagnosis Codes:

_____

_____

Procedure Codes:

_____

_____

MS-DRG:

_____

_____

Answers and Rationale

Preoperative diagnosis:
Transitional cell carcinoma of the bladder

Postoperative diagnosis:
Transitional cell carcinoma of the bladder[1]

Procedure performed:
Cystoscopy with fulguration of greater than 5 cm of bladder tumor

Indications:
This is an 46-year-old male with a long history of transitional cell carcinoma with multiple recurrences and multiple resections. The patient's last procedure was 10 weeks ago when early in the resection his bladder was perforated and the procedure was terminated without completion of tumor resection. The patient presents now for complete resection.

Procedure description:
The patient was taken to the operating room where he received spinal anesthesia. However, as we were setting up the patient it was obvious that the spinal anesthesia had failed and at that time a general anesthetic with LMA was administered. The patient was then placed in the dorsal lithotomy position and prepped and draped in the usual sterile fashion.

A 21-French cystoscope was then inserted with the finding of a soft bulbar stricture, which was easily passed with the scope. Prostatic urethra was opened. Upon entering the bladder, there was a fairly large area of tumor evident on the posterior aspect extending up onto the dome and some at the anterior and right lateral bladder neck.[1-3] This all appeared fairly superficial. We then switched to the resectoscope with the roller bar electrode through the resectoscope. We then proceeded to fulgurate all areas of evident tumor.[2,3]

The patient tolerated this well. At the end of the case, a 16-French Foley catheter was inserted and the patient's urine was draining light pink. Drains consist only of a 16-French Foley catheter. There were no complications. The patient was extubated and taken to the post-anesthesia care unit in stable condition and then transferred to the floor for observation.

Diagnosis Codes

C67.8   **Malignant neoplasm of overlapping sites of bladder[1]**

Rationale for Diagnosis Codes
The transitional cell carcinoma is specified as being on the posterior aspect extending up onto the dome and some at the anterior and right lateral bladder neck. The diagnosis code should reflect that these are considered "overlapping" sites of the bladder in ICD-10-CM.

Procedure Codes

ØT5B8ZZ   **Destruction of Bladder, Via Natural or Artificial Opening Endoscopic[2]**

ØT5C8ZZ   **Destruction of Bladder Neck, Via Natural or Artificial Opening Endoscopic[3]**

Rationale for Procedure Codes
It is important to note that the cystoscopy is not reported separately as it is done as part of the procedure. *Destruction* is the most appropriate root operation for a fulguration, according to the ICD-10-PCS index. Two codes are required to fully report the procedure because the areas involved are represented by two separate body part character values, B, *Bladder*, and C, *Bladder Neck*, as explained in *ICD-10-PCS Official Guidelines for Coding and Reporting* section B3.2.a. The cystoscope and resectoscope were both inserted via the urethra, making the approach *Via Natural or Artificial Opening Endoscopic*. As the physician already knew the lesion was transitional cell carcinoma, this was not a diagnostic procedure and a seventh character of X would be incorrect.

MS-DRG

670	Transurethral Procedures without CC/MCC	RW 0.9207

If the incorrect approach character value of Ø, *Open*, 3, *Percutaneous*, or 4, *Percutaneous Endoscopic* is used, the resulting MS-DRG would be incorrect.

🕯️ **CODING AXIOM**

ICD-10-PCS Official Guidelines for Coding and Reporting

Section B3.2.a:

During the same operative episode, multiple procedures are coded if:

- The same root operation is performed on different body parts as defined by distinct values of the body part character.

Section B3.11a:

Inspection of a body part(s) performed in order to achieve the objective of a procedure is not coded separately.

OPERATIVE REPORT MDC 11—#5

Preoperative diagnosis:
Benign prostatic hypertrophy

Postoperative diagnosis:
Benign prostatic hypertrophy

Procedure performed:
Transurethral microwave thermal therapy

Indications:
This is an 56-year-old male with BPH who is experiencing slow stream and urinary frequency.

Procedure description:
Moderate sedation was performed per moderate sedation protocol with EKG, pulse oximetry, and blood pressure monitoring. The patient underwent Prostaprobe insertion. Prostate ultrasound was performed. The patient's intraoperative verification was performed using both transabdominal and prostate ultrasound. The patient had no other evidence for abnormality. Initiated low wattage therapy using the 3.5 30 minute protocol on the Prostatron. The patient's tolerance was excellent. The Prostaprobe was removed with no complications or overt bleeding. The patient was sent to the recovery area in good condition.

Code all relevant ICD-10-CM diagnosis and ICD-10-PCS procedure codes in accordance with official guidelines and coding conventions.

Diagnosis Codes:

_____

_____

Procedure Codes:

_____

_____

MS-DRG:

_____

_____

Answers and Rationale

Preoperative diagnosis:
Benign prostatic hypertrophy

Postoperative diagnosis:
Benign prostatic hypertrophy[1]

Procedure performed:
Transurethral microwave thermal therapy[4]

Indications:
This is an 56-year-old male with BPH who is experiencing slow stream[2] and urinary frequency.[3]

Procedure description:
Moderate sedation was performed per moderate sedation protocol with EKG, pulse oximetry, and blood pressure monitoring. The patient underwent Prostaprobe insertion. Prostate ultrasound was performed. The patient's intraoperative verification was performed using both transabdominal and prostate ultrasound. The patient had no other evidence for abnormality. Initiated low wattage therapy using the 3.5 30 minute protocol on the Prostatron.[4] The patient's tolerance was excellent. The Prostaprobe was removed with no complications or overt bleeding. The patient was sent to the recovery area in good condition.

Diagnosis Codes

N40.1	**Enlarged prostate with lower urinary tract symptoms[1]**
R39.12	**Poor urinary stream[2]**
R35.0	**Frequency of micturition[3]**

Rationale for Diagnosis Codes
The terms "Hypertrophy, prostate" in the ICD-10-CM index directs the coder to see "Enlarged, Enlargement, Prostate." The coder then must choose whether the patient also has LUTS (lower urinary tract symptoms), which in this case he does, described by the documentation as slow stream and frequency. Therefore code N40.1 should be used. Additional codes should be reported for the specified LUTS according to the instructional note under N40.1.

Procedure Codes

0V507ZZ	**Destruction of Prostate, Via Natural or Artificial Opening[4]**

Rationale for Procedure Codes
When a portion of a body part is eradicated by the use of energy or force, the root operation is *Destruction*. In this case, the prostatic tissue was eradicated using microwave thermal therapy. The probe that delivers the microwave thermal therapy is inserted via the urethra with no mention of an endoscope, making the approach value 7, *Via Natural or Artificial Opening*.

MS-DRG

667	Prostatectomy without CC/MCC	RW 0.9964

DEFINITIONS

LUTS. Lower urinary tract symptoms.

micturition. Urination.

OPERATIVE REPORT MDC 11—#6

Preoperative diagnosis:
Stress urinary incontinence

Postoperative diagnosis:
Stress urinary incontinence

Procedure performed:
Pubovaginal sling

Indications:
The patient is a 45-year-old female with stress urinary incontinence.

Procedure description:
The patient was premedicated and received preoperative antibiotics. She was delivered to the operating room and spinal anesthesia was induced. She was placed in the dorsal lithotomy position and prepped and draped in the usual sterile fashion.

A weighted vaginal speculum was placed. A Lone Star retractor was positioned and a Foley catheter placed for drainage. The bladder was emptied. After the vaginal epithelium was infiltrated, an inverted U-shaped incision was made with the apex halfway between the bladder neck and the urethral meatus. The vaginal flap was developed all the way down to the bladder neck. Dissection was then carried down laterally at the level of the bladder neck and the retropubic space was entered bluntly. This space was enlarged and the Microvasive applicator was then used to place nickel titanium bone screws with #1 monofilament line.

The Foley catheter was removed. Standard cystoscopy was carried out to ensure the integrity of the bladder. A 2 x 8 cm segment of Repliform dermal graft was then prepared. The ends were folded over and tacked in place with 5-0 Vicryl. The suspension sutures were delivered through the folded-over ends using 19-gauge needle. The right side of the graft was first tied securely. The graft was then swung over and positioned properly with appropriate amount of support for the bladder neck. Throughout the procedure the surgical sites were irrigated with antibiotic solution.

There was no excessive tension on the urethra and bladder neck. I could easily pass an instrument between the urethra and the graft. After completing the suspension sutures, the edges of the graft were secured to the periurethral tissue with interrupted sutures of 5-0 Vicryl. The vaginal flap was then closed with running locking suture of 3-0 Vicryl antibiotic ointment soaked packing was placed per vagina.

The patient tolerated the procedure well and left the operating room in satisfactory condition.

Code all relevant ICD-10-CM diagnosis and ICD-10-PCS procedure codes in accordance with official guidelines and coding conventions.

Diagnosis Codes:

_____

_____

Procedure Codes:

_____

_____

MS-DRG:

_____

_____

Answers and Rationale

Preoperative diagnosis:
Stress urinary incontinence

Postoperative diagnosis:
Stress urinary incontinence[1]

Procedure performed:
Pubovaginal sling

Indications:
The patient is a 45-year-old female with stress urinary incontinence.

Procedure description:
The patient was premedicated and received preoperative antibiotics. She was delivered to the operating room and spinal anesthesia was induced. She was placed in the dorsal lithotomy position and prepped and draped in the usual sterile fashion.

A weighted vaginal speculum was placed. A Lone Star retractor was positioned and a Foley catheter placed for drainage. The bladder was emptied. After the vaginal epithelium was infiltrated, an inverted U-shaped incision was made with the apex halfway between the bladder neck and the urethral meatus. The vaginal flap was developed all the way down to the bladder neck. Dissection was then carried down laterally at the level of the bladder neck and the retropubic space was entered bluntly. This space was enlarged and the Microvasive applicator was then used to place nickel titanium bone screws with #1 monofilament line.

The Foley catheter was removed. Standard cystoscopy was carried out to ensure the integrity of the bladder. A 2 x 8 cm segment of Repliform dermal graft was then prepared. The ends were folded over and tacked in place with 5-0 Vicryl. The suspension sutures were delivered through the folded-over ends using 19-gauge needle. The right side of the graft was first tied securely. The graft was then swung over and positioned properly with appropriate amount of support for the bladder neck.[2] Throughout the procedure the surgical sites were irrigated with antibiotic solution.

There was no excessive tension on the urethra and bladder neck. I could easily pass an instrument between the urethra and the graft. After completing the suspension sutures, the edges of the graft were secured to the periurethral tissue with interrupted sutures of 5-0 Vicryl. The vaginal flap was then closed with running locking suture of 3-0 Vicryl antibiotic ointment soaked packing was placed per vagina.

The patient tolerated the procedure well and left the operating room in satisfactory condition.

Diagnosis Codes

N39.3   Stress incontinence (female) (male)[1]

Rationale for Diagnosis Codes
The coding of stress urinary incontinence is straightforward when looking up "Incontinence" in the ICD-10-CM index.

Procedure Codes

ØTUCØJZ   Supplement Bladder Neck with Synthetic Substitute, Open Approach[2]

Rationale for Procedure Codes
Although the term "Sling" in the ICD-10-PCS index leads the coder to the root operation *Reposition*, the operation does not include the placement of the graft. Because the graft was left in place at the end of the procedure, the root operation must reflect that a device was inserted. In this case, the root operation *Supplement* fits the scenario as the graft was put into place to reinforce the bladder neck. The procedure was performed via an *Open* approach. The graft used was a Repliform dermal graft, which is a synthetic substitute.

MS-DRG

664   Minor Bladder Procedures without CC/MCC   RW 1.2987

OPERATIVE REPORT MDC 11—#7

Pre- and postoperative diagnoses

- End-stage renal disease
- Type 1 diabetes

Operative procedure:

Creation of left radiocephalic arteriovenous fistula for dialysis access.

Procedure description:

After informed consent was obtained, the patient was taken to the operating room. The patient was placed in the supine position and received a regional nerve block and intravenous sedation. The left arm was prepped and draped in the usual sterile fashion.

A small transverse incision was made in the right cubital fossa. The cephalic vein was identified and mobilized proximally and distally. The fascia was incised, and the radial artery was also identified and mobilized proximally and distally. A good pulse was noted. The radial artery and cephalic vein were clamped. A longitudinal incision was made in the radial artery, and a longitudinal incision was made in the cephalic vein. The vessels were then sewn in a side-to-side fashion using a running 7-0 Prolene suture. The area was irrigated, and the anastomosis was then completed. We then ligated the cephalic vein beyond the arteriovenous anastomosis and divided it. This surrounded the anastomosis as an end-to-side functionally. Hemostasis was secured. We then closed the wound using interrupted PDS sutures for the fascia and a running 4-0 Monocryl subcuticular suture for the skin. Sterile dry dressing was applied. The patient tolerated the procedure well. There were no operative complications. The patient was transferred to the recovery room in satisfactory condition. A great thrill was felt in the fistula completion. There was also a palpable radial pulse distally.

Code all relevant ICD-10-CM diagnosis and ICD-10-PCS procedure codes in accordance with official guidelines and coding conventions.

Diagnosis Codes:

_____

_____

Procedure Codes:

_____

_____

MS-DRG:

_____

_____

Answers and Rationale

Pre- and postoperative diagnoses:

- End-stage renal disease[1]
- Type 1 diabetes[2]

Operative procedure:

Creation of left radiocephalic arteriovenous fistula for dialysis access.[3]

Procedure description:

After informed consent was obtained, the patient was taken to the operating room. The patient was placed in the supine position and received a regional nerve block and intravenous sedation. The left arm was prepped and draped in the usual sterile fashion.

A small transverse incision was made in the right cubital fossa. The cephalic vein was identified and mobilized proximally and distally. The fascia was incised, and the radial artery was also identified and mobilized proximally and distally. A good pulse was noted. The radial artery and cephalic vein were clamped. A longitudinal incision was made in the radial artery, and a longitudinal incision was made in the cephalic vein. The vessels were then sewn in a side-to-side fashion using a running 7-0 Prolene suture. The area was irrigated, and the anastomosis was then completed. We then ligated the cephalic vein beyond the arteriovenous anastomosis and divided it. This surrounded the anastomosis as an end-to-side functionally.[3] Hemostasis was secured. We then closed the wound using interrupted PDS sutures for the fascia and a running 4-0 Monocryl subcuticular suture for the skin. Sterile dry dressing was applied. The patient tolerated the procedure well. There were no operative complications. The patient was transferred to the recovery room in satisfactory condition. A great thrill was felt in the fistula completion. There was also a palpable radial pulse distally.

Diagnosis Codes:

N18.6   **End stage renal disease[1]**

E10.9   **Type 1 diabetes mellitus without complications[2]**

Rationale for Diagnosis Codes

The end-stage renal disease is the reason for the procedure. The documentation describes the creation of the fistula but does not specify that the patient had been on dialysis or was dialysis-dependent. Therefore, the coder cannot assume that the criteria are met to assign the code Z99.2 Dependence on renal dialysis. There is no documented connection between the diabetes and the renal disease, so the code for Type 1 diabetes uncomplicated should be reported in this instance.

Procedure Codes

031C0ZF   **Bypass Left Radial Artery to Lower Arm Vein, Open Approach[3]**

Rationale for Procedure Codes

The key to coding the creation of an arteriovenous fistula is to ascertain which vessel was bypassed to and which bypassed from, which determines whether the code is constructed from the upper artery or upper vein table. AHA's *Coding Clinic for ICD-10-CM and ICD-10-PCS* first quarter 2013, page 28, states, "In the context of hemodialysis access, blood flow is generally bypassed from the artery to the vein (high pressure system to low pressure system)." The procedure was performed with an open approach and no device was used.

MS-DRG

675	Other Kidney and Urinary Tract Procedures without CC/MCC	RW 1.5595

MDC 12 Diseases and Disorders of the Male Reproductive System

Operative Report MDC 12—#1

Preoperative diagnoses:
Desired sterilization

Postoperative diagnoses:
Same

Procedure description:
Vasectomy

Procedure description:
The patient was placed in a supine position on the procedure table, and the surgical assistant cleaned the scrotal area with iodine. The assistant placed elastic around the penis and clipped the elastic to the patient's shirt to expose the scrotum. The patient was then draped in the usual manner. No needle anesthetic (nna) was administered. Once the area was frozen, the physician located the vas deferens tubes one at a time. The physician gently held each vas tube between his fingertips, grasping them with a specially designed ringed clamp. Using special forceps, the physician made one tiny puncture into the skin on the scrotum. Using the same instrument, the first vas tube was lifted gently out through this opening. Once the vas was lifted out of the scrotum, it was cut and both ends were cauterized. The fascial sheath was tied around one end of the cut tube, creating a natural barrier between the two cut ends. The testicular end was left open to reduce the risk of post-vasectomy pain. The separated and blocked ends were returned to the scrotum, and the same procedure was done through the same small opening on the other side. The opening was finally covered with a gauze pad. The one small skin opening will close itself without stitches.

Code all relevant ICD-10-CM diagnosis and ICD-10-PCS procedure codes in accordance with official guidelines and coding conventions.

Diagnosis Codes:

_____

_____

Procedure Codes:

_____

_____

MS-DRG:

_____

_____

Definitions

no needle anesthetic (nna). An air jet injector that delivers a spray of anesthetic under high pressure through the skin.

Answers and Rationale

Preoperative diagnoses:
Desired sterilization[1]

Postoperative diagnoses:
Same

Procedure description:
Vasectomy[2]

Procedure description:
The patient was placed in a supine position on the procedure table, and the surgical assistant cleaned the scrotal area with iodine. The assistant placed elastic around the penis and clipped the elastic to the patient's shirt to expose the scrotum. The patient was then draped in the usual manner. No needle anesthetic (nna) was administered. Once the area was frozen, the physician located the vas deferens tubes one at a time. The physician gently held each vas tube between his fingertips, grasping them with a specially designed ringed clamp. Using special forceps, the physician made one tiny puncture into the skin on the scrotum. [2] Using the same instrument, the first vas tube was lifted gently out through this opening. Once the vas was lifted out of the scrotum, it was cut and both ends were cauterized. The fascial sheath was tied around one end of the cut tube, creating a natural barrier between the two cut ends. The testicular end was left open to reduce the risk of post-vasectomy pain. The separated and blocked ends were returned to the scrotum, and the same procedure was done through the same small opening on the other side. [2] The opening was finally covered with a gauze pad. The one small skin opening will close itself without stitches.

Diagnosis Codes

Z30.2   Encounter for sterilization[1]

Rationale for Diagnosis Codes

The patient presented for a sterilization procedure, found in the ICD-10-CM index under the term "Encounter" and the subterm "Sterilization." The coding guidelines state that Z codes may be used as principal diagnoses when applicable.

Procedure Codes

0VBQ3ZZ   Excision of Bilateral Vas Deferens, Percutaneous Approach[2]

Rationale for Procedure Codes

The term "Vasectomy" in the ICD-10-PCS index directs the coder to the root operation *Excision*. Although it is not necessary to consult the index in ICD-10-PCS, it can help locate the appropriate root operation. Because both vas deferens were treated, the bilateral body part character must be reported. The approach is a small incision, described as a puncture, which coincides with the definition of *Percutaneous* in ICD-10-PCS.

MS-DRG

730	Other Male Reproductive System Diagnoses without CC/MCC	RW 0.6036

The procedure in this case is not considered an operating room procedure and therefore does not qualify for a surgical MS-DRG.

🕯️ CODING AXIOM

ICD-10-CM Official Guidelines for Coding and Reporting Section I.C.21.a:

Z codes are for use in any healthcare setting. Z codes may be used as either a first-listed (principal diagnosis code in the inpatient setting) or secondary code, depending on the circumstances of the encounter. Certain Z codes may only be used as first-listed or principal diagnosis.

ICD-10-PCS Official Guidelines for Coding and Reporting Section A7:

It is not required to consult the index first before proceeding to the tables to complete the code. A valid code may be chosen directly from the tables.

OPERATIVE REPORT MDC 12—#2

Preoperative diagnoses:
Elevated PSA, suspect malignancy

Postoperative diagnoses:
Prostatic adenofibroma

Procedures:
Transrectal ultrasound needle biopsy of the prostate

Procedure description:
The patient is prepped and draped in the left lateral position. Ultrasonography reveals no hypoechoic areas. Then 2 ml of 1% lidocaine are injected at the base of the seminal vesicles and the prostate. Volumetrics are then performed, revealing a 33 cubic centimeter prostate. Six biopsies were then taken on each side of the prostate from the base to apex, medially, and laterally. The patient tolerated the procedure well. There was no evidence of bleeding at the conclusion.

Code all relevant ICD-10-CM diagnosis and ICD-10-PCS procedure codes in accordance with official guidelines and coding conventions.

Diagnosis Codes:

_____

_____

Procedure Codes:

_____

_____

MS-DRG:

_____

_____

CODING AXIOM

ICD-10-CM Official Guidelines for Coding and Reporting Section I.A.12.a:

Excludes1

A type 1 Excludes note is a pure excludes note. It means "NOT CODED HERE!" An Excludes1 note indicates that the code excluded should never be used at the same time as the code above the Excludes1 note. An Excludes1 is used when two conditions cannot occur together, such as a congenital form versus an acquired form of the same condition.

Answers and Rationale

Preoperative diagnoses:
Elevated PSA, suspect malignancy

Postoperative diagnoses:
Prostatic adenofibroma[1]

Procedures:
Transrectal ultrasound needle biopsy of the prostate[2]

Procedure description:
The patient is prepped and draped in the left lateral position. Ultrasonography reveals no hypoechoic areas. Then 2 ml of 1% lidocaine are injected at the base of the seminal vesicles and the prostate. Volumetrics are then performed, revealing a 33 cubic centimeter prostate. Six biopsies were then taken on each side of the prostate from the base to apex, medially, and laterally. [2] The patient tolerated the procedure well. There was no evidence of bleeding at the conclusion.

Diagnosis Codes

D29.1   Benign neoplasm of prostate[1]

Rationale for Diagnosis Codes
An adenofibroma is a benign tumor also known as a fibroadenoma. The terms "Adenofibroma, Prostate" in the ICD-10-CM index refer the coder to see "Enlarged, Enlargement, Prostate," which leads to code range N40- (enlarged prostate). However, the Excludes 1 note under N40 states that benign neoplasms of the prostate are coded to D29.1.

Procedure Codes

0VB03ZX   Excision of Prostate, Percutaneous Approach, Diagnostic[2]

Rationale for Procedure Codes
A biopsy is, by ICD-10-PCS root operation definition, a *Diagnostic* (character 7, the qualifier) *Excision* (character 3, the root operation). Although the procedure is performed transrectally, a needle must puncture the tissue, making the approach for this procedure *Percutaneous* rather than *Via natural or artificial opening*.

MS-DRG

| 730 | Other Male Reproductive System Diagnoses without CC/MCC | RW 0.6036 |

If the coder mistakenly assigned the procedure as a therapeutic instead of a diagnostic excision, the resulting MS-DRG would be a surgical DRG and therefore higher weighted. As this is a diagnostic biopsy, this MS-DRG is non-surgical and grouped based on the principal diagnosis assigned.

OPERATIVE REPORT MDC 12—#3

Preoperative diagnosis:
Left inguinal hernia, possible left spermatocele

Postoperative diagnosis:
Left spermatocele

Procedure performed:
Exploration of the left groin, spermatocelectomy

Procedure description:
The patient was brought to the operating room, placed under general endotracheal anesthesia. The groin area was shaved, prepped, and adequately draped; 1% Xylocaine with Marcaine was administered. An oblique incision starting from the pubic tubercle toward the iliac spine, carried for 4 cm and then carried through the subcutaneous tissue. The fascia was divided; the cord was isolated; a Penrose drain was placed around it. Exploration around the cord in the internal ring did not reveal evidence of any indirect or direct hernia. As a result of this finding, a left spermatocelectomy was done.

An incision was made over the spermatocele, and the spermatocele sac was exposed and excised, taking care not to injure the cord. Bleeders were cauterized. Skin was closed with subcuticular sutures of 2.0 chromic catgut. Dermabond was applied to the skin. The external oblique was closed with a continuous suture of 2-0 Vicryl, making sure not to incorporate any nerves. The subcutaneous tissue was closed with a continuous suture of 4-0 Vicryl and reinforced with Steri-strips. Dressing was applied. The patient left the operating room in good condition.

Code all relevant ICD-10-CM diagnosis and ICD-10-PCS procedure codes in accordance with official guidelines and coding conventions.

Diagnosis Codes:

_____

_____

Procedure Codes:

_____

_____

MS-DRG:

_____

_____

DEFINITIONS

inguinal. Within the groin region.

spermatocele. Noncancerous accumulation of fluid and dead sperm cells normally located at the head of the epididymis that exhibits itself as a hard, smooth scrotal mass and do not normally require treatment unless they become enlarged or cause pain.

Answers and Rationale

Preoperative diagnosis:
Left inguinal hernia, possible left spermatocele

Postoperative diagnosis:
Left spermatocele[1]

Procedure performed:
Exploration of the left groin, spermatocelectomy

Procedure description:
The patient was brought to the operating room, placed under general endotracheal anesthesia. The groin area was shaved, prepped, and adequately draped; 1% Xylocaine with Marcaine was administered. An oblique incision starting from the pubic tubercle toward the iliac spine, carried for 4 cm and then carried through the subcutaneous tissue.[3] The fascia was divided; the cord was isolated; a Penrose drain was placed around it. Exploration around the cord in the internal ring did not reveal evidence of any indirect or direct hernia.[1,3] As a result of this finding, a left spermatocelectomy was done.

An incision was made over the spermatocele, and the spermatocele sac was exposed and excised,[2] taking care not to injure the cord. Bleeders were cauterized. Skin was closed with subcuticular sutures of 2.0 chromic catgut. Dermabond was applied to the skin. The external oblique was closed with a continuous suture of 2-0 Vicryl, making sure not to incorporate any nerves. The subcutaneous tissue was closed with a continuous suture of 4-0 Vicryl and reinforced with Steri-strips. Dressing was applied. The patient left the operating room in good condition.

Diagnosis Codes

N43.41   **Spermatocele of epididymis, single[1]**

Rationale for Diagnosis Codes

The most important factor to note in this scenario is that the procedure revealed there was no inguinal hernia, meaning that a code for the hernia would not be reported.

The operative note implies but does not specifically state that there is only a single spermatocele, making N43.41 the most appropriate ICD-10-CM code to report.

Procedure Codes

ØVBKØZZ   **Excision of Left Epididymis, Open Approach[2]**

ØYJ6ØZZ   **Inspection of Left Inguinal Region, Open Approach[3]**

Rationale for Procedure Codes

The excision of a spermatocele is an excision of a portion of the epididymis . It is also important to note that the inspection of the left groin (inguinal) area is separately reportable as this part of the procedure was *not* the operative approach for the spermatocelectomy. Documentation clearly states that a second incision was made to access the spermatocele.

MS-DRG

712   **Testes Procedures without CC/MCC**   **RW 0.9475**

🕯 **CODING AXIOM**

ICD-10-PCS Official Guidelines for Coding and Reporting Section B3.1b:

Procedural steps necessary to reach the operative site and close the operative site are also not coded separately.

OPERATIVE REPORT MDC 12—#4

Preoperative diagnosis:
Peyronie's disease

Postoperative diagnosis:
Same

Procedure performed:
Implantation of inflatable penile prosthesis

Procedure description:
The patient was brought to the operative suite and placed in the supine position. General endotracheal intubation was initiated and he was prepped and draped in the usual sterile fashion. An incision was made below the scrotum and carried down into the dartos muscle. Care was taken during the dissection to minimize bleeding secondary to the fact that Bovie cautery cannot be used due to the patient's cardiac pacemaker. The corpora cavernosa was identified and dissected free, and the soft tissues were retracted to allow direct and full access to the contralateral corpora cavernosa. A small vertical incision was made between the corpora. The lumen was dilated proximally and distally, first using Metzenbaum scissors followed by Hegar dilators up to 13. The corpora cavernosa were measured at 17 cm total with 8 cm distal and 7 cm proximal. We chose a 13 cm prosthesis with 4 cm extensions and 12 mm caliber. With the insertion device, the proximal prosthesis was placed into the proximal corpora cavernosa. After inspecting for proper positioning, the prosthesis was tested and produced satisfactory results with no leaking or kinking. The device was deflated.

Attention was turned to inserting the 65 mL reservoir. Using the Metzenbaum scissors, the transversalis fascia was punctured for access to the retroperitoneal space. The reservoir was placed and filled. The pump was then positioned in the pocket formed in the subcutaneous tissue of the subdartos area, and the unit was connected. The prosthesis was tested in its entirety and showed again satisfactory performance. A Blake drain was placed into the subdartos space. The tissues were closed in layers using interrupted 3-0 chromic sutures. Sterile dressings were applied and stretch tape was placed over the scrotum. The patient tolerated the procedure well and was taken to the recovery room in good condition.

Code all relevant ICD-10-CM diagnosis and ICD-10-PCS procedure codes in accordance with official guidelines and coding conventions.

Diagnosis Codes:

_____

_____

Procedure Codes:

_____

_____

MS-DRG:

_____

_____

Answers and Rationale

Preoperative diagnosis:
Peyronie's disease[1]

Postoperative diagnosis:
Same

Procedure performed:
Implantation of inflatable penile prosthesis[3]

Procedure description:
The patient was brought to the operative suite and placed in the supine position. General endotracheal intubation was initiated and he was prepped and draped in the usual sterile fashion. An incision was made below the scrotum and carried down into the dartos muscle. Care was taken during the dissection to minimize bleeding secondary to the fact that Bovie cautery cannot be used due to the patient's cardiac pacemaker.[2] The corpora cavernosa was identified and dissected free, and the soft tissues were retracted to allow direct and full access to the contralateral corpora cavernosa. A small vertical incision was made between the corpora. The lumen was dilated proximally and distally, first using Metzenbaum scissors followed by Hegar dilators up to 13. The corpora cavernosa were measured at 17 cm total with 8 cm distal and 7 cm proximal. We chose a 13 cm prosthesis with 4 cm extensions and 12 mm caliber. With the insertion device, the proximal prosthesis was placed into the proximal corpora cavernosa. After inspecting for proper positioning, the prosthesis was tested and produced satisfactory results with no leaking or kinking. The device was deflated. Attention was turned to inserting the 65 mL reservoir. Using the Metzenbaum scissors, the transversalis fascia was punctured for access to the retroperitoneal space. The reservoir was placed and filled. The pump was then positioned in the pocket formed in the subcutaneous tissue of the subdartos area, and the unit was connected. The prosthesis was tested in its entirety and showed again satisfactory performance.[3] A Blake drain was placed into the subdartos space. The tissues were closed in layers using interrupted 3-0 chromic sutures. Sterile dressings were applied and stretch tape was placed over the scrotum. The patient tolerated the procedure well and was taken to the recovery room in good condition.

Diagnosis Codes

N48.6	Induration penis plastica[1]
Z95.Ø	Presence of cardiac pacemaker[2]

Rationale for Diagnosis Codes

The reason for the procedure is Peyronie's disease, which has a specific code that can be located easily in the ICD-10-CM index followed up by verification in the tabular. It is also important to report the pacemaker mentioned in the body of the operative report as it impacted how the surgery was performed.

Procedure Codes

ØVUSØJZ	Supplement Penis with Synthetic Substitute, Open Approach[3]

Rationale for Procedure Codes

The purpose of the prosthesis is to augment or reinforce the function of the penis. This objective coincides with the ICD-10-PCS definition of *Supplement*. It is important to note that a prosthesis of this nature is considered a synthetic substitute.

MS-DRG

710	Penis Procedures without CC/MCC	RW 1.4170

📖 **DEFINITIONS**

---

supplement. Putting in or on biological or synthetic material that physically reinforces and/or augments the function of a portion of a body part.

MDC 13 Diseases and Disorders of the Female Reproductive System

OPERATIVE REPORT MDC 13—#1

Preoperative diagnoses:
Chronic pelvic pain, dysmenorrhea

Postoperative diagnoses:
Endometriosis of the posterior cul-de-sac and ovary, chronic pelvic pain, dysmenorrhea

Procedure description:
Patient was taken to the operating room; prepped and draped in normal sterile fashion. Attention was turned to the abdomen. A 5 mm skin incision was made in the patient's umbilicus with scalpel. Veress needle was inserted and pneumoperitoneum was achieved. A 5 mm trocar was inserted, and the scope confirmed placement in the peritoneal cavity. A separate 7-8 mm incision was made in the lower abdomen, and a 7-8 mm trocar was inserted through the incision under direct visualization. A probe was inserted, and the pelvic cavity was explored. The anterior cul-de-sac was normal. The posterior cul-de-sac showed 2 areas of endometriosis close to the uterosacral ligaments on both sides, which were cauterized with the bipolar cautery. Another area of endometriosis was noted on the patient's left ovary, and this was cauterized as well. All instruments were removed from the abdomen. Excellent hemostasis was noted. Sponge, lap, and needle counts were correct. The patient tolerated the procedure well and was taken to the recovery room in stable condition.

Code all relevant ICD-10-CM diagnosis and ICD-10-PCS procedure codes in accordance with official guidelines and coding conventions.

Diagnosis Codes:

_____

_____

Procedure Codes:

_____

_____

MS-DRG:

_____

_____

DEFINITIONS

cul-de-sac. Blind pouch, or cavity, such as the pouch of Douglas (retro uterine) or the conjunctival fornix, which is the loose pocket of conjunctiva between the eyelid and the eyeball that permits the eyeball to rotate freely.

CODING AXIOM

ICD-10-CM Official Guidelines for Coding and Reporting Section I.C.6.b.1:

A code from category G89 (Pain, not elsewhere classified) should not be assigned if the underlying (definitive) diagnosis is known, unless the reason for the encounter is pain control/ management and not management of the underlying condition.

Answers and Rationale

Preoperative diagnoses:
Chronic pelvic pain, dysmenorrhea

Postoperative diagnoses:
Endometriosis of the posterior cul-de-sac and ovary,[1,2] chronic pelvic pain, dysmenorrhea

Procedure description:
Patient was taken to the operating room; prepped and draped in normal sterile fashion. Attention was turned to the abdomen. A 5 mm skin incision was made in the patient's umbilicus with scalpel. Veress needle was inserted and pneumoperitoneum was achieved. A 5 mm trocar and the laparoscope[3,4] were inserted. A separate 7-8 mm incision was made in the lower abdomen, ad a 7-8 mm trocar was inserted through the incision. A probe was inserted, and the pelvic cavity was explored. The anterior cul-de-sac was normal. The posterior cul-de-sac showed 2 areas of endometriosis close to the uterosacral ligaments on both sides, which were cauterized with the bipolar cautery.[2,4] Another area of endometriosis was noted on the patient's left ovary, and this was cauterized as well.[1,3] All instruments were removed from the abdomen. Excellent hemostasis was noted. Sponge, lap, and needle counts were correct. The patient tolerated the procedure well and was taken to the recovery room in stable condition.

Diagnosis Codes

N80.1	**Endometriosis of ovary**[1]
N80.3	**Endometriosis of pelvic peritoneum**[2]

Rationale for Diagnosis Codes
The operative note specifies that the endometriosis discovered is in the posterior cul-de-sac and on the left ovary. According to the index for ICD-10-CM, the posterior cul-de-sac is coded to pelvic peritoneum. The chronic pelvic pain is not reported, according to guidelines section I.C.6.b.1, which states that codes from the G89 category (Pain, not elsewhere classified) should not be reported if the definitive diagnosis is known. It is also inappropriate to report the dysmenorrhea as this is routinely associated with endometriosis (section I.B.6).

Procedure Codes

0U514ZZ	**Destruction of Left Ovary, Percutaneous Endoscopic Approach**[3]
0U5F4ZZ	**Destruction of Cul-de-sac, Percutaneous Endoscopic Approach**[4]

Rationale for Procedure Codes
The procedures were performed using a laparoscope, making the approach character value 4. Two codes are necessary to report the cauterization of the endometriosis because two separate anatomical sites were treated. In the index, "Cauterization" refers to *Destruction* or "physical eradication of all or a portion of a body part by direct use of energy, force or a destructive agent."

MS-DRG

743	**Uterine and Adnexa Procedures for Nonmalignancy without CC/MCC**	**RW 1.0090**

Both the diagnosis of endometriosis and the procedure for the cauterization of the ovary lesion drive the assignment of this MS-DRG. If only the procedure on the lesion of the cul-de-sac was reported, the result would be lower-weighted MS-DRG 747 Vagina, Cervix and Vulva Procedures without CC/MCC.

OPERATIVE REPORT MDC 13—#2

Preoperative diagnoses:
Desires permanent sterility

Postoperative diagnoses:
Desires permanent sterility

Procedure description:
Patient was taken to the operating room; prepped and draped in normal sterile fashion. Attention was turned to the abdomen. A 5 mm skin incision was made in the patient's umbilicus with scalpel. Veress needle was inserted and pneumoperitoneum was achieved. A 5 mm trocar was inserted, and the scope confirmed placement in the peritoneal cavity. A separate 7-8 mm incision was made in the lower abdomen, and a 7-8 mm trocar was inserted through the incision. The Falope ring applicator was inserted into the pelvic cavity. The left fallopian tube was grasped with the applicator and the ring applied. A 3 cm knuckle of blanched white tissue was noted on the fallopian tube. The Falope ring was then used to grab the right fallopian tube and apply the ring; however, the tube appeared to tear somewhat. Therefore, this area was then cauterized to achieve full bilateral tubal ligation.

All instruments were removed from the abdomen. Excellent hemostasis was noted. Sponge, lap, and needle counts were correct. The patient tolerated the procedure well and was taken to the recovery room in stable condition.

Code all relevant ICD-10-CM diagnosis and ICD-10-PCS procedure codes in accordance with official guidelines and coding conventions.

Diagnosis Codes:

_____

_____

Procedure Codes:

_____

_____

MS-DRG:

_____

_____

Answers and Rationale

Preoperative diagnoses:

Desires permanent sterility

Postoperative diagnoses:

Desires permanent sterility[1]

Procedure description:

Patient was taken to the operating room; prepped and draped in normal sterile fashion. Attention was turned to the abdomen. A 5 mm skin incision was made in the patient's umbilicus with scalpel. Veress needle was inserted and pneumoperitoneum was achieved. A 5 mm trocar and laparoscope were inserted.[2,3] A separate 7-8 mm incision was made in the lower abdomen, and a 7-8 mm trocar was inserted through the incision. The Falope ring applicator was inserted into the pelvic cavity. The left fallopian tube was grasped with the applicator and the ring applied. [3] A 3 cm knuckle of blanched white tissue was noted on the fallopian tube. The Falope ring was then used to grab the right fallopian tube and apply the ring; however, the tube appeared to tear somewhat. Therefore, this area was then cauterized to achieve full bilateral tubal ligation. [2] All instruments were removed from the abdomen. Excellent hemostasis was noted. Sponge, lap, and needle counts were correct. The patient tolerated the procedure well and was taken to the recovery room in stable condition.

Diagnosis Codes

Z30.2   **Encounter for sterilization**[1]

Rationale for Diagnosis Codes

The term "Sterilization" in the index states to "see—Encounter (for), sterilization," which lists the complete code Z30.2. This is the only diagnosis code required for this encounter.

Procedure Codes

ØUL54ZZ   **Occlusion of Right Fallopian Tube, Percutaneous Endoscopic Approach**[2]

ØUL64CZ   **Occlusion of Left Fallopian Tube with Extraluminal Device, Percutaneous Endoscopic Approach**[3]

Rationale for Procedure Codes

Two codes are needed to specify that the left fallopian tube was occluded differently from the right. According to the operative report, a Falope ring was applied to the left fallopian tube but due to tearing one was not applied to the right tube. The physician did attempt to apply the device to the right fallopian tube, but *ICD-10-PCS Official Guidelines for Coding and Reporting* section B6.1a states that "a device is only coded if a device remains after the procedure is completed. If no device remains, the device value No Device (Z) is coded." It is also important to note that a Falope ring is applied to the exterior of the fallopian tubes, making it an extraluminal device. The procedures were performed using a laparoscope, making the approach character value 4 for both procedures.

MS-DRG

743	**Uterine and Adnexa Procedures for Nonmalignancy without CC/MCC**	**RW 1.0090**

In this scenario, because the identical procedure was not performed bilaterally, the MS-DRG does not map to lower-weighted 745 D&C, Conization, Laparoscopy and Tubal Interruption without CC/MCC. For the procedure codes to map to the sterilization MS-DRG, the body part character value must be 7, *Bilateral Fallopian Tubes.*

🕯️ **CODING AXIOM**

ICD-10-PCS Official Guidelines for Coding and Reporting Section B6.1a:

A device is only coded if a device remains after the procedure is completed. If no device remains, the device value No Device (Z) is coded.

OPERATIVE REPORT MDC 13—#3

Preoperative diagnosis:
Endometriosis stage 4

Postoperative diagnosis:
Same

Procedure performed:
TAH-BSO

Procedure description:
The patient was taken to the operating suite, placed in the dorsal supine position, prepped and draped in the routine fashion. An incision was made and the abdomen opened. Abdominal exploration was done. The retractor was placed and bowel packed away. Kelly clamps were placed on the round ligaments; #1 chromic suture placed laterally. The round ligaments were divided and the anterior peritoneum incised in an elliptical fashion. The bladder was pushed down. Clamps were placed across the adnexa, and the pedicles were sutured with figure-of-eight #1 chromic and a free tie of #1 chromic.

The posterior peritoneum was incised to the uterosacral ligament, skeletonizing the uterine vessels, which were grasped with an Allis clamp and sutured with #1 chromic. Heaney clamps were placed on either side of the ligature, the vessels divided and again suture-ligated with #1 chromic. The vagina was entered anteriorly, cervix excised in toto. Figure-of-eight #1 chromic sutures were placed to the lateral vaginal cuff, incorporating this with the cardinal ligament. The cuff was then reefed using continuous interlocking #1 chromic. Adequate hemostasis was assured as the visceroperitoneum was closed with continuous 0 chromic gut. The retractor and packs were removed. Sponge and instrument counts were correct. The abdominal peritoneum was closed with continuous 0 chromic gut, continuous on the recti muscles.

The fascia was closed with continuous interlocking 0 Vicryl. The fat was closed with continuous #2-0 plain, and the skin closed with staples. The patient tolerated the procedure well and left the operating suite in satisfactory condition. The uterus, tubes, and ovaries were sent to pathology.

Code all relevant ICD-10-CM diagnosis and ICD-10-PCS procedure codes in accordance with official guidelines and coding conventions.

Diagnosis Codes:

_____

_____

Procedure Codes:

_____

_____

MS-DRG:

_____

_____

DEFINITIONS

TAH BSO. Total abdominal hysterectomy, bilateral salpingo-oophorectomy.

Answers and Rationale

Preoperative diagnosis:
Endometriosis stage 4[1]

Postoperative diagnosis:
Same

Procedure performed:
TAH-BSO[2-4]

Procedure description:
The patient was taken to the operating suite, placed in the dorsal supine position, prepped and draped in the routine fashion. An incision was made and the abdomen opened. Abdominal exploration was done. The retractor was placed and bowel packed away. Kelly clamps were placed on the round ligaments; #1 chromic suture placed laterally. The round ligaments were divided and the anterior peritoneum incised in an elliptical fashion. The bladder was pushed down. Clamps were placed across the adnexa, and the pedicles were sutured with figure-of-eight #1 chromic and a free tie of #1 chromic.[3,4]

The posterior peritoneum was incised to the uterosacral ligament, skeletonizing the uterine vessels, which were grasped with an Allis clamp and sutured with #1 chromic. Heaney clamps were placed on either side of the ligature, the vessels divided and again suture-ligated with #1 chromic.[2-4] The vagina was entered anteriorly, cervix excised in toto.[5] Figure-of-eight #1 chromic sutures were placed to the lateral vaginal cuff, incorporating this with the cardinal ligament. The cuff was then reefed using continuous interlocking #1 chromic. Adequate hemostasis was assured as the visceroperitoneum was closed with continuous 0 chromic gut. The retractor and packs were removed. Sponge and instrument counts were correct. The abdominal peritoneum was closed with continuous 0 chromic gut, continuous on the recti muscles.

The fascia was closed with continuous interlocking 0 Vicryl. The fat was closed with continuous #2-0 plain, and the skin closed with staples. The patient tolerated the procedure well and left the operating suite in satisfactory condition. The uterus, tubes, and ovaries were sent to pathology.[2-4]

Diagnosis Codes

N80.9	**Endometriosis, unspecified[1]**

Rationale for Diagnosis Codes

Usually the default code, listed next to the main term in the ICD-10-CM index, must be used when the documentation is vague or basic. In this case, the documentation does not specify where the endometriosis is, but anatomical site is how the index divides the category. The specificity the documentation provides (stage 4) is not relevant to code assignment. Therefore, the default code, N80.9, should be reported.

Procedure Codes

0UT90ZZ	**Resection of Uterus, Open Approach[2]**
0UT20ZZ	**Resection of Bilateral Ovaries, Open Approach[3]**
0UT70ZZ	**Resection of Bilateral Fallopian Tubes, Open Approach[4]**
0UTC7ZZ	**Resection of Cervix, Via Natural or Artificial Opening[5]**

Rationale for Procedure Codes

ICD-10-PCS requires four codes to report a total abdominal hysterectomy with bilateral salpingo-oophorectomy (TAH-BSO). The first code reports the resection of the uterus, the second the bilateral ovaries, the third the bilateral fallopian tubes, and the fourth the removal of the cervix. The root operation is *Resection* for each site as the entire organ was removed. The procedure was performed via an abdominal incision and therefore should be reported with an approach character value of 0, *Open*. AHA *Coding Clinic for ICD-10-CM and ICD-10-PCS*, third quarter 2013, page 28, confirms that two codes are required for the total hysterectomy, one for the removal of the uterus and the other for the removal of the cervix.

MS-DRG

743	**Uterine and Adnexa Procedures for Nonmalignancy without CC/MCC**	**RW 1.0090**

OPERATIVE REPORT MDC 13—#4

Preoperative diagnosis:
Vaginal stricture

Postoperative diagnosis:
Same

Procedure performed:
Release of stricture

Indications:
Scarring and vaginal stricture as a result of vaginal trauma. Risks and benefits were discussed, and the patient indicated a desire for the procedure. Informed consent was obtained.

Findings:
Approximately 1.5 cm wide stricture that is approximately 1.5 cm high and extends from approximately the 9 o'clock position to the 3 o'clock position posterior across the vagina approximately 3 cm inside the introitus.

Procedure description:
With the patient in the dorsolithotomy position and under adequate anesthesia, three V-shaped incisions were made at the 4, 8, and 6 o'clock positions. A small portion of scar tissue was excised in each of these locations. The mucosa was oversewn with running, locked sutures for hemostasis. Rectal examination was performed to verify that there was no compromise to the rectovaginal septum. Vaseline-saturated gauze pack was placed in the vagina at the close of this portion of the procedure. The patient was taken to the post-anesthesia care unit in good condition.

Code all relevant ICD-10-CM diagnosis and ICD-10-PCS procedure codes in accordance with official guidelines and coding conventions.

Diagnosis Codes:

_____

_____

Procedure Codes:

_____

_____

MS-DRG:

_____

_____

CODING AXIOM

ICD-10-PCS Official Guidelines for Coding and Reporting Section I.A.9:

- "Other" codes—Codes titled "other" or "other specified" are for use when the information in the medical record provides detail for which a specific code does not exist. Alphabetic Index entries with NEC in the line designate "other" codes in the Tabular List. These Alphabetic Index entries represent specific disease entities for which no specific code exists so the term is included within an "other" code.

- "Unspecified" codes—Codes titled "unspecified" are for use when the information in the medical record is insufficient to assign a more specific code. For those categories for which an unspecified code is not provided, the "other specified" code may represent both other and unspecified.

CODING AXIOM

ICD-10-CM Official Guidelines for Coding and Reporting Section I.B.10:

A sequela is the residual effect (condition produced) after the acute phase of an illness or injury has terminated. There is no time limit on when a sequela code can be used. The residual may be apparent early, such as in cerebral infarction, or it may occur months or years later, such as that due to a previous injury. Coding of sequela generally requires two codes sequenced in the following order: The condition or nature of the sequela is sequenced first. The sequela code is sequenced second.

Answers and Rationale

Preoperative diagnosis:
Vaginal stricture

Postoperative diagnosis:
Same

Procedure performed:
Release of stricture[4]

Indications:
Scarring[2] and vaginal stricture[1] as a result of vaginal trauma.[3] Risks and benefits were discussed, and the patient indicated a desire for the procedure. Informed consent was obtained.

Findings:
Approximately 1.5 cm wide stricture that is approximately 1.5 cm high and extends from approximately the 9 o'clock position to the 3 o'clock position posterior across the vagina approximately 3 cm inside the introitus.

Procedure description:
With the patient in the dorsolithotomy position and under adequate anesthesia, three V-shaped incisions were made at the 4, 8, and 6 o'clock positions. A small portion of scar tissue was excised in each of these locations. The mucosa was oversewn with running, locked sutures for hemostasis.[4] Rectal examination was performed to verify that there was no compromise to the rectovaginal septum. Vaseline-saturated gauze pack was placed in the vagina at the close of this portion of the procedure. The patient was taken to the post-anesthesia care unit in good condition.

Diagnosis Codes

N89.5	Stricture and atresia of vagina[1]
N89.8	Other specified noninflammatory disorders of vagina[2]
S39.93XS	Unspecified injuries of pelvis, sequela[3]

Rationale for Diagnosis Codes

The stricture and the scarring are due to a previous trauma, calling for a sequela code, a code with a seventh character representing sequela (also known as late effects). In this case the ICD-10-CM index refers the coder to "Injury, vagina," which assigns code S39.93-Unspecified injury of pelvis. *ICD-10-CM Official Guidelines for Coding and Reporting* sections I.B.10 and I.C.19.a discuss that the sequela code should be reported as a secondary code following the manifestations of that injury, in this case the stricture and scarring.

Procedure Codes

0UNG7ZZ	Release Vagina, Via Natural or Artificial Opening[4]

Rationale for Procedure Codes

The procedure performed aimed to release the stricture/scar tissue, coinciding with the ICD-10-PCS root operation *Release*. Since the procedure note does not mention the use of any endoscope or devices, the approach character value is 7, *Via Natural or Artificial Opening*.

MS-DRG

747	Vagina, Cervix and Vulva Procedures without CC/MCC	RW 0.9099

If the sequela code is incorrectly sequenced as principal diagnosis, the resulting MS-DRG becomes higher weighted 909 Other O.R. Procedures for Injuries without CC/MCC (RW 1.2992).

MDC 14 Pregnancy, Childbirth and the Puerperium

OPERATIVE REPORT MDC 14—#1

Preoperative diagnosis:
Embryonic demise, 10 weeks

Postoperative diagnosis:
Embryonic demise, 10 weeks and posterior uterine perforation

Procedure performed:
Operative laparoscopy, dilation of cervix, uterine suction, cauterization of uterine perforation

Indications:
This is a 29-year-old, gravida 3, para 1, abortions 1, with embryonic demise at 10 weeks gestational age.

Procedure description:
The patient was taken to the operating room where general anesthesia was provided and found to be adequate. She was cleansed and draped in the usual fashion and Foley catheter was inserted for bladder drainage.

With a sterile speculum, the cervix was exposed, grasped with a single-tooth tenaculum and dilated using the Hegar dilators. Using a #9 suction catheter, the uterine contents were evacuated and sharp curettage of the uterine cavity was done until a gritty sensation was felt. At this time a uterine perforation was suspected and immediate attention was turned to the umbilical area. The abdomen was cleansed and draped appropriately and a 1 cm skin incision was made, Veress needle inserted and 3 liters of CO_2 gas were used to fill the abdominal cavity.

A 10 mm trocar and sleeve were inserted through the umbilical incision and 10 mm laparoscope was used to perform a diagnostic laparoscopy; the suspicion of perforation was confirmed. A 5 mm secondary incision was made in the lower abdomen, the 5 mm trocar and sleeve were introduced under direct visualization, and then the trocar was removed. The patient was placed in reverse Trendelenburg position, and the 200 ml hemoperitoneum was suctioned. Irrigation of the abdominal cavity was then performed, after which a small 1 cm to 2 cm posterior wall uterine perforation was visualized. Bipolar cauterization at setting 40 of the power measurement of a Kleppinger instrument was used to cauterize the uterine perforation. Good hemostasis was achieved, and a small piece of Surgicel was placed laparoscopically over the posterior uterine wall perforation. Irrigation was again performed and good hemostasis confirmed with no sign of any additional bleeding from the uterine wall.

The abdominal contents were again visualized, and no signs of any bleeding from the bowel or bladder were noted. The CO_2 gas was evacuated, and both laparoscopic sleeves were removed. The fascial and skin incisions were repaired using #0 and #4-0 Vicryl sutures, respectively. Since the procedure was stopped immediately after the uterine perforation was noticed, a vaginal ultrasound was performed, which showed only a moderate amount of fluid in the abdominal cavity as is expected after laparoscopy and massive irrigation. No products of conception were visualized inside the uterus. The endometrial tissue was sent to the pathology department.

The patient was then taken to the recovery room where she was observed for 4 hours, with adequate heart rate and normal blood pressure. She was told of the intraoperative complication and informed of all precautions, including any abdominal pain, nausea, vomiting, fever, or excessive vaginal bleeding. She will be followed up in the office in 7 days.

Code all relevant ICD-10-CM diagnosis and ICD-10-PCS procedure codes in accordance with official guidelines and coding conventions.

Diagnosis Codes:

_____

_____

Procedure Codes:

_____

_____

MS-DRG:

_____

_____

Answers and Rationale

Preoperative diagnosis:
Embryonic demise, 10 weeks

Postoperative diagnosis:
Embryonic demise,[1] 10 weeks[3] and posterior uterine perforation[2]

Procedure performed:
Operative laparoscopy, dilation of cervix, uterine suction, cauterization of uterine perforation

Indications:
This is a 29-year-old, gravida 3, para 1, abortions 1, with embryonic demise at 10 weeks gestational age.

Procedure description:
The patient was taken to the operating room where general anesthesia was provided and found to be adequate. She was cleansed and draped in the usual fashion and Foley catheter was inserted for bladder drainage.

With a sterile speculum, the cervix was exposed, grasped with a single-tooth tenaculum and dilated using the Hegar dilators. Using a #9 suction catheter, the uterine contents were evacuated and sharp curettage of the uterine cavity was done[4] until a gritty sensation was felt. At this time a uterine perforation was suspected[2] and immediate attention was turned to the umbilical area. The abdomen was cleansed and draped appropriately and a 1 cm skin incision was made, Veress needle inserted and 3 liters of CO_2 gas were used to fill the abdominal cavity.

A 10 mm trocar and sleeve were inserted through the umbilical incision and 10 mm laparoscope was used to perform a diagnostic laparoscopy;[4-6] the suspicion of perforation was confirmed.[2] A 5 mm secondary incision was made in the lower abdomen, the 5 mm trocar and sleeve were introduced under direct visualization, and then the trocar was removed. The patient was placed in reverse Trendelenburg position, and the 200 ml hemoperitoneum was suctioned.[5] Irrigation of the abdominal cavity was then performed, after which a small 1 cm to 2 cm posterior wall uterine perforation was visualized. Bipolar cauterization at setting 40 of the power measurement of a Kleppinger instrument was used to cauterize the uterine perforation. Good hemostasis was achieved, and a small piece of Surgicel was placed laparoscopically over the posterior uterine wall perforation. [6] Irrigation was again performed and good hemostasis confirmed with no sign of any additional bleeding from the uterine wall.

The abdominal contents were again visualized, and no signs of any bleeding from the bowel or bladder were noted. The CO_2 gas was evacuated, and both laparoscopic sleeves were removed. The fascial and skin incisions were repaired using #0 and #4-0 Vicryl sutures, respectively. Since the procedure was stopped immediately after the uterine perforation was noticed, a vaginal ultrasound was performed, which showed only a moderate amount of fluid in the abdominal cavity as is expected after laparoscopy and massive irrigation. No products of conception were visualized inside the uterus. The endometrial tissue was sent to the pathology department.

The patient was then taken to the recovery room where she was observed for 4 hours, with adequate heart rate and normal blood pressure. She was told of the intraoperative complication and informed of all precautions, including any abdominal pain, nausea, vomiting, fever, or excessive vaginal bleeding. She will be followed up in the office in 7 days.

Diagnosis Codes

O02.1	Missed abortion[1]
N99.71	Accidental puncture and laceration of a genitourinary system organ or structure during a genitourinary system procedure[2]
Z3A.1Ø	1Ø weeks gestation of pregnancy[3]

Rationale for Diagnosis Codes

An embryonic demise is also known as an abortion. A missed abortion occurs when the uterus does not expel the products of conception and must be treated surgically. The accidental puncture should also be reported as this prompted the surgeon to perform additional surgery and intervention. A code from category Z3A should also be reported as an additional diagnosis, according to the "code also" note at the beginning of chapter 15 in ICD-10-CM.

 DEFINITIONS

missed abortion. Retention of a dead fetus within the uterus in cases where fetal demise occurred before completion of 20 weeks of gestation. Abortion in this context refers to retained products of conception from the death of a normal fetus that does not follow spontaneous or induced abortion, or missed delivery.

Procedure Codes

1ØD17ZZ	Extraction of Products of Conception, Retained, Via Natural or Artificial Opening[4]
ØW9G4ZZ	Drainage of Peritoneal Cavity, Percutaneous Endoscopic Approach[5]
ØUQ94ZZ	Repair Uterus, Percutaneous Endoscopic Approach[6]

Rationale for Procedure Codes

According to ICD-10-PCS guideline C2, if the procedure is performed to remove retained products of conception (missed abortion), the procedure is coded from the *Obstetric* section with a root operation of *Extraction*. The dilation of the cervix would not be reported separately as this is considered part of the approach; coding guidelines section B3.1b states that procedural steps taken to reach the operative site are not coded separately. The drainage of the hemoperitoneum and the cauterization and Surgicel application to repair the uterine perforation should be reported separately, however, as they are different root operations, with different objectives, performed on different body parts.

MS-DRG

770	Abortion with D&C, Aspiration Curettage or Hysterotomy	RW 0.8272

OPERATIVE REPORT MDC 14—#2

Preoperative diagnosis:
Active labor

Postoperative diagnosis:
Same

Indications:
A 32-year-old female presents in active late-stage labor. She is at 38 weeks gestation and is gravida 2, para 1, abortus 0. This pregnancy has been complicated by cervical shortening, requiring frequent monitoring. At the 16th week of gestation, cervical measurements of 20 mm necessitated high-risk surveillance to minimize the risk of premature delivery.

Procedure description:
Upon full dilation and cervical effacement, the obstetrician assisted the patient in spontaneous delivery of a full-term, single liveborn infant. Manual assisted delivery was performed by gentle manual traction in coordination with uterine contractions. Soft tissue resistance at the vaginal opening necessitated midline episiotomy to accommodate delivery of the fetal head, prevent obstetric tear, and to ensure optimal healing. Under local anesthesia, a sharp midline perineal incision was made, extending into the perineal soft tissues. Upon incision, it was noted that the perineal muscle and soft tissues were abnormally rigid. Upon delivery of the fetal head, a spontaneous second degree tear occurred in extension of the episiotomy. The episiotomy and perineal tear were reapproximated with sutures.

Code all relevant ICD-10-CM diagnosis and ICD-10-PCS procedure codes in accordance with official guidelines and coding conventions.

Diagnosis Codes:

_____

_____

Procedure Codes:

_____

_____

MS-DRG:

_____

_____

Answers and Rationale

Preoperative diagnosis:
Active labor

Postoperative diagnosis:
Same

Indications:
A 32-year-old female presents in active late-stage labor. She is at 38 weeks gestation[4] and is gravida 2, para 1, abortus 0. This pregnancy has been complicated by cervical shortening, requiring frequent monitoring.[2] At the 16th week of gestation, cervical measurements of 20 mm necessitated high-risk surveillance to minimize the risk of premature delivery.

Procedure description:
Upon full dilation and cervical effacement, the obstetrician assisted the patient in spontaneous delivery of a full-term, single liveborn infant.[3] Manual assisted delivery was performed[5] by gentle manual traction in coordination with uterine contractions. Soft tissue resistance at the vaginal opening necessitated midline episiotomy to accommodate delivery of the fetal head, prevent obstetric tear, and to ensure optimal healing. Under local anesthesia, a sharp midline perineal incision was made, extending into the perineal soft tissues.[7] Upon incision, it was noted that the perineal muscle and soft tissues were abnormally rigid. Upon delivery of the fetal head, a spontaneous second degree tear occurred in extension of the episiotomy.[1] The episiotomy and perineal tear were reapproximated with sutures.[6]

Diagnosis Codes

O70.1	Second degree perineal laceration during delivery[1]
O26.873	Cervical shortening, third trimester[2]
Z37.0	Single live birth[3]
Z3A.38	38 weeks gestation of pregnancy[4]

Rationale for Diagnosis Codes

ICD-10-CM Official Guidelines for Coding and Reporting Section I.C.15.b.4 dictates that the main complication of the delivery be sequenced first when a vaginal delivery occurs. In this case, the patient had a perineal laceration during the delivery. The cervical shortening is important as well, as it is making the patient's pregnancy high risk. It is important to note that the sixth character for the cervical shortening represents the third trimester based on guidelines section I.C.15.a.3. This guideline gives the instructions to use the trimester coinciding with the physician's documentation of gestation when there is no selection for *in childbirth* for complications that are still present during delivery. A code from category Z37 should always be reported on the maternal record when there has been a delivery during the encounter (guidelines section I.C.15.b.5). A final code is required to specify the weeks of gestation (category Z3A), according to the "code also" note found in the beginning of chapter 15 of ICD-10-CM.

Procedure Codes

10E0XZZ	Delivery of Products of Conception, External Approach[5]
0KQM0ZZ	Repair of perineum muscle, open approach[6]
0W8NXZZ	Division of Female Perineum, External Approach[7]

Rationale for Procedure Codes

The only procedures reported in the *Obstetrics* section of ICD-10-PCS are those performed on the *products of conception* or fetus. This means that only the delivery code comes from this section. The codes for the episiotomy (root operation *Division*) and the repair of the laceration (root operation *Repair*) should be constructed from the tables outside of the obstetrics section. Based on advice from *AHA Coding Clinic for ICD-10-CM and ICD-10-PCS* (fourth quarter 2014, page 43), a second degree perineal laceration is considered to involve tearing of the perineal muscle. The documentation of repair of second degree laceration alone warrants the use of repair of perineum muscle.

MS-DRG

775	Vaginal Delivery without Complicating Diagnoses	RW 0.5865

CODING AXIOM

ICD-10-PCS Official Guidelines for Coding and Reporting Section C1:

Procedures performed on the products of conception are coded to the Obstetrics section. Procedures performed on the pregnant female other than the products of conception are coded to the appropriate root operation in the Medical and Surgical section.

OPERATIVE REPORT MDC 14—#3

Preoperative diagnosis:
Acute abdomen, rule out ectopic pregnancy

Postoperative diagnosis:
Ectopic pregnancy

Procedure performed:
Diagnostic laparoscopy, a right salpingectomy

Procedure description:
The patient was taken to the operating room. After general endotracheal anesthesia was induced, the patient was prepped and draped in the usual sterile fashion. An examination under anesthesia revealed an anteverted, anteflexed, small, nontender uterus, a right adnexal mass, and a fullness in the vagina, consistent with hyperperitoneum.

At that point, a small incision was made in the umbilicus and a 10 mm trocar was inserted directly into the abdomen. After the intra-abdominal contents were visualized, a pneumoperitoneum was created with 3.5 liters of CO_2. The hemoperitoneum was noticed, and a second 10 mm laparoscopic port was placed to a 3 cm suprapubic incision, under direct visualization. Two 5 mm laparoscopic ports were also placed under direct visualization, both in the right and left lower quadrants, lateral to epigastric vessels, without complications. These laparoscopic ports were then secured using 0 silk suture. At that point in time, the hemoperitoneum was reduced with irrigator/aspirator. The abnormal gestation was demonstrated on the right side. The right fallopian tube and adhesions to the right pelvic sidewall were taken down, both bluntly and sharply, using forceps and Kleppinger monopolar electrocurrent. Once the distal fallopian tube was freed from the pelvic sidewall and the path of the ureter noted to be out of the way, the fallopian tube, which was thought to be dilated, distended, and beyond repair, was doubly ligated with two pre-tied chromic surgical Endoloops. This specimen was then delivered from the operative field through a 10 mm port. At that point in time, an Endo catch was placed through the 10 mm port and 300 to 400 cc of clot were placed in the Endo catch, and this was removed through the 10 mm fascial defect noted at the suprapubic port. Several more adhesions were then noted lower down in the pelvis, on the right side of the cul-de-sac, and these were taken down both bluntly and sharply. The distal end of the fimbria was noted to still be present, and this was taken down bluntly and sharply, and the pedicle doubly ligated with two Endoloops of 0 chromic suture. This was also delivered from the operative field. After adequate inspection of the abdomen, adequate hemostasis was noted.

The laparoscopic ports were then removed under direct visualization, as well as the pneumoperitoneum being lost. The fascial defects were closed with 0 Vicryl, and the skin was closed with 4-0 Dexon. The patient was then extubated, and went to the Recovery Room in stable condition.

Code all relevant ICD-10-CM diagnosis and ICD-10-PCS procedure codes in accordance with official guidelines and coding conventions.

Diagnosis Codes:

_____

_____

Procedure Codes:

_____

_____

MS-DRG:

_____

_____

DEFINITIONS

ectopic pregnancy. Fertilized ovum that implants and develops outside the uterus. The ovum may implant itself in different sites, such as the fallopian tube, the ovary, the abdomen, or the cervix.

hemoperitoneum. Effusion of blood into the peritoneal cavity, the space between the continuous membrane lining the abdominopelvic walls and encasing the visceral organs.

Answers and Rationale

Preoperative diagnosis:
Acute abdomen, rule out ectopic pregnancy

Postoperative diagnosis:
Ectopic pregnancy[1]

Procedure performed:
Diagnostic laparoscopy, a right salpingectomy

Procedure description:
The patient was taken to the operating room. After general endotracheal anesthesia was induced, the patient was prepped and draped in the usual sterile fashion. An examination under anesthesia revealed an anteverted, anteflexed, small, nontender uterus, a right adnexal mass, and a fullness in the vagina, consistent with hyperperitoneum.

At that point, a small incision was made in the umbilicus and a 10 mm trocar was inserted directly into the abdomen.[3-5] After the intra-abdominal contents were visualized, a pneumoperitoneum was created with 3.5 liters of CO_2. The hemoperitoneum was noticed,[2] and a second 10 mm laparoscopic port was placed to a 3 cm suprapubic incision, under direct visualization. Two 5 mm laparoscopic ports were also placed under direct visualization, both in the right and left lower quadrants, lateral to epigastric vessels, without complications. These laparoscopic ports were then secured using 0 silk suture. At that point in time, the hemoperitoneum was reduced with irrigator/aspirator.[5] The abnormal gestation was demonstrated on the right side.[1] The right fallopian tube and adhesions to the right pelvic sidewall were taken down, both bluntly and sharply, using forceps and Kleppinger monopolar electrocurrent. Once the distal fallopian tube was freed from the pelvic sidewall and the path of the ureter noted to be out of the way, the fallopian tube, which was thought to be dilated, distended, and beyond repair, was doubly ligated with two pre-tied chromic surgical Endoloops.[1,3-4] This specimen was then delivered from the operative field through a 10 mm port. At that point in time, an Endo catch was placed through the 10 mm port and 300 to 400 cc of clot were placed in the Endo catch, and this was removed through the 10 mm fascial defect noted at the suprapubic port. Several more adhesions were then noted lower down in the pelvis, on the right side of the cul-de-sac, and these were taken down both bluntly and sharply. The distal end of the fimbria was noted to still be present, and this was taken down bluntly and sharply, and the pedicle doubly ligated with two Endoloops of 0 chromic suture.[4] This was also delivered from the operative field. After adequate inspection of the abdomen, adequate hemostasis was noted.

The laparoscopic ports were then removed under direct visualization, as well as the pneumoperitoneum being lost. The fascial defects were closed with 0 Vicryl, and the skin was closed with 4-0 Dexon. The patient was then extubated, and went to the Recovery Room in stable condition.

Diagnosis Codes

O00.1	Tubal pregnancy[1]
K66.1	Hemoperitoneum[2]

Rationale for Diagnosis Codes

The terms "Pregnancy, Ectopic" in the ICD-10-CM index lists various subterms. The operative note mentions that the ectopic pregnancy is in the right fallopian tube, making the appropriate code O00.1. The hemoperitoneum, which the body of the operative note describes as being aspirated, should also be reported.

Procedure Codes

10T24ZZ	Resection of Products of Conception, Ectopic, Percutaneous Endoscopic Approach[3]
0UT54ZZ	Resection of Right Fallopian Tube, Percutaneous Endoscopic Approach[4]
0W9G4ZZ	Drainage of Peritoneal Cavity, Percutaneous Endoscopic Approach[5]

Rationale for Procedure Codes

Because the procedure is being performed to remove ectopic products of conception, the code should come from the *Obstetrics* section of ICD-10-PCS. The entire pregnancy, including the tube, was removed, making the root operation *Resection*. The only body part character available in this table is *Products of Conception, Ectopic*. The procedure was performed via laparoscope, making the approach character value 4. There was no device and no qualifier to report. A second code should be reported to address the resection of the entire right fallopian tube, not just the products of conception.

In addition to the salpingectomy, it should be noted that the hemoperitoneum was reduced or drained using an aspirator. A code for the drainage of the peritoneal cavity should be reported for this portion of the procedure.

MS-DRG

777	**Ectopic Pregnancy**	**RW 0.9386**

OPERATIVE REPORT MDC 14—#4

Preoperative diagnosis:
Thirteen-plus week intrauterine pregnancy with incompetent cervix

Postoperative diagnosis:
Same

Procedure performed:
McDonald cerclage placement

Procedure description:
The patient was taken to the operating room where spinal anesthesia was placed. The patient was placed in a dorsal lithotomy position and prepped and draped in the usual sterile fashion.

The cervix was examined and noted to be approximately 3 cm in length. The external os was 1 cm and was closed. Retractors were placed and the anterior and posterior lip of the cervix was grasped with ring forceps. A mersilene band was then placed in a counterclockwise fashion circumferentially, approximately 2.5-3.0 cm superior to the external os and then tied. The cervix was examined and was closed after tying of the cerclage. A Prolene suture was tied to the Mersilene band for easy detection at term. Sponge and needle count was correct. The patient tolerated the procedure well.

Code all relevant ICD-10-CM diagnosis and ICD-10-PCS procedure codes in accordance with official guidelines and coding conventions.

Diagnosis Codes:

_____

_____

Procedure Codes:

_____

_____

MS-DRG:

_____

_____

Answers and Rationale

Preoperative diagnosis:

Thirteen-plus week[2] intrauterine pregnancy with incompetent cervix[1]

Postoperative diagnosis:

Same

Procedure performed:

McDonald cerclage placement

Procedure description:

The patient was taken to the operating room where spinal anesthesia was placed. The patient was placed in a dorsal lithotomy position and prepped and draped in the usual sterile fashion.

The cervix was examined and noted to be approximately 3 cm in length. The external os was 1 cm and was closed. Retractors were placed and the anterior and posterior lip of the cervix was grasped with ring forceps. A mersilene band was then placed in a counterclock-wise fashion circumferentially, approximately 2.5-3.0 cm superior to the external os and then tied.[3] The cervix was examined and was closed after tying of the cerclage. A Prolene suture was tied to the Mersilene band for easy detection at term. Sponge and needle count was correct. The patient tolerated the procedure well.

Diagnosis Codes

O34.31   **Maternal care for cervical incompetence, first trimester**[1]

Z3A.13   **13 weeks gestation of pregnancy**[2]

Rationale for Diagnosis Codes

It is important to know the weeks that make up each trimester of pregnancy. In ICD-10-CM, 13 weeks is the end of the first trimester. This bit of information is needed to correctly complete the partial code O34.3, listed in the ICD-10-CM index under the terms "Incompetence, Cervix, Cervical (os), In Pregnancy." It is also required to report the gestational weeks, if known, using a code from category Z3A according to the "code also" note at the beginning of chapter 15 in ICD-10-CM. In this case, the physician specified 13 plus weeks.

Procedure Codes

0UVC7ZZ   **Restriction of Cervix, Via Natural or Artificial Opening**[3]

Rationale for Procedure Codes

Although the title of the procedure, McDonald cerclage placement, implies the insertion of a device, a cerclage is in fact a suture of the cervix to close it. According to *ICD-10-PCS Official Guidelines for Coding and Reporting* section B6.1b, sutures are not considered a device and therefore are not coded as such. With that in mind, the root operation that best describes the objective of the procedure is *Restriction* of the cervix performed via a natural approach with no device and no qualifier.

MS-DRG

782	Other Antepartum Diagnoses without Medical Complications	RW 0.5454

DEFINITIONS

trimester. Normal pregnancy has a duration of approximately 40 weeks and is grouped into three-month periods consisting of three trimesters. ICD-10-CM counts trimesters from the first day of the last menstrual period as follows: 1st trimester less than 14 weeks and 0 days. 2nd trimester 14 weeks, 0 days to less than 28 weeks and 0 days. 3rd trimester 28 weeks and 0 days until delivery.

OPERATIVE REPORT MDC 14—#5

Diagnoses:
41-week gestation; VBAC failed due to fetal decelerations

Procedure performed:
Primary low transverse cesarean section; insertion of IUD

Procedure description:
After informed consent was obtained, the patient was taken to the operating suite and an adequate anesthetic level was confirmed. A Foley catheter had been previously placed or was placed in the operating suite. The patient was placed in the supine position, left lateral tilt, and prepped and draped in the usual sterile fashion for cesarean section.

A Pfannenstiel skin incision was made and carried down sharply through the subcutaneous tissues. The fascia was incised in the midline and extended laterally and elliptically. Sharp and blunt dissection was then used to separate the fascia from the underlying rectus muscles. The rectus muscles were divided in the midline, and the peritoneum was entered using sharp dissection. The peritoneal incision was extended superiorly and inferiorly down to the level of the dome of the bladder. The uterus was noted to be midline.

The vesicouterine peritoneum was then incised, and sharp and blunt dissection was then used to separate the bladder from the lower uterine segment. A transverse incision was made in the lower uterine segment and carried down sharply until the amniotic membranes were ruptured and this confirmed clear fluid. The incision was then extended until the fetal head was exposed. The head was grasped, flexed, and delivered through the incision. The infant's nose and mouth were suctioned. The rest of the infant was delivered. The cord was doubly clamped and cut. The placenta was then manually extracted. A Mirena intrauterine device was then placed within the uterus. The placement was confirmed by vaginal digital examination. The string was trimmed to an acceptable length.

The uterus incision was inspected and noted to be free of extensions. It was then closed in a single layer of running locking #1 chromic suture, and hemostasis was confirmed. The uterus was returned to the intra-abdominal site. The peritoneum was then reapproximated using running 3-0 Vicryl suture. The fascia was reapproximated using 2-0 PDS suture. The subcutaneous tissues were repaired using electrocautery and the skin with staples. The patient tolerated the procedure well. All counts were correct x3, and the patient was transferred to the recovery room in good condition.

Code all relevant ICD-10-CM diagnosis and ICD-10-PCS procedure codes in accordance with official guidelines and coding conventions.

Diagnosis Codes:

_____

_____

Procedure Codes:

_____

_____

MS-DRG:

_____

_____

Answers and Rationale

Diagnoses:

41-week gestation;[4] VBAC[1,3] failed[3] due to fetal decelerations[2]

Procedure performed:

Primary low transverse cesarean section;[5] insertion of IUD[6]

Procedure description:

After informed consent was obtained, the patient was taken to the operating suite and an adequate anesthetic level was confirmed. A Foley catheter had been previously placed or was placed in the operating suite. The patient was placed in the supine position, left lateral tilt, and prepped and draped in the usual sterile fashion for cesarean section.

A Pfannenstiel skin incision was made and carried down sharply through the subcutaneous tissues. The fascia was incised in the midline and extended laterally and elliptically. Sharp and blunt dissection was then used to separate the fascia from the underlying rectus muscles. The rectus muscles were divided in the midline, and the peritoneum was entered using sharp dissection. The peritoneal incision was extended superiorly and inferiorly down to the level of the dome of the bladder. The uterus was noted to be midline.

The vesicouterine peritoneum was then incised, and sharp and blunt dissection was then used to separate the bladder from the lower uterine segment. A transverse incision was made in the lower uterine segment and carried down sharply until the amniotic membranes were ruptured and this confirmed clear fluid. The incision was then extended until the fetal head was exposed. The head was grasped, flexed, and delivered through the incision.[6] The infant's nose and mouth were suctioned.[5] The rest of the infant was delivered.[6] The cord was doubly clamped and cut. The placenta was then manually extracted. A Mirena intrauterine contraceptive device was then placed within the uterus.[7] The placement was confirmed by vaginal digital examination. The string was trimmed to an acceptable length.

The uterus incision was inspected and noted to be free of extensions. It was then closed in a single layer of running locking #1 chromic suture, and hemostasis was confirmed. The uterus was returned to the intra-abdominal site. The peritoneum was then reapproximated using running 3-0 Vicryl suture. The fascia was reapproximated using 2-0 PDS suture. The subcutaneous tissues were repaired using electrocautery and the skin with staples. The patient tolerated the procedure well. All counts were correct x3, and the patient was transferred to the recovery room in good condition.

Diagnosis Codes

O34.21	**Maternal care for scar from previous cesarean delivery[1]**
O76	**Abnormality in fetal heart rate and rhythm complicating labor and delivery[2]**
O66.41	**Failed attempted vaginal birth after previous cesarean delivery[3]**
Z3A.41	**41 weeks gestation of pregnancy[4]**
Z37.Ø	**Single live birth[5]**

Rationale for Diagnosis Codes

The reason for admission (VBAC) should be sequenced as the principal diagnosis according to coding guidelines. The reason for the cesarean section (fetal heart decelerations) is sequenced as a secondary diagnosis. A code identifying that the VBAC failed should also be assigned (O66.41). The coder is instructed to report a code from both categories Z3A and Z37 when a delivery occurs.

Procedure Codes

1ØDØØZ1	**Extraction of Products of Conception, Low Cervical, Open Approach[6]**
ØUH97HZ	**Insertion of Contraceptive Device into Uterus, Via Natural or Artificial Opening[7]**

Rationale for Procedure Codes

The cesarean section is reported using a code from the obstetrics section of the ICD-10-PCS manual. The approach is open, and the type of incision (or qualifier) is low classical, also known as low transverse. The physician also inserts an IUD at the same time. The ICD-10-PCS manual does not have a code to report an *Open* insertion of an IUD and therefore AHA *Coding Clinic for ICD-10-CM and ICD-10-PCS*, second quarter 2013, page 34, clarifies that the approach of "via natural and artificial opening" will suffice in this scenario.

MS-DRG

766	**Cesarean Section without CC/MCC**	**RW 0.7807**

CODING AXIOM

ICD-10-CM Official Coding Guidelines for Coding and Reporting Section I.C.15.b.4:

When a delivery occurs, the principal diagnosis should correspond to the main circumstances or complication of the delivery. In cases of cesarean delivery, the selection of the principal diagnosis should be the condition established after study that was responsible for the patient's admission. If the patient was admitted with a condition that resulted in the performance of a cesarean procedure, that condition should be selected as the principal diagnosis. If the reason for the admission/encounter was unrelated to the condition resulting in the cesarean delivery, the condition related to the reason for the admission/encounter should be selected as the principal diagnosis.

MDC 15 Newborns and Other Neonates with Conditions Originating in the Perinatal Period

OPERATIVE REPORT MDC 15—#1

Preoperative diagnosis:
Scalp abscess

Postoperative diagnosis:
Scalp abscess

Procedure performed:
Puncture aspiration of abscess

Indications:
The patient is a 2-day-old newborn female. During delivery (earlier in this encounter), the patient's scalp was scratched by the forceps. Over the course of the last two days the area has become red and indurated. Empiric antibiotics have been started, and the pediatrician believes draining the abscess is the most appropriate course of action. The risks and benefits were explained to the parents, and they elected to proceed with the procedure.

Procedure description:
The area was prepped and draped in the usual sterile fashion. Topical lidocaine was introduced to the area, followed by intramuscular introduction. The abscess was then punctured using a 16 gauge needle, and 30 ccs of fluid were aspirated. The fluid was sent for culture and sensitivity. A sterile dressing was applied to the wound. The patient tolerated the procedure well. Infectious disease and immunology consultants are to follow up prior to discharge.

Findings:
The culture and sensitivity returned positive for MRSA. The patient has been placed in isolation in the NICU and started on Vancomycin.

Code all relevant ICD-10-CM diagnosis and ICD-10-PCS procedure codes in accordance with official guidelines and coding conventions.

Diagnosis Codes:

_____

_____

Procedure Codes:

_____

_____

MS-DRG:

_____

_____

Answers and Rationale

Preoperative diagnosis:
Scalp abscess

Postoperative diagnosis:
Scalp abscess[3,4]

Procedure performed:
Puncture aspiration of abscess

Indications:
The patient is a 2-day-old newborn female. During delivery (earlier in this encounter),[1] the patient's scalp was scratched by the forceps.[2] Over the course of the last two days the area has become red and indurated. Empiric antibiotics have been started, and the pediatrician believes draining the abscess is the most appropriate course of action. The risks and benefits were explained to the parents, and they elected to proceed with the procedure.

Procedure description:
The area was prepped and draped in the usual sterile fashion. Topical lidocaine was introduced to the area, followed by intramuscular introduction. The abscess was then punctured using a 16 gauge needle, and 30 ccs of fluid were aspirated.[6] The fluid was sent for culture and sensitivity.[6] A sterile dressing was applied to the wound. The patient tolerated the procedure well. Infectious disease and immunology consultants are to follow up prior to discharge.

Findings:
The culture and sensitivity returned positive for MRSA.[5] The patient has been placed in isolation in the NICU and started on Vancomycin.

Diagnosis Codes

Z38.00	**Single liveborn infant, delivered vaginally**[1]
P12.89	**Other birth injuries to scalp**[2]
P39.4	**Neonatal skin infection**[3]
L02.811	**Cutaneous abscess of head (any part, except face)**[4]
B95.62	**Methicillin resistant Staphylococcus aureus infection as the cause of diseases classified elsewhere**[5]

Rationale for Diagnosis Codes

Since the patient was delivered during this encounter, the first-listed code must be a code from category Z38. The documentation notes that the patient was delivered vaginally using forceps. The patient developed the abscess due to a scratch from forceps, identified by code P12.89. The abscess first must be represented by a code from chapter 16 ("Conditions Originating in the Perinatal Period"), followed by codes from the other chapters to further identify the condition according to the "use additional code" note under category P39. The abscess is of the scalp and is found to be caused by MRSA.

Procedure Codes

0J903ZX	**Drainage of Scalp Subcutaneous Tissue and Fascia, Percutaneous Approach, Diagnostic**[6]

Rationale for Procedure Codes

The objective of the procedure is to aspirate the abscess, which is adequately represented by the root operation *Drainage* in ICD-10-PCS. Because the section *Skin and Breast* does not have a code that represents the *Percutaneous* approach, the *Subcutaneous Tissue and Fascia* section should be used as the puncture of the site with a needle is by ICD-10-PCS definition a *Percutaneous* approach. Lastly, the seventh character value should be X, *Diagnostic* as the specimen was sent for culture and sensitivity to further diagnose the infection.

MS-DRG

793	**Full Term Neonate with Major Problems**	**RW 3.6692**

CODING AXIOM

ICD-10-CM Official Guidelines for Coding and Reporting

Section I.C.16.a.2:

When coding the birth episode in a newborn record, assign a code from category Z38, Liveborn infants according to place of birth and type of delivery, as the principal diagnosis.

Section I.C.16.a.3:

Codes from other chapters may be used with codes from chapter 16 if the codes from the other chapters provide more specific detail. Codes for signs and symptoms may be assigned when a definitive diagnosis has not been established. If the reason for the encounter is a perinatal condition, the code from chapter 16 should be sequenced first.

DEFINITIONS

drainage. Taking or letting out fluids and/or gases from a body part.

DEFINITIONS

foreskin. Prepuce.

prepuce. Fold of penile skin covering the glans.

OPERATIVE REPORT MDC 15—#2

Preoperative diagnosis:
Parents desire circumcision

Postoperative diagnosis:
Same

Procedure performed:
Routine neonate circumcision

Indications:
The parents desired circumcision of their premature 36-week gestation infant delivered via spontaneous vaginal delivery on this encounter. Prior to the procedure the infant was examined and has no signs of hypospadias or illness. The risks, benefits, and alternatives were discussed with the parents prior to the procedure, and consent was obtained.

Procedure description:
The area was prepped and draped in the usual sterile fashion. Topical anesthesia was applied, followed by an injection of 1% lidocaine. After allowing the appropriate time for the anesthesia to be effective, a Plastibell circumcision device was applied and the foreskin trimmed away. The area was examined for cosmetic appearance and was found to be satisfactory. Vaseline gauze was applied. The patient tolerated the procedure well and there were no complications. The baby was returned to the mother's room in excellent condition. Further instructions were given to the parents.

Code all relevant ICD-10-CM diagnosis and ICD-10-PCS procedure codes in accordance with official guidelines and coding conventions.

Diagnosis Codes:
_____
_____

Procedure Codes:
_____
_____

MS-DRG:
_____
_____

Answers and Rationale

Preoperative diagnosis:
Parents desire circumcision

Postoperative diagnosis:
Same

Procedure performed:
Routine neonate circumcision

Indications:
The parents desired circumcision of their premature 36 week gestation infant delivered via spontaneous vaginal delivery on this encounter.[1,2] Prior to the procedure the infant was examined and has no signs of hypospadias or illness. The risks, benefits, and alternatives were discussed with the parents prior to the procedure, and consent was obtained.

Procedure description:
The area was prepped and draped in the usual sterile fashion. Topical anesthesia was applied, followed by an injection of 1% lidocaine. After allowing the appropriate time for the anesthesia to be effective, a Plastibell circumcision device was applied and the foreskin trimmed away.[3] The area was examined for cosmetic appearance and was found to be satisfactory. Vaseline gauze was applied. The patient tolerated the procedure well and there were no complications. The baby was returned to the mother's room in excellent condition. Further instructions were given to the parents.

Diagnosis Codes

Z38.00   **Single liveborn infant, delivered vaginally[1]**

P07.39   **Preterm newborn, gestational age 36 completed weeks[2]**

Rationale for Diagnosis Codes
The principal diagnosis for an encounter with a delivery must be represented by a code from category Z38 on the newborns chart. Because the physician documents that the patient had a 36-week gestation, this should be reported based on ICD-10-CM *Official Guidelines for Coding and Reporting* Section I.C.16.d.

Procedure Codes

0VBTXZZ   **Excision of Prepuce, External Approach[3]**

Rationale for Procedure Codes
The foreskin is removed in a circumcision, this part of the anatomy is also known as the prepuce. Because it is only the extra skin of the prepuce being removed, this procedure is assigned the root operation of *Excision*.

MS-DRG

792	Prematurity without Major Problems	RW 2.1552

If the secondary code P07.39 is not assigned, the MS-DRG groups to lower-weighted 795 Normal Newborn (RW 0.1758).

CODING AXIOM

ICD-10-CM Official Guidelines for Coding and Reporting Section I.C.16.d:

Providers utilize different criteria in determining prematurity. A code for prematurity should not be assigned unless it is documented. Assignment of codes in categories P05 Disorders of newborn related to slow fetal growth and fetal malnutrition, and P07 Disorders of newborn related to short gestation and low birth weight, not elsewhere classified, should be based on the recorded birth weight and estimated gestational age. Codes from category P05 should not be assigned with codes from category P07.

When both birth weight and gestational age are available, two codes from category P07 should be assigned, with the code for birth weight sequenced before the code for gestational age.

MDC 16 Diseases and Disorders of the Blood and Blood-Forming Organs and Immunological Disorders

DEFINITIONS

lymphadenitis. Inflammation of the lymph nodes.

OPERATIVE REPORT MDC 16—#1

Preoperative diagnosis:
Acute lymphadenitis

Postoperative diagnosis:
Same

Procedure performed:
Incision and drainage

Procedure description:
The left inguinal area was prepped and draped in the usual sterile fashion. Local anesthesia was obtained using lidocaine 1%. Using a #11 scalpel, a 3 cm incision was made through the skin and subcutaneous tissue to the swollen lymph glands. These were palpated, then incised, draining 4 cc of purulent material. This material was sent for analysis for further diagnostic work-up. The wound was copiously irrigated, and the wound was closed using 5-0 Prolene. Sterile dressings were applied. The patient tolerated the procedure well with no complications.

Code all relevant ICD-10-CM diagnosis and ICD-10-PCS procedure codes in accordance with official guidelines and coding conventions.

Diagnosis Codes:

_____

_____

Procedure Codes:

_____

_____

MS-DRG:

_____

_____

Answers and Rationale

Preoperative diagnosis:
Acute lymphadenitis[1]

Postoperative diagnosis:
Same

Procedure performed:
Incision and drainage

Procedure description:
The left inguinal area[1,2] was prepped and draped in the usual sterile fashion. Local anesthesia was obtained using lidocaine 1%. Using a #11 scalpel, a 3 cm incision was made through the skin and subcutaneous tissue to the swollen lymph glands. These were palpated, then incised, draining 4 cc of purulent material. This material was sent for analysis for further diagnostic work-up.[2] The wound was copiously irrigated, and the wound was closed using 5-0 Prolene. Sterile dressings were applied. The patient tolerated the procedure well with no complications.

Diagnosis Codes

L04.1   **Acute lymphadenitis of trunk[1]**

Rationale for Diagnosis Codes

The terms "Lymphadenitis, Acute" in the ICD-10-CM index specify the anatomical site. In this case, the operative note discusses the left inguinal (groin) area. The index does not provide an entry for "Groin" but does for "Trunk" or "Leg." When the tabular is consulted, it must be noted that there is an Excludes 2 note under L04.3 Acute lymphadenitis of lower limb, to note that acute lymphadenitis of the groin is reported with L04.1.

Procedure Codes

Ø79JØZX   **Drainage of Left Inguinal Lymphatic, Open Approach, Diagnostic[2]**

Rationale for Procedure Codes

The drainage of a lymph node is reported using a table from the section *Lymphatic and Hemic System* of ICD-10-PCS rather than from the section *Subcutaneous Tissue and Fascia* because the lymph node was actually incised. Since the incision was made through the subcutaneous tissue, this would be considered an *Open* approach. It is also important to note that the purulent material is being sent for further diagnostic testing, which implies that the procedure is diagnostic and should have a qualifier seventh character value of X.

MS-DRG

804   **Other O.R. Procedures of the Blood and Blood-Forming**   **RW 1.1715**
             Organs without CC/MCC

 CODING AXIOM

ICD-10-CM Official Guidelines for Coding and Reporting Section I.A.12.b:

A type 2 excludes note represents "Not included here." An Excludes2 note indicates that the condition excluded is not part of the condition represented by the code, but a patient may have both conditions at the same time. When an Excludes2 note appears under a code, it is acceptable to use both the code and the excluded code together, when appropriate.

OPERATIVE REPORT MDC 16—#2

Preoperative diagnosis:
Mass lesion, left lower pole of thymus

Postoperative diagnosis:
Enlarged and lymphatic-appearing thymus gland and large left lower pole of thymus

Procedure performed:
Transsternal radical thymectomy; diagnostic bronchoscopy

Indications:
The patient is a 49-year-old female who obtained a chest x-ray several months ago for an unrelated reason. It was essentially negative. A CT scan was obtained and showed a 4 cm mass lesion in the left anterior mediastinum in the position of the left lobe of thymus.

Procedure description:
The patient was brought in the operating suite and placed on the operating table in a supine position. Compression boots were placed on both lower extremities and set in motion prior to induction of general anesthesia. The patient was intubated with a single lumen endotracheal tube. An epidural catheter was placed. Due to the presence of a possible anterior mediastinal tumor, the patient's airways were explored with a diagnostic bronchoscope. Airways were found to be normal.

The chest and abdomen were prepped and draped in a sterile manner. A time-out was called, and the patient's identity was confirmed by all. Everyone agreed the patient was in the operating room for transsternal resection of mediastinal mass. The anterior mediastinum was explored through a standard midline sternotomy. Vancomycin paste was used to control marrow bleeding. The sternum was separated using a sternal retractor, and the mediastinum was explored. The thymus gland had a very "lymphatic" appearance instead of being replaced by fat. There was a significant difference in character and color between the thymus and surrounding fat. The thymus gland was enlarged. The left lower lobe of thymus was quite enlarged, thus giving the appearance of a left lower lobe mass lesion. Ligaments attaching the thymus to the pericardium were taken down. The thymic vein was identified and ligated with free ties of 2-0 silk. The innominate vein was skeletonized. The superior pole was the larger of the two and was directly attached to the inferior pole of the thyroid. The thyrothymic ligament was transected and clipped. The remainder of the thymus was then removed, including the enlarged left lower pole. The left upper pole was not as large and came out quite nicely. The thymus was sent to pathology for analysis. Tissue from the left upper mediastinum was then resected and sent to pathology for analysis.

The operative site was inspected and showed no signs of bleeding. A #28 French straight Argyle chest tube was placed into the left pleural space while the mediastinum was drained with a similar tube. The sternum was reapproximated using five #5 stainless steel wire sutures in a figure-of-eight fashion. The linea alba was reapproximated with running simple stitch of 0 Vicryl. The subcutaneous tissue and fascia were closed with a running simple stitch of 2-0 Vicryl while the skin was closed with running subcuticular stitch of 4-0 Vicryl. Steri-Strips were applied, sterile dressing was placed, chest tubes were placed for seal suction, and the procedure was terminated. The patient tolerated the procedure well and was returned to the thoracic ICU in satisfactory condition. Instrument and sponge counts were correct at the end of the procedure. Estimated blood loss was approximately 50 ml.

Code all relevant ICD-10-CM diagnosis and ICD-10-PCS procedure codes in accordance with official guidelines and coding conventions.

Diagnosis Codes:

_____

_____

Procedure Codes:

_____

_____

MS-DRG:

_____

_____

Answers and Rationale

Preoperative diagnosis:

Mass lesion, left lower pole of thymus

Postoperative diagnosis:

Enlarged and lymphatic-appearing thymus gland and large left lower pole of thymus[1]

Procedure performed:

Transsternal radical thymectomy; diagnostic bronchoscopy

Indications:

The patient is a 49-year-old female who obtained a chest x-ray several months ago for an unrelated reason. It was essentially negative. A CT scan was obtained and showed a 4 cm mass lesion in the left anterior mediastinum in the position of the left lobe of thymus.

Procedure description:

The patient was brought in the operating suite and placed on the operating table in a supine position. Compression boots were placed on both lower extremities and set in motion prior to induction of general anesthesia. The patient was intubated with a single lumen endotracheal tube. An epidural catheter was placed. Due to the presence of a possible anterior mediastinal tumor, the patient's airways were explored with a diagnostic bronchoscope.[3] Airways were found to be normal.

The chest and abdomen were prepped and draped in a sterile manner. A time-out was called, and the patient's identity was confirmed by all. Everyone agreed the patient was in the operating room for transsternal resection of mediastinal mass. The anterior mediastinum was explored through a standard midline sternotomy.[2,4] Vancomycin paste was used to control marrow bleeding. The sternum was separated using a sternal retractor, and the mediastinum was explored. The thymus gland had a very "lymphatic" appearance instead of being replaced by fat. There was a significant difference in character and color between the thymus and surrounding fat. The thymus gland was enlarged. The left lower lobe of thymus was quite enlarged, thus giving the appearance of a left lower lobe mass lesion.[1] Ligaments attaching the thymus to the pericardium were taken down. The thymic vein was identified and ligated with free ties of 2-0 silk. The innominate vein was skeletonized. The superior pole was the larger of the two and was directly attached to the inferior pole of the thyroid. The thyrothymic ligament was transected and clipped. The remainder of the thymus was then removed, including the enlarged left lower pole. The left upper pole was not as large and came out quite nicely.[2] The thymus was sent to pathology for analysis.

Tissue from the left upper mediastinum was then resected and sent to pathology for analysis.[4]

The operative site was inspected and showed no signs of bleeding. A #28 French straight Argyle chest tube was placed into the left pleural space while the mediastinum was drained with a similar tube. The sternum was reapproximated using five #5 stainless steel wire sutures in a figure-of-eight fashion. The linea alba was reapproximated with running simple stitch of 0 Vicryl. The subcutaneous tissue and fascia were closed with a running simple stitch of 2-0 Vicryl while the skin was closed with running subcuticular stitch of 4-0 Vicryl. Steri-Strips were applied, sterile dressing was placed, chest tubes were placed for seal suction, and the procedure was terminated. The patient tolerated the procedure well and was returned to the thoracic ICU in satisfactory condition. Instrument and sponge counts were correct at the end of the procedure. Estimated blood loss was approximately 50 mL.

Diagnosis Codes

E32.0   Persistent hyperplasia of thymus[1]

Rationale for Diagnosis Codes

The preoperative diagnosis states that there is a lesion. However, this is not an appropriate diagnosis to report as the body of the operative note and the postoperative diagnosis state that there is no mass, just that the thymus is enlarged, particularly the left lower pole. Therefore, the only correct code to report with the documentation provided is that for the enlarged thymus gland.

Procedure Codes

07TM0ZZ   Resection of Thymus, Open Approach[2]

0BJ08ZZ   Inspection of Tracheobronchial Tree, Via Natural or Artificial Opening Endoscopic[3]

0WBC0ZX   Excision of Mediastinum, Open Approach, Diagnostic[4]

Rationale for Procedure Codes

First and foremost, the main procedure was to inspect and remove the entire thymus, making the correct principal procedure *Resection* of the thymus gland. Following the resection, a biopsy was done of the mediastinum, which is a separately reportable procedure as it has a distinct objective of its own. Because it was a biopsy, the qualifier character value has to be X, *Diagnostic*. Both of these procedures were performed via a sternotomy, which is an *Open* approach. It is also important to note that a bronchoscopy was performed to inspect the patient's airways. Although it is described as a diagnostic bronchoscopy, there were no tissue samples taken and so it should be reported with a qualifier of Z.

MS-DRG

804	Other O.R. Procedures of the Blood and Blood-Forming Organs without CC/MCC	RW 1.1715

MDC 17 Myeloproliferative Diseases and Disorders and Poorly Differentiated Neoplasms

OPERATIVE REPORT MDC 17—#1

Preoperative diagnosis:
Non-Hodgkin's lymphoma

Postoperative diagnosis:
Non-Hodgkin's lymphoma

Procedure performed:
Port placement

Indications:
Vascular port placement requested for chemotherapy access for this 57-year-old male patient with non-Hodgkin's lymphoma

Procedure description:
Intravenous sedation was administered. 3 mg Versed and 100 mcg Fentanyl IV. Vital signs and sedation monitored by nursing staff under interventional radiologist's supervision. Limited jugular ultrasound documented jugular vein patency.

The right neck and upper chest were prepped and draped in the usual sterile fashion. 10:1 volume mixture of 1% lidocaine without epinephrine buffered with 8.4% bicarbonate solution was used for local anesthesia. Under ultrasound guidance, right internal jugular venotomy was made with a micropuncture needle. Permanent copy of the image documenting the vein was entered into the patient's record.

Under fluoroscopic guidance, the micropuncture needle was exchanged over the guidewire for the micropuncture sheath. Catheter length was measured with the 0.018 guidewire. Micropuncture sheath saline locked. A subcutaneous pocket was created for the port over the right anterior chest using a combination of sharp and blunt dissection. The pocket was liberally irrigated with 1 gm Ancef solution. Catheter was subcutaneously tunneled from the right anterior chest pocket to the right internal jugular venotomy site. Catheter was cut to length. Micropuncture sheath exchanged over guidewire for the peel-away sheath and advanced under fluoroscopic guidance to the superior vena cava. Peel-away sheath removed. Port aspirated and flushed adequately. Port secured with a single 2-0 PDS II suture around the catheter. The right anterior chest incision was closed with 4-0 Vicryl interrupted suture, a running 4-0 Monocryl subcuticular suture, and Dermabond. Right internal jugular venotomy site closed with Dermabond. Port accessed and then heparin locked with 100:1 heparin solution. No immediate complication.

Impression:
6 French single-lumen Bard PowerPort placed. Tip in the superior vena cava. Port left accessed, heparin locked, and ready for use.

Code all relevant ICD-10-CM diagnosis and ICD-10-PCS procedure codes in accordance with official guidelines and coding conventions.

Diagnosis Codes:

_____

_____

Procedure Codes:

_____

_____

MS-DRG:

_____

_____

Answers and Rationale

Preoperative diagnosis:
Non-Hodgkin's lymphoma

Postoperative diagnosis:
Non-Hodgkin's lymphoma[1]

Procedure performed:
Port placement

Indications:
Vascular port placement requested for chemotherapy access for this 57-year-old male patient with non-Hodgkin's lymphoma

Procedure description:
Intravenous sedation was administered. 3 mg Versed and 100 mcg Fentanyl IV. Vital signs and sedation monitored by nursing staff under interventional radiologist's supervision. Limited jugular ultrasound documented jugular vein patency.

The right neck and upper chest were prepped and draped in the usual sterile fashion. 10:1 volume mixture of 1% lidocaine without epinephrine buffered with 8.4% bicarbonate solution was used for local anesthesia. Under ultrasound guidance, right internal jugular venotomy was made with a micropuncture needle. Permanent copy of the image documenting the vein was entered into the patient's record.

Under fluoroscopic guidance, the micropuncture needle was exchanged over the guidewire for the micropuncture sheath. Catheter length was measured with the 0.018 guidewire. Micropuncture sheath saline locked. A subcutaneous pocket was created for the port over the right anterior chest using a combination of sharp and blunt dissection.[3] The pocket was liberally irrigated with 1 gm Ancef solution. Catheter was subcutaneously tunneled from the right anterior chest pocket to the right internal jugular venotomy site. Catheter was cut to length. Micropuncture sheath exchanged over guidewire for the peel-away sheath and advanced under fluoroscopic guidance to the superior vena cava.[2] Peel-away sheath removed. Port aspirated and flushed adequately. Port secured with a single 2-0 PDS II suture around the catheter.[3] The right anterior chest incision was closed with 4-0 Vicryl interrupted suture, a running 4-0 Monocryl subcuticular suture, and Dermabond. Right internal jugular venotomy site closed with Dermabond. Port accessed and then heparin locked with 100:1 heparin solution. No immediate complication.

Impression:
6 French single-lumen Bard PowerPort placed. Tip in the superior vena cava. Port left accessed, heparin locked, and ready for use.

Diagnosis Codes

C85.9Ø   **Non-Hodgkin lymphoma, unspecified, unspecified site**[1]

Rationale for Diagnosis Codes
The reason for the port insertion is the non-Hodgkin's lymphoma, this makes this diagnosis the first-listed diagnosis for this procedure. It would be inappropriate to report Z45.2 Encounter for adjustment and management of vascular access device, for this scenario because the device is being inserted rather than adjusted or managed.

Procedure Codes

Ø2HV33Z   **Insertion of infusion device into superior vena cava, percutaneous approach**[2]

ØJH6ØXZ   **Insertion of Vascular Access Device into Chest Subcutaneous Tissue and Fascia, Open Approach**[3]

Rationale for Procedure Codes
The port placement consists of two parts and therefore requires two codes to describe it. One code describes the percutaneous insertion of the catheter with the tip of the infusion device residing in the superior vena cava. The second is for the open insertion of the vascular access device (port) into the subcutaneous tissue of the anterior chest wall. This is consistent with advice from *AHA Coding Clinic for ICD-10-CM and ICD-10-PCS*, second quarter 2015, page 29.

MS-DRG

| 842 | Lymphoma and Nonacute Leukemia without CC/MCC | RW 1.1167 |

Reporting V45.2 incorrectly as a principal diagnosis would result in much lower weighted MS-DRG 950 Aftercare without CC/MCC (RW 0.5798). Neither the insertion of the vascular access device (port) nor the insertion of the infusion device is considered an operating room procedure in ICD-10-PCS and therefore this scenario groups to a medical MS-DRG driven by the principal diagnosis.

OPERATIVE REPORT MDC 17—#2

Preoperative diagnosis:
Splenomegaly of unknown etiology, rule out lymphoma

Postoperative diagnosis:
Same

Procedure performed:
Splenectomy with mesenteric lymph node biopsies

Findings:
There were extensive retroperitoneal and mesenteric lymph nodes, and the spleen was very enlarged consistent with lymphoma. A minimal amount of ascites was encountered. The rest of the anatomy was without any obvious abnormalities.

Procedure description:
The patient was placed supine on the operating table. After induction of general anesthesia, the abdomen was prepped and draped in the usual sterile fashion. Midline incision was made. The skin, subcutaneous layers, and fascia were divided using electrocautery. The abdomen was entered and the spleen was visualized. This was extremely large. We pulled the spleen down and medially to begin dissection. Starting at the inferior pole near the splenorenal ligament using a combination of cautery and clamps moving superiorly, the superior pole of the spleen was dissected free. The hilar structures were visualized. The remaining vessels were divided until the spleen was free. This was then removed and sent to pathology. Hemostasis was obtained, and the abdomen was thoroughly irrigated. The peritoneal cavity was then explored, revealing extensive nodal disease within the retroperitoneum and the mesentery of the small bowel and colon. A lymph node from the small bowel mesentery was excised and sent to pathology in addition to the spleen. The fascia was closed with a #1 Maxon suture. The subcutaneous tissue and skin closed with staples. Sterile dressings were applied, and the patient was transported to the recovery room in stable condition.

Addendum:
The pathology report was reviewed by the surgeon. The lymph node biopsy came back positive for lymphoblastic B-cell lymphoma.

Code all relevant ICD-10-CM diagnosis and ICD-10-PCS procedure codes in accordance with official guidelines and coding conventions.

Diagnosis Codes:

_____

_____

Procedure Codes:

_____

_____

MS-DRG:

_____

_____

Answers and Rationale

Preoperative diagnosis:

Splenomegaly of unknown etiology, rule out lymphoma

Postoperative diagnosis:

Same

Procedure performed:

Splenectomy with mesenteric lymph node biopsies

Findings:

There were extensive retroperitoneal and mesenteric lymph nodes, and the spleen was very enlarged consistent with lymphoma. A minimal amount of ascites was encountered.[2] The rest of the anatomy was without any obvious abnormalities.

Procedure description:

The patient was placed supine on the operating table. After induction of general anesthesia, the abdomen was prepped and draped in the usual sterile fashion. Midline incision was made.[3,4] The skin, subcutaneous layers, and fascia were divided using electrocautery. The abdomen was entered and the spleen was visualized. This was extremely large. We pulled the spleen down and medially to begin dissection. Starting at the inferior pole near the splenorenal ligament using a combination of cautery and clamps moving superiorly, the superior pole of the spleen was dissected free. The hilar structures were visualized. The remaining vessels were divided until the spleen was free. This was then removed and sent to pathology.[3] Hemostasis was obtained, and the abdomen was thoroughly irrigated. The peritoneal cavity was then explored, revealing extensive nodal disease within the retroperitoneum and the mesentery of the small bowel and colon. A lymph node from the small bowel mesentery was excised and sent to pathology in addition to the spleen.[1,4] The fascia was closed with a #1 Maxon suture. The subcutaneous tissue and skin closed with staples. Sterile dressings were applied, and the patient was transported to the recovery room in stable condition.

Addendum:

The pathology report was reviewed by the surgeon. The lymph node biopsy came back positive for lymphoblastic B-cell lymphoma.[1]

Diagnosis Codes

C83.53   Lymphoblastic (diffuse) lymphoma, intra-abdominal lymph nodes[1]

R18.8   Other ascites[2]

Rationale for Diagnosis Codes

The pathology report came back positive for lymphoblastic B-cell lymphoma, making a code from category C83.5 appropriate. The lymph node sampled and diagnosed was from the mesenteric lymph nodes, which are in the abdominal area, as are the retroperitoneal lymph nodes, making the correct fifth character 3. The splenomegaly should not be reported separately, according to *ICD-10-CM Official Guidelines for Coding and Reporting* section I.B.4, as it is commonly seen in lymphoma and was included in the diagnosis.

Procedure Codes

Ø7TPØZZ   Resection of Spleen, Open Approach[3]

Ø7BBØZX   Excision of Mesenteric Lymphatic, Open Approach, Diagnostic[4]

Rationale for Procedure Codes

The removal of the spleen was complete, resulting in the ICD-10-PCS root operation *Resection*. Due to the incision as the approach, both the splenectomy and the lymph node procedure are performed via an *Open* approach. The biopsy of the lymph nodes is reported as an *Excision*. The seventh character value of X, *Diagnostic*, reflects that the procedure is a biopsy.

MS-DRG

821   Lymphoma and Leukemia with Major O.R. Procedure with CC   RW 2.3113

If the encounter is coded incorrectly, with the symptom of splenomegaly as principal diagnosis, the result is higher-weighted MS-DRG 800 Splenectomy with CC (RW 2.7364). It is imperative to follow coding guidelines to avoid unnecessary risk of an audit.

DEFINITIONS

lymphoma. Tumors occurring in the lymphoid tissues that are most commonly malignant.

mesentery. Two layers of peritoneum that fold to surround the organs and attach to the abdominal wall.

CODING AXIOM

ICD-10-CM Official Guidelines for Coding and Reporting Section I.B.4:

Codes that describe symptoms and signs, as opposed to diagnoses, are acceptable for reporting purposes when a related definitive diagnosis has not been established (confirmed) by the provider. Chapter 18 of ICD-10-CM, "Symptoms, Signs, and Abnormal Clinical and Laboratory Findings, Not Elsewhere Classified" (codes RØØ.Ø–R99) contains many, but not all codes for symptoms.

OPERATIVE REPORT MDC 17—#3

Preoperative diagnosis:
Hodgkin's lymphoma

Postoperative diagnosis:
Hodgkin's lymphoma

Procedure performed:
Bone marrow biopsy

Procedure description:
The patient was placed in the prone position, and her right posterior superior iliac spine was cleaned with Betadine and anesthetized with 1% lidocaine. A bone marrow biopsy was performed, and the specimen was sent for biopsy.

Preliminary report of the aspirate shows no evidence of abnormal cells, suggesting lymphoma per the pathologist's preliminary report; therefore, flow and cytogenetics were not sent. The patient tolerated the procedure well.

Code all relevant ICD-10-CM diagnosis and ICD-10-PCS procedure codes in accordance with official guidelines and coding conventions.

Diagnosis Codes:

_____

_____

Procedure Codes:

_____

_____

MS-DRG:

_____

_____

Answers and Rationale

Preoperative diagnosis:
Hodgkin's lymphoma

Postoperative diagnosis:
Hodgkin's lymphoma[1]

Procedure performed:
Bone marrow biopsy[2]

Procedure performed:
The patient was placed in the prone position, and her right posterior superior iliac spine was cleaned with Betadine and anesthetized with 1% lidocaine. A bone marrow biopsy was performed, and the specimen was sent for biopsy.[2]

Preliminary report of the aspirate shows no evidence of abnormal cells, suggesting lymphoma per the pathologist's preliminary report; therefore, flow and cytogenetics were not sent. The patient tolerated the procedure well.

Diagnosis Codes

C81.9Ø   **Hodgkin lymphoma, unspecified, unspecified site**[1]

Rationale for Diagnosis Codes

Because there is no further documentation of the site of the lymphoma, the most appropriate code that reflects the documentation is C81.90. A code for the lymphoma is still assigned although the preliminary reports came back negative as that was the documented reason for the test. Without the rest of the medical record, it is not known if this is a follow-up for Hodgkin's lymphoma or an initial encounter. Therefore, the documentation must be interpreted as is.

Procedure Codes

Ø7DR3ZX   **Extraction of Iliac Bone Marrow, Percutaneous Approach, Diagnostic**[2]

Rationale for Procedure Codes

Bone marrow biopsies can be located in the index under the root operation *Extraction*. It is also listed in the ICD-10-PCS coding guideline B3.4a.

MS-DRG

842   **Lymphoma and Nonacute Leukemia without CC/MCC**   RW 1.1167

 CODING AXIOM

ICD-10-PCS Official Guidelines for Coding and Reporting Section B3.4a:

Biopsy procedures are coded using the root operations Excision, Extraction, or Drainage and the qualifier Diagnostic.

Examples: Fine needle aspiration biopsy of lung is coded to the root operation Drainage with the qualifier Diagnostic. Biopsy of bone marrow is coded to the root operation Extraction with the qualifier Diagnostic. Lymph node sampling for biopsy is coded to the root operation Excision with the qualifier Diagnostic.

 CODING AXIOM

Biopsy of bone marrow and endometrium are found under the root operation *Extraction*.

OPERATIVE REPORT MDC 17—#4

Preoperative diagnosis:
Swollen inguinal lymph node

Postoperative diagnosis:
Metastatic melanoma

Procedure performed:
Excision of lymph nodes

Indications:
The patient is a 32-year-old female with a history of melanoma of the skin of the right shoulder that has been removed and chemotherapy completed 13 months ago. The patient has swelling in the groin area, which after examination was determined to be a palpable lymph node. Biopsy confirmed metastatic disease.

Procedure description:
The patient was brought to the operating suite and general anesthesia was induced. The left inguinal area was prepped and draped in the usual sterile fashion. The area was infiltrated with lidocaine for local block. A #8 scalpel was used to make an incision through all of the tissue layers until the superficial lymph nodes were identified. These were carefully dissected free, the lymph channels clamped, and the nodes excised. The incision was carried down to the deeper lymph nodes, and these were removed in the same fashion. The area was further explored for any remaining lymph node tissue. None was encountered. All of the specimens were labeled and sent to pathology. The wound was irrigated thoroughly and hemostasis was confirmed. The wound was closed in layers using 3-0 Prolene. Sterile dressings were applied. There were no complications.

Code all relevant ICD-10-CM diagnosis and ICD-10-PCS procedure codes in accordance with official guidelines and coding conventions.

Diagnosis Codes:

_____

_____

Procedure Codes:

_____

_____

MS-DRG:

_____

_____

Answers and Rationale

Preoperative diagnosis:
Swollen inguinal lymph node

Postoperative diagnosis:
Metastatic melanoma[1]

Procedure performed:
Excision of lymph nodes

Indications:
The patient is a 32-year-old female with a history of melanoma of the skin of the right shoulder that has been removed and chemotherapy completed 13 months ago.[2] The patient has swelling in the groin area, which after examination was determined to be a palpable lymph node. Biopsy confirmed metastatic disease.

Procedure description:
The patient was brought to the operating suite and general anesthesia was induced. The left inguinal area[3] was prepped and draped in the usual sterile fashion. The area was infiltrated with lidocaine for local block. A #8 scalpel was used to make an incision through all of the tissue layers until the superficial lymph nodes were identified. These were carefully dissected free, the lymph channels clamped, and the nodes excised. The incision was carried down to the deeper lymph nodes, and these were removed in the same fashion. The area was further explored for any remaining lymph node tissue. None was encountered.[3] All of the specimens were labeled and sent to pathology. The wound was irrigated thoroughly and hemostasis was confirmed. The wound was closed in layers using 3-0 Prolene. Sterile dressings were applied. There were no complications.

Diagnosis Codes

C77.4   **Secondary and unspecified malignant neoplasm of inguinal and lower limb lymph nodes[1]**

Z85.820   **Personal history of malignant melanoma of skin[2]**

Rationale for Diagnosis Codes

Two concepts are key when assigning the codes for this scenario. The first is that when treatment is directed at a secondary malignancy rather than the primary, the secondary (inguinal lymph node) is sequenced first. The second concept is that when there is no further treatment directed at a malignancy, it should be reported using a code representing personal history from category Z85 Personal history of malignant neoplasm.

In the index, the terms "Melanoma, metastatic" list a code for other specified site: C79.89 Secondary malignant neoplasm of other specified sites. However, the site of the neoplasm is known and therefore should be reported rather than an "other specified" code according to *ICD-10-CM Official Coding Guidelines for Coding and Reporting*, section I.A.9.a. The code for the metastatic melanoma of the lymph nodes can be located using the Neoplasm Table in ICD-10-CM. The code from the secondary column opposite the term "Lymph Node or Gland" is reported. To locate the correct code for the history of melanoma, the terms "History, Personal, Melanoma" should be consulted.

Procedure Codes

07TJ0ZZ   **Resection of Left Inguinal Lymphatic, Open Approach[3]**

Rationale for Procedure Codes

The body of the operative report notes that the procedure is being performed on the left inguinal lymph nodes. It also specifies that the lymph tissue was removed in its entirety, which translates to the ICD-10-PCS root operation *Resection*. The procedure was performed via an *Open* approach, as can be determined by the incision to reach the operative field. There was no device involved and no qualifier necessary.

MS-DRG

822   **Lymphoma and Leukemia with Major O.R. Procedure without CC/MCC**   **RW 1.2851**

 CODING AXIOM

ICD-10-CM Official Guidelines for Coding and Reporting

Section I.C.2.b:

When a patient is admitted because of a primary neoplasm with metastasis and treatment is directed toward the secondary site only, the secondary neoplasm is designated as the principal diagnosis even though the primary malignancy is still present.

Section I.C.2.l.2:

When an encounter is for a primary malignancy with metastasis and treatment is directed toward the metastatic (secondary) site(s) only, the metastatic site(s) is designated as the principal/first-listed diagnosis. The primary malignancy is coded as an additional code.

Section I.C.2.m:

When a primary malignancy has been excised but further treatment, such as an additional surgery for the malignancy, radiation therapy or chemotherapy is directed to that site, the primary malignancy code should be used until treatment is completed.

When a primary malignancy has been previously excised or eradicated from its site, there is no further treatment (of the malignancy) directed to that site, and there is no evidence of any existing primary malignancy, a code from category Z85, Personal history of malignant neoplasm, should be used to indicate the former site of the malignancy.

MDC 18 Infectious and Parasitic Diseases

OPERATIVE REPORT MDC 18—#1

Preoperative diagnoses:
Suspected wound abscess

Postoperative diagnoses:
E. coli muscle abscess s/p lymph node excision

History of illness:
This 36-year-old female was admitted to the hospital for postoperative wound exploration following an excision of a 1 cm mass in the right posterior triangle of her neck, mid-point, behind the sternocleidomastoid approximately three weeks ago. The pathology of the mass was determined to be a necrotic lymph node with no evidence of malignancy. Ten days post procedure, the patient was seen for suture removal. At this time, it was noted that the wound site was inflamed and tender. The patient was started on antibiotics. In spite of treatment with antibiotics, the patient returned to the office complaining of a fever and increased inflammation and tenderness at the operative site. The patient is now admitted for postoperative wound exploration with possible incision and drainage of a suspected wound abscess.

Procedure description:
The previous incision site was opened. On exploration of the previous operative site, an abscess was noted in the sternocleidomastoid muscle. The abscess was incised and 10 cc of purulent material was aspirated and sent to the lab for culture and sensitivity. The area was copiously irrigated with normal saline, and the wound was closed in layers. The patient was discharged to postanesthesia recovery in good condition. The culture results came back positive for *Escherichia coli*.

Code all relevant ICD-10-CM diagnosis and ICD-10-PCS procedure codes in accordance with official guidelines and coding conventions.

Diagnosis Codes:
_____

_____

Procedure Codes:
_____

_____

MS-DRG:
_____

_____

Answers and Rationale

Preoperative diagnoses:
Suspected wound abscess

Postoperative diagnoses:
E. coli muscle abscess s/p lymph node excision[1,2,3]

History of illness:
This 36-year-old female was admitted to the hospital for postoperative wound exploration following an excision of a 1 cm mass in the right posterior triangle of her neck,[4] mid-point, behind the sternocleidomastoid approximately three weeks ago. The pathology of the mass was determined to be a necrotic lymph node with no evidence of malignancy. Ten days post procedure, the patient was seen for suture removal. At this time, it was noted that the wound site was inflamed and tender. The patient was started on antibiotics. In spite of treatment with antibiotics, the patient returned to the office complaining of a fever and increased inflammation and tenderness at the operative site. The patient is now admitted for postoperative wound exploration[1] with possible incision and drainage of a suspected wound abscess.

Procedure description:
The previous incision site was opened. [5] On exploration of the previous operative site, an abscess was noted in the sternocleidomastoid muscle.[2,5] The abscess was incised and 10 cc of purulent material was aspirated and sent to the lab for culture and sensitivity. [5] The area was copiously irrigated with normal saline, and the wound was closed in layers. The patient was discharged to postanesthesia recovery in good condition. The culture results came back positive for *Escherichia coli*. [3]

Diagnosis Codes

T81.4XXA   Infection following a procedure, initial encounter[1]

M60.08   Infective myositis, other site[2]

B96.20   Unspecified Escherichia coli [E. coli] as the cause of diseases classified elsewhere[3]

Y83.8   Other surgical procedures as the cause of abnormal reaction of the patient, or of later complication, without mention of misadventure at the time of the procedure[4]

Rationale for Diagnosis Codes
The documentation specifies that this is an abscess of the sternocleidomastoid muscle postoperatively. The terms "Infection, postoperative" in the ICD-10-CM index directs the coder to T81.4. This is the initial encounter and therefore a seventh character of A should be added (preceded by the placeholder X twice). There is an instructional note under T81 that directs the coder to "code also" the infection. In this case, the infection is of the sternocleidomastoid muscle, part of the neck, which codes to M60.08. Under category M60 there is an instructional note directing the coder to identify the organism if known by using a code from the range of B95-B97. *E. coli* is specified by code B96.2, but the tabular indicates a fifth-digit requirement for B96.2. The documentation provides no additional detail on the type of *E. coli,* so the appropriate code would be B96.20. Code Y83.8 should be reported to identify the external cause status.

Procedure Codes

0K920ZX   Drainage of Right Neck Muscle, Open Approach, Diagnostic[5]

Rationale for Procedure Codes
The purpose of the procedure was to drain the purulent material from the muscle and send it to pathology. Based on the Body Park Key, this is classified as a drainage of the right neck muscle. The approach was *Open*, as the previous incision was reopened to access the site. There is no device used. The qualifier is X Diagnostic, as the material was sent to pathology for further diagnostic testing.

MS-DRG

857   **Postoperative or Post-Traumatic Infections**   **RW 2.0516**
   with O.R. Procedure with CC

It is important to follow the sequencing guidelines in this case. If the infection code is reported as the principal diagnosis instead of the complication T code, the MS-DRG changes to 501 Soft Tissue Procedures with CC (RW 1.6064), or if the T code is omitted entirely, the lower-weighted MS-DRG 502 Soft Tissue Procedures without CC/MCC (RW 1.1752), would be assigned.

OPERATIVE REPORT MDC 18—#2

Preoperative diagnosis :
Postoperative infected seroma

Postoperative diagnosis:
Same

Procedure performed:
Incision and drainage

Indications:
The patient is a 55-year-old male who previously underwent a repair of a large abdominal hernia on the left side. The herniorrhaphy required extensive subcutaneous undermining. Three months following the procedure, the patient noted increased swelling and pain at the wound site. This was identified as a seroma and was aspirated. The patient presented for drainage but was found to be febrile. The patient was subsequently admitted for an incision and drainage and IV antibiotics for a recurrent seroma positive for staphylococcal infection.

Procedure description:
The patient was brought to the operating room and given general anesthesia. He was prepped and draped in the usual sterile fashion. The previous incision was reopened using electrocautery. The swelling was noted to be below the aponeurosis and anterior layer of the rectus sheath, which were further dissected until the seroma pocket was encountered within the rectus abdominus muscle. This was drained and thoroughly irrigated using a mixture of warmed normal saline and Cefazolin . Hemostasis was ensured by visual inspection. The fascia was closed with a #1 Maxon suture. The subcutaneous tissue and skin were closed with staples. Sterile dressings were applied and the patient was transported to the recovery room in stable condition.

Code all relevant ICD-10-CM diagnosis and ICD-10-PCS procedure codes in accordance with official guidelines and coding conventions.

Diagnosis Codes:

_____

_____

Procedure Codes:

_____

_____

MS-DRG:

_____

_____

Answers and Rationale

Preoperative diagnosis:
Postoperative infected seroma[1,2]

Postoperative diagnosis:
Same

Procedure performed:
Incision and drainage

Indications:
The patient is a 55-year-old male who previously underwent a repair of a large abdominal hernia on the left side.[5] The herniorrhaphy required extensive subcutaneous undermining. Three months following the procedure, the patient noted increased swelling and pain at the wound site. This was identified as a seroma and was aspirated.[4] The patient presented for drainage but was found to be febrile. The patient was subsequently admitted for an incision and drainage and IV antibiotics for a recurrent seroma positive for staphylococcal infection.[3]

Procedure description:
The patient was brought to the operating room and given general anesthesia. He was prepped and draped in the usual sterile fashion. The previous incision was reopened using electrocautery.[5] The swelling was noted to be below the aponeurosis and anterior layer of the rectus sheath, which were further dissected until the seroma pocket was encountered within the rectus abdominus muscle.[2,5] This was drained and thoroughly irrigated using a mixture of warmed normal saline and Cefazolin. Hemostasis was ensured by visual inspection. The fascia was closed with a #1 Maxon suture. The subcutaneous tissue and skin were closed with staples. Sterile dressings were applied and the patient was transported to the recovery room in stable condition.

Diagnosis Codes

T81.4XXA **Infection following a procedure, initial encounter[1]**

M96.83Ø **Postprocedural hemorrhage and hematoma of a musculoskeletal structure following a musculoskeletal system procedure[2]**

B95.8 **Unspecified staphylococcus as the cause of diseases classified elsewhere[3]**

Y83.8 **Other surgical procedures as the cause of abnormal reaction of the patient, or of later complication, without mention of misadventure at the time of the procedure[4]**

Rationale for Diagnosis Codes
The term "Seroma" in the ICD-10 index directs the coder to T79.2 (Traumatic secondary and recurrent hemorrhage) or to see the entry for "Hematoma." The excludes notes under category T79 in the tabular indicate that complications following a procedure are coded to categories T80-T88. As the infected seroma occurred after the procedure, code T81.4- is the most appropriate. The "use additional code" notes for T81.4 states that the type of infection, or the seroma, also must be reported. Therefore, the coder should follow the index's reference to see the term "Hematoma." The term "Hematoma," subterm "postoperative" direct the coder to *see Complication, postprocedural, hemorrhage*. At this point, the location of the hematoma (the muscle) and type of previous surgery (nonorthopaedic) factor into code selection. The code B95.8 is appropriate to report to distinguish that the infecting organism is known and is staphylococcal in nature. Finally, code Y83.8 should be reported in addition to identify the external cause status.

Procedure Codes

ØK9LØZZ **Drainage of Left Abdomen Muscle, Open Approach[5]**

Rationale for Procedure Codes
Because the objective of the procedure is to drain the seroma, the root operation is *Drainage*. The seroma was located in the left abdominal muscles and was incised, making the approach *Open*.

MS-DRG

857 **Postoperative or Posttraumatic Infections with O.R. Procedure with CC** **RW 2.0516**

☙ CODING AXIOM

ICD-10-CM Official Guidelines for Coding and Reporting Section I.B.7:

"Use additional code" notes are found in the Tabular List at codes that are not part of an etiology/manifestation pair where a secondary code is useful to fully describe a condition. The sequencing rule is the same as the etiology/manifestation pair, "use additional code" indicates that a secondary code should be added.

OPERATIVE REPORT MDC 18—#3

Diagnosis:
Crohn's disease with rectal abscess

Indications:
The patient is a 48-year-old native American male with a known history of Crohn's disease of the small intestine who presented with severe sepsis thought to be secondary to a rectal abscess.

Procedure:
Incision and drainage

Procedure description:
The patient was taken to the operating room after obtaining an informed consent. Prior to prepping, I performed a digital rectal examination that showed no pathology. I found some small internal hemorrhoids and no fistulous tracts. A spinal anesthetic was given, and the patient was prepped and draped in the usual fashion.

I proceeded to insert an anoscope. The abscess area, which was in the left side, was incised with a cruciate incision and drained. All necrotic tissue was debrided. The cavity was explored and found to have no communication to any deeper structures. The cavity was irrigated with saline.

Estimated blood loss was minimal. The patient tolerated the procedure well and was sent for recovery in satisfactory condition.

Code all relevant ICD-10-CM diagnosis and ICD-10-PCS procedure codes in accordance with official guidelines and coding conventions.

Diagnosis Codes:

_____

_____

Procedure Codes:

_____

_____

MS-DRG:

_____

_____

Answers and Rationale

Diagnosis:

Crohn's disease with rectal abscess[4]

Indications:

The patient is a 48-year-old native American male with a known history of Crohn's disease of the small intestine[3] who presented with severe sepsis thought to be secondary to a rectal abscess.[1,2,4]

Procedure:

Incision and drainage

Procedure description:

The patient was taken to the operating room after obtaining an informed consent. Prior to prepping, I performed a digital rectal examination that showed no pathology. I found some small internal hemorrhoids[5] and no fistulous tracts. A spinal anesthetic was given, and the patient was prepped and draped in the usual fashion.

I proceeded to insert an anoscope. The abscess area, which was in the left side, was incised with a cruciate incision and drained. All necrotic tissue was debrided.[6] The cavity was explored and found to have no communication to any deeper structures. The cavity was irrigated with saline.

Estimated blood loss was minimal. The patient tolerated the procedure well and was sent for recovery in satisfactory condition.

Diagnosis Codes

A41.9	Sepsis, unspecified organism[1]
R65.20	Severe sepsis without septic shock[2]
K50.014	Crohn's disease of small intestine with abscess[3]
K61.1	Rectal abscess[4]
K64.8	Other hemorrhoids[5]

Rationale for Diagnosis Codes

The indications section discusses the patient's diagnosis of severe sepsis, which is reported using a minimum of two codes. When present with a localized infection, the sepsis is sequenced first, followed by a code for the localized infection. Since the abscess is in a patient with Crohn's disease, a code for the Crohn's with an abscess and an additional code for the location of the abscess should be reported. This is consistent with the advice given in AHA's *Coding Clinic for ICD-10-CM and ICD-10-PCS*, fourth quarter 2012, page 104. Finally, a code for the findings of hemorrhoids should be reported.

Procedure Codes

0D9P8ZZ	Drainage of Rectum, Via Natural or Artificial Opening Endoscopic[6]

Rationale for Procedure Codes

The incision and drainage of the rectal tissue was performed using an anoscope, which is an approach of *Natural or Artificial Opening Endoscopic.*

MS-DRG

854	Infectious and Parasitic Diseases with O.R. Procedure with CC	RW 2.3804

CODING AXIOM

ICD-10-CM Official Guidelines for Coding and Reporting

Section I.C.1.d.1.b:

The coding of severe sepsis requires a minimum of two codes: first a code for the underlying systemic infection, followed by a code from subcategory R65.2, Severe sepsis. If the causal organism is not documented, assign code A41.9, Sepsis, unspecified organism, for the infection.

Section I.C.1.d.4:

If the reason for admission is both sepsis or severe sepsis and a localized infection, such as pneumonia or cellulitis, a code(s) for the underlying systemic infection should be assigned first and the code for the localized infection should be assigned as a secondary diagnosis. If the patient has severe sepsis, a code from subcategory R65.2 should also be assigned as a secondary diagnosis. If the patient is admitted with a localized infection, such as pneumonia, and sepsis/severe sepsis doesn't develop until after admission, the localized infection should be assigned first, followed by the appropriate sepsis/severe sepsis codes.

MDC 19 Mental Diseases and Disorders

OPERATIVE REPORT MDC 19—#1

Preoperative diagnosis:
Severe mental disabilities

Postoperative diagnosis:
Severe mental disabilities

Procedure performed:
Insertion of PEG tube

Indications:
The patient is a 15-year-old female who resides in a skilled nursing facility. She was transferred for PEG tube insertion due to a decrease in p.o. intake secondary to her intellectual disabilities. The patient is also a quadriplegic.

Procedure description:
The patient was taken to the operating room and placed in the supine position. After adequate IV sedation was obtained, esophagogastroduodenoscopy was performed. The esophagus, stomach, and duodenum were visualized without any abnormalities. The appropriate location for the tube insertion was marked on the skin of the abdomen. The area was then prepped and draped in the sterile fashion. This area was infiltrated with 1% lidocaine for local anesthesia, and a needle was used to enter the stomach under visualization by the endoscope. A guidewire was then passed and the needle was then withdrawn. An incision was made and dilated to the size of the tube. The guidewire and dilator were then removed and the PEG tube was placed. The lumen of the stomach was examined and proper placement of the tube was ensured. The endoscope was removed. The tube was then connected to the skin using Prolene sutures. Sterile dressings were applied. The patient was transferred to recovery in a stable condition.

Code all relevant ICD-10-CM diagnosis and ICD-10-PCS procedure codes in accordance with official guidelines and coding conventions.

Diagnosis Codes:

_____

_____

Procedure Codes:

_____

_____

MS-DRG:

_____

_____

Answers and Rationale

Preoperative diagnosis:
Severe mental disabilities

Postoperative diagnosis:
Severe mental disabilities[1]

Procedure performed:
Insertion of PEG tube[3]

Indications:
The patient is a 15-year-old female who resides in a skilled nursing facility. She was transferred for PEG tube insertion due to a decrease in p.o. intake[3] secondary to her intellectual disabilities.[1] The patient is also a quadriplegic.[2]

Procedure description:
The patient was taken to the operating room and placed in the supine position. After adequate IV sedation was obtained, esophagogastroduodenoscopy was performed. The esophagus, stomach, and duodenum were visualized without any abnormalities. The appropriate location for the tube insertion was marked on the skin of the abdomen. The area was then prepped and draped in the sterile fashion. This area was infiltrated with 1% lidocaine for local anesthesia, and a needle was used to enter the stomach under visualization by the endoscope. A guidewire was then passed and the needle was then withdrawn. An incision was made and dilated to the size of the tube. The guidewire and dilator were then removed and the PEG tube was placed.[4] The lumen of the stomach was examined and proper placement of the tube was ensured. The endoscope was removed. The tube was then connected to the skin using Prolene sutures. Sterile dressings were applied. The patient was transferred to recovery in a stable condition.

Diagnosis Codes

F72	**Severe intellectual disabilities**[1]
G82.5Ø	**Quadriplegia, unspecified**[2]
R63.3	**Feeding difficulties**[3]

Rationale for Diagnosis Codes
The procedure is being performed for the patient's severe intellectual disabilities, making this the appropriate principal diagnosis. The quadriplegia is an additional diagnosis that should be reported as it increases nursing care and resources.

Procedure Codes

ØDH63UZ   Insertion of Feeding Device into Stomach, Percutaneous Approach[4]

Rationale for Procedure Codes
A percutaneous endoscopic gastrostomy (PEG) tube insertion is reported using the root operation *Insertion* as there is a device being placed into the stomach. The approach is via a percutaneous puncture and represented by percutaneous approach. The visualization by the endoscope is not coded separately. This is consistent with the advice given in the *AHA Coding Clinic for ICD-10-CM and ICD-10-PCS*, fourth quarter, 2013, page 117. The device placed is a feeding device.

MS-DRG

884	**Organic Disturbances and Mental Retardation**	RW 1.1483

 CODING AXIOM

ICD-10-PCS Official Guidelines for Coding and Reporting Section B6.1a:

A device is coded only if a device remains after the procedure is completed. If no device remains, the device value No Device is coded.

OPERATIVE REPORT MDC 19—#2

Preoperative diagnosis:
Dyspareunia

Postoperative diagnosis:
Psychogenic dyspareunia

Procedure performed:
Diagnostic hysteroscopy

Indications:
The patient is a 36-year-old female who experiences deep pelvic pain during and after intercourse. The patient has been examined, and blood work has been negative for any obvious reason for the pain. It was decided to perform a hysteroscopy to examine the internal structures. The procedure was discussed in length including risks, benefits, and complications that could occur. The patient agreed and her signed informed consent is present in the medical record.

Procedure description:
The patient was taken to the operating room and general anesthesia was initiated. After this was satisfactory, the patient was placed in dorsal lithotomy position. The patient was prepped and draped in the usual sterile fashion, and an external manual examination of the vulva was performed and all anatomy was normal. An internal examination of the vagina was performed and the anatomy was found to be normal. A weighted speculum was then placed in the vaginal vault, and the anterior lip of the cervix was grasped. The cervix was dilated to 5 mm using a #16 Hanks dilator. Then, using normal saline within the uterus for distention, a 5 mm diagnostic hysteroscope was inserted. The uterus was visualized intact and grossly normal. Photographs were taken and the scope was removed. The speculum and tenaculum were removed from the vagina. There was a routine amount of bleeding from the cervix, but this should be self-limited. The patient was transported to the recovery room in stable condition.

Code all relevant ICD-10-CM diagnosis and ICD-10-PCS procedure codes in accordance with official guidelines and coding conventions.

Diagnosis Codes:

_____

_____

Procedure Codes:

_____

_____

MS-DRG:

_____

_____

Answers and Rationale

Preoperative diagnosis:
Dyspareunia

Postoperative diagnosis:
Psychogenic dyspareunia[1]

Procedure performed:
Diagnostic hysteroscopy

Indications:
The patient is a 36-year-old female who experiences deep pelvic pain during and after intercourse. The patient has been examined, and blood work has been negative for any obvious reason for the pain. It was decided to perform a hysteroscopy to examine the internal structures. The procedure was discussed in length including risks, benefits, and complications that could occur. The patient agreed and her signed informed consent is present in the medical record.

Procedure description:
The patient was taken to the operating room and general anesthesia was initiated. After this was satisfactory, the patient was placed in dorsal lithotomy position. The patient was prepped and draped in the usual sterile fashion, and an external manual examination of the vulva was performed[4] and all anatomy was normal. An internal examination of the vagina was performed[3] and the anatomy was found to be normal. A weighted speculum was then placed in the vaginal vault, and the anterior lip of the cervix was grasped. The cervix was dilated to 5 mm using a #16 Hanks dilator. Then, using normal saline within the uterus for distention, a 5 mm diagnostic hysteroscope was inserted. The uterus was visualized intact and grossly normal.[2] Photographs were taken and the scope was removed. The speculum and tenaculum were removed from the vagina. There was a routine amount of bleeding from the cervix, but this should be self-limited. The patient was transported to the recovery room in stable condition.

Diagnosis Codes

F52.6	**Dyspareunia not due to a substance or known physiological condition**[1]

Rationale for Diagnosis Codes

The postoperative diagnosis further describes the dyspareunia as "psychogenic."

Procedure Codes

0UJD8ZZ	**Inspection of Uterus and Cervix, Via Natural or Artificial Opening Endoscopic**[2]
0UJH7ZZ	**Inspection of Vagina and Cul-de-sac, Via Natural or Artificial Opening**[3]
0UJMXZZ	**Inspection of Vulva, External Approach**[4]

Rationale for Procedure Codes

The hysteroscopy is only a portion of the procedure performed. In addition, the vulva and vagina were manually inspected as well. These should be reported separately as they are not part of the approach. The cervical dilation, however, would not be reported as it was necessary for inserting the hysteroscope.

MS-DRG

887	**Other Mental Disorder Diagnoses**	**RW 0.9939**

☼ CODING AXIOM

ICD-10-PCS Official Guidelines for Coding and Reporting Section B3.1b:

Components of a procedure specified in the root operation definition and explanation are not coded separately. Procedural steps necessary to reach the operative site and close the operative site are also not coded separately.

MDC 21 Injury, Poisoning and Toxic Effects of Drugs

OPERATIVE REPORT MDC 21—#1

Preoperative diagnosis:
SFA laceration

Postoperative diagnosis:
Same

Procedure performed:
Repair of the superficial femoral artery

Indications:
The patient is a 42-year-old male who was the passenger involved in an MVA. He sustained a major laceration to his right superficial femoral artery that requires emergent repair. A temporary tourniquet was placed by EMS prior to arrival.

Procedure description:
Sedation and spinal anesthesia were initiated with adequate response by the patient. He was then placed supine on the operating table, and his right leg was prepped and draped. The wound leading to the lacerated artery was extended longitudinally, and the laceration was visualized utilizing copious amounts of normal saline. Loose particulates of dirt and debris were washed away. The arterial wound edges were debrided back to healthy arterial tissue. Both the proximal and distal ends of the laceration were flushed with heparinized saline solution, and the patient received 5000 units of heparin. Using Monofilament 6-0, an arterial patch graft was sutured into place over the injury. The tourniquet was released and the site checked for hemostasis. The synthetic patch graft was determined to be patent, and attention was then turned to the soft tissue injury. This was irrigated using normal saline and closely examined. The wound was then closed in layers. The patient tolerated the procedure well and was transported to the recovery room in guarded condition.

Code all relevant ICD-10-CM diagnosis and ICD-10-PCS procedure codes in accordance with official guidelines and coding conventions.

Diagnosis Codes:

_____

_____

Procedure Codes:

_____

_____

MS-DRG:

_____

Answers and Rationale

Preoperative diagnosis:
SFA laceration

Postoperative diagnosis:
Same

Procedure performed:
Repair of the superficial femoral artery

Indications:
The patient is a 42-year-old male who was the passenger involved in an MVA.[3] He sustained a major laceration to his right superficial femoral artery[1,4] that requires emergent repair. A temporary tourniquet was placed by EMS prior to arrival.

Procedure description:
Sedation and spinal anesthesia were initiated with adequate response by the patient. He was then placed supine on the operating table, and his right leg was prepped and draped. The wound leading to the lacerated artery was extended longitudinally, and the laceration was visualized utilizing copious amounts of normal saline. Loose particulates of dirt and debris were washed away.[2] The arterial wound edges were debrided back to healthy arterial tissue. Both the proximal and distal ends of the laceration were flushed with heparinized saline solution, and the patient received 5000 units of heparin. Using Monofilament 6-0, an arterial patch graft was sutured into place over the injury.[4] The tourniquet was released and the site checked for hemostasis. The synthetic patch graft[4] was determined to be patent, and attention was then turned to the soft tissue injury. This was irrigated using normal saline and closely examined. The wound was then closed in layers. The patient tolerated the procedure well and was transported to the recovery room in guarded condition.

Diagnosis Codes

S75.021A   Major laceration of femoral artery, right leg, initial encounter[1]

S71.121A   Laceration with foreign body, right thigh[2]

V49.50XA   Passenger injured in collision with unspecified motor vehicles in traffic accident, initial encounter[3]

Rationale for Diagnosis Codes

The right superficial femoral artery had a major laceration per the documentation, making the selection of the injury code straightforward. According to the "code also" instructional note under S75, the associated open wound is reported and specified as with foreign body due to the dirt and debris. It is especially important to apply the seventh character of A *Initial Encounter*, to the code. Also code V49.50XA should be reported to signify that the patient was a passenger in a car that was involved in a motor vehicle accident with an unspecified type of vehicle.

Procedure Codes

04UK0JZ   Supplement Right Femoral Artery with Synthetic Substitute, Open Approach[4]

Rationale for Procedure Codes

Although the dictation refers to this procedure as a repair, it is clear that the objective was to place the patch graft to reinforce the area that was lacerated. This objective coincides with the root operation *Supplement*. The procedure was performed via an *Open* approach, although through a wound, the wound was extended to reach the site of the laceration. The patch graft is of synthetic material per the body of the operative report.

MS-DRG

909	Other O.R. Procedures for Injuries without CC/MCC	RW 1.2992

CODING AXIOM

ICD-10-CM Official Guidelines for Coding and Reporting Section I.C.19.b.2:

When a primary injury results in minor damage to peripheral nerves or blood vessels, the primary injury is sequenced first with additional code(s) for injuries to nerves and spinal cord (such as category S04), and/or injury to blood vessels (such as category S15). When the primary injury is to the blood vessels or nerves, that injury should be sequenced first.

OPERATIVE REPORT MDC 21—#2

Preoperative diagnosis:
Alcohol poisoning

Postoperative diagnosis:
Same

Procedure performed:
Gastric lavage

Indications:
A 22-year-old female college student consumed an unknown amount or type of alcoholic beverages. She was brought to the hospital after experiencing seizures and becoming cool, pale, and diaphoretic. She was also in and out of consciousness. Due to this, the patient required intubation and IV sedation in order to safely perform the procedure.

Procedure description:
The patient was taken to the endoscopy suite, and an endotracheal tube was inserted and IV sedation was administered by anesthesia. The patient was placed in the Semi-Fowler's position. The nasogastric tube was inserted and manipulated down into the stomach. The positioning of the tube was confirmed via portable x-ray. Normal saline was used to irrigate the stomach. This was then aspirated out. This continued until the fluid returned clear and we were certain there were no remaining stomach contents. The NG tube was removed and the patient was extubated. She was transferred to a room on the general medical floor in mildly guarded condition.

Code all relevant ICD-10-CM diagnosis and ICD-10-PCS procedure codes in accordance with official guidelines and coding conventions.

Diagnosis Codes:
_____

_____

Procedure Codes:
_____

_____

MS-DRG:
_____

_____

Answers and Rationale

Preoperative diagnosis:
Alcohol poisoning[1]

Postoperative diagnosis:
Same

Procedure performed:
Gastric lavage

Indications:
A 22-year-old female college student consumed an unknown amount or type of alcoholic beverages.[1] She was brought to the hospital after experiencing seizures[2] and becoming cool, pale, and diaphoretic. She was also in and out of consciousness.[3] Due to this, the patient requires intubation and IV sedation in order to safely perform the procedure.

Procedure description:
The patient was taken to the endoscopy suite, and an endotracheal tube was inserted and IV sedation was administered by anesthesia. The patient was placed in the Semi-Fowler's position. The nasogastric tube was inserted and manipulated down into the stomach.[4] The positioning of the tube was confirmed via portable x-ray. Normal saline was used to irrigate the stomach. This was then aspirated out. This continued until the fluid returned clear and we were certain there were no remaining stomach contents.[4] The NG tube was removed and the patient was extubated. She was transferred to a room on the general medical floor in mildly guarded condition.

Diagnosis Codes

T51.0X1A Toxic effect of ethanol, accidental (unintentional), initial encounter[1]

R56.9 Unspecified convulsions[2]

R40.4 Transient alteration of awareness[3]

Rationale for Diagnosis Codes
The patient presented for alcohol poisoning secondary to alcoholic beverages. The Table of Drugs and Chemicals in ICD-10-CM leads the coder to T51.0X1. The seventh character of "A" should be added to indicate that this is the initial encounter. Category T51 has a "use additional code" instructional note requiring that any manifestations of the poisoning be reported in addition to T51.0X1A. Those conditions, according to the documentation provided, are seizures and transient consciousness. Because the seizures are not described further, the default code of R56.9 is the most appropriate. The unconsciousness is described as being "in and out," which by definition is transient consciousness or alteration of awareness, best described by R40.4.

Procedure Codes

3E1G78Z Irrigation of Upper GI using Irrigating Substance, Via Natural or Artificial Opening[4]

Rationale for Procedure Codes
The term "Lavage" in the index directs the coder to the root operation *Irrigation*. The stomach is part of the upper gastrointestinal system (from mouth to jejunum). The *Irrigation* table in the *Administration* section of ICD-10-PCS assigns the fourth character G and specifies that the procedure was performed via a natural orifice without the use of an endoscope (fifth character 7).

MS-DRG

918 Poisoning and Toxic Effects of Drugs without MCC RW 0.6859

DEFINITIONS

irrigation. To wash out or cleanse a body cavity, wound, or tissue with water or other fluid.

lavage. Washing.

CODING AXIOM

Note under category T51–T65

When no intent is indicated code to accidental. Undetermined intent is only for use when there is specific documentation in the record that the intent of the toxic effect cannot be determined.

OPERATIVE REPORT MDC 21—#3

Preoperative diagnosis:
Infected mesh from previous incisional hernia repair

Postoperative diagnosis:
Same

Procedure performed:
Debridement of abdominal necrotized soft tissue with removal of mesh

Procedure description:
The patient was placed on the operative table in the supine position. The abdomen was prepped and draped in a routine manner. Local anesthetic was infiltrated into the site of the previous incision of the lower abdomen. A transverse incision was made through the old scar and carried down to the mesh. Adhesions were lysed from the mesh using blunt and sharp dissection. Necrotized tissue and the mesh were excised from the muscle attachments. The wound was thoroughly irrigated with antibiotic solution. Final exploration revealed no remaining necrotized tissue. Subcutaneous tissue was closed with running 3-0 Vicryl, and the skin was closed with running subcuticular 4-0 Monocryl. Estimated blood loss was less than 5 ccs. A dressing was applied and the patient was released to the recovery room in satisfactory condition. Follow-up in the office in 7 days.

Code all relevant ICD-10-CM diagnosis and ICD-10-PCS procedure codes in accordance with official guidelines and coding conventions.

Diagnosis Codes:

_____

_____

Procedure Codes:

_____

_____

MS-DRG:

_____

_____

Answers and Rationale

Preoperative diagnosis:
Infected mesh from previous incisional hernia repair[1]

Postoperative diagnosis:
Same

Procedure performed:
Debridement of abdominal necrotized soft tissue[2] with removal of mesh[4]

Procedure description:
The patient was placed on the operative table in the supine position. The abdomen was prepped and draped in a routine manner. Local anesthetic was infiltrated into the site of the previous incision of the lower abdomen. A transverse incision was made through the old scar and carried down to the mesh.[4,5] Adhesions were lysed[3] from the mesh using blunt and sharp dissection. Necrotized tissue[2,5] and the mesh were excised from the muscle attachments.[4] The wound was thoroughly irrigated with antibiotic solution. Final exploration revealed no remaining necrotized tissue. Subcutaneous tissue was closed with running 3-0 Vicryl, and the skin was closed with running subcuticular 4-0 Monocryl. Estimated blood loss was less than 5 ccs. A dressing was applied and the patient was released to the recovery room in satisfactory condition. Follow-up in the office in 7 days.

Diagnosis Codes

T85.79XA   **Infection and inflammatory reaction due to other internal prosthetic devices, implants and grafts, initial encounter**[1]

I96   **Gangrene, not elsewhere classified**[2]

K66.0   **Peritoneal adhesions (postprocedural) (postinfection)** [3]

Rationale for Diagnosis Codes

The principal diagnosis in this case is the infection of the mesh. Category T85.7 has an instructional note specifying that a secondary code should be used to report the infection. In this case, an infection is not documented but necrosis of the abdominal wall soft tissue is. The term "Necrosis" in the index does not list a coinciding subterm for the abdominal wall, but there is a "see also Gangrene" instructional note. The term "Gangrene" does have a subterm for "Abdominal Wall," which leads to code I96. The adhesions should also be reported as these were inhibiting the removal of the mesh.

Procedure Codes

0WPF0JZ   **Removal of Synthetic Substitute from Abdominal Wall, Open Approach**[4]

0WBF0ZZ   **Excision of Abdominal Wall, Open Approach**[5]

Rationale for Procedure Codes

The immediate objective of the procedure is to remove the mesh (synthetic substitute of the abdominal wall), which would include the lysis of adhesions as those are a routine and expected pathology after such abdominal surgery. Guidelines section B3.1b discusses that procedural steps taken to reach the operative field (such as adhesiolysis) are not reported separately. However, the debridement of the necrotic tissue is not included in the device removal as it was not necessary to reach the operative site. The codes should reflect that both procedures were performed via an *Open* approach.

MS-DRG

908   **Other O.R. Procedures for Injuries with CC**   **RW 1.9904**

If the code for the abdominal wall necrosis is not reported, there is no longer a CC and the MS-DRG changes to lower-weighted 909 Other O.R. Procedures for Injuries without CC/MCC (RW 1.2992).

CODING AXIOM

ICD-10-CM Official Guidelines for Coding and Reporting Section I.A.16:

The "see" instruction following a main term in the Alphabetic Index indicates that another term should be referenced. It is necessary to go to the main term referenced with the "see" note to locate the correct code.

A "see also" instruction following a main term in the Alphabetic Index instructs that there is another main term that may also be referenced that may provide additional Alphabetic Index entries that may be useful. It is not necessary to follow the "see also" note when the original main term provides the necessary code.

MDC 22 Burns

OPERATIVE REPORT MDC 22—#1

Preoperative diagnoses:
Full-thickness burns of torso and both lower extremities

Postoperative diagnoses:
Same

Procedure description:
A 7-year-old male victim of a house fire at his grandparents' mobile home is taken to the operating suite for skin grafting of extensive full-thickness burns covering approximately 65 percent of his body. Due to the extensive nature of the burns on his torso, thighs, and lower legs, there is a lack of autologous donor sites available for large area wound coverage to be carried out in a permanent manner at the present time. It is determined that Integra brand acellular dermal replacement should be used to cover the burns on the abdomen, chest, lower back, and legs, and the skin substitute is applied.

Code all relevant ICD-10-CM diagnosis and ICD-10-PCS procedure codes in accordance with official guidelines and coding conventions.

Diagnosis Codes:

_____

_____

Procedure Codes:

_____

_____

MS-DRG:

_____

_____

Answers and Rationale

Preoperative diagnoses:
Full-thickness[1-5] burns of torso and both lower extremities

Postoperative diagnoses:
Same

Procedure description:
A 7-year-old male victim of a house fire at his grandparents' mobile home[7,8] is taken to the operating suite for skin grafting of extensive full-thickness burns covering approximately 65 percent of his body.[6, 9-15] Due to the extensive nature of the burns on his torso, thighs,[12,13] and lower legs,[14,15] there is a lack of autologous donor sites available for large area wound coverage to be carried out in a permanent manner at the present time. It is determined that Integra brand acellular dermal replacement[9-15] should be used to cover the burns on the abdomen,[2,11] chest,[1,9] lower back,[3,10] and legs[4,5,12-15], and the skin substitute is applied.

Diagnosis Codes

T21.31XA Burn of third degree of chest wall, initial encounter[1]

T21.32XA Burn of third degree of abdominal wall, initial encounter[2]

T21.34XA Burn of third degree of lower back, initial encounter[3]

T24.391A Burn of third degree of multiple sites of right lower limb, except ankle and foot, initial encounter[4]

T24.392A Burn of third degree of multiple sites of left lower limb, except ankle and foot, initial encounter[5]

T31.66 Burns involving 60-69% of body surface with 60-69% third degree burns[6]

X00.0 Exposure to flames in uncontrolled fire in building or structure[7]

Y92.029 Unspecified place in mobile home as the place of occurrence of the external cause[8]

Rationale for Diagnosis Codes

There are multiple coding guidelines pertaining to burn codes. The first is section I.C.19.d, which states that "burns are classified by depth as … third degree (full-thickness involvement)"; because the documentation states full thickness, the coder can assume the burns are third degree. *ICD-10-CM Official Guidelines for Coding and Reporting* section I.C.19.d.5 states that a code should be assigned for each burn site if there are multiple sites; thus the multiple code assignment seen above. Section I.C.19.d.6 points out that a code from section T31 should be assigned but is most appropriate when greater than 20 percent of the body is involved. Lastly, guidelines section I.C.19.d.9 discusses the use of external cause codes.

Procedure Codes

0HR5XK3 Replacement of Chest Skin with Nonautologous Tissue Substitute, Full Thickness, External Approach[9]

0HR6XK3 Replacement of Back Skin with Nonautologous Tissue Substitute, Full Thickness, External Approach[10]

0HR7XK3 Replacement of Abdomen Skin with Nonautologous Tissue Substitute, Full Thickness, External Approach[11]

0HRHXK3 Replacement of Right Upper Leg Skin with Nonautologous Tissue Substitute, Full Thickness, External Approach[12]

0HRJXK3 Replacement of Left Upper Leg Skin with Nonautologous Tissue Substitute, Full Thickness, External Approach[13]

0HRKXK3 Replacement of Right Lower Leg Skin with Nonautologous Tissue Substitute, Full Thickness, External Approach[14]

0HRLXK3 Replacement of Left Lower Leg Skin with Nonautologous Tissue Substitute, Full Thickness, External Approach[15]

Rationale for Procedure Codes

The most important thing to remember when coding a procedure in which the same operation is performed on multiple body parts is that *ICD-10-PCS Official Guidelines for Coding and Reporting* section B3.2.a states that the procedure should be reported separately for each body site. Since Integra acellular dermal replacement is biologically

KEY POINT

Rule of Nines

The rule of nines is a rapid measurement system used to calculate the total body surface area (TBSA) involved in burns, based upon dividing the total area into segments as multiples of 9 percent. The perineum or external genitals are 1 percent; each arm is 9 percent; the front and back of the trunk, and each leg are separately counted as 18 percent; and the head is another 9 percent in adults. For infants and children, the head is 18 percent involvement and the legs are 14 percent each, due to the larger surface area of a child's head in proportion to the body.

CODING AXIOM

ICD-10-CM Official Guidelines for Coding and Reporting Section I.C.19.b:

A combination code for an injury should be assigned when available rather than separate codes for each injury. Such as T24.391A and T24.392A.

derived, the appropriate device value would be nonautologous tissue substitute. This is consistent with the advice given in the *AHA Coding Clinic for ICD-10-CM and ICD-10-PCS*, second quarter, 2014, page 5.

MS-DRG

927	Extensive Burns or Full Thickness Burns with Mechanical Ventilation 96+ Hours with Skin Graft	RW 15.9672

Multiple components are required to qualify for this high-weighted MS-DRG. First, a code from category T31 or T32 must report that at least 20 percent of the body surface is burned with 10 percent being third degree. A procedure code also must report skin grafting. Without both of these codes on the claim, the MS-DRG would be lower weighted.

MDC 24 Multiple Significant Trauma

OPERATIVE REPORT MDC 24—#1

Preoperative diagnosis:
Traumatic brain injury

Postoperative diagnosis:
Same

Procedure performed:
Decompressive craniectomy with evacuation of hematoma

Indications:
A 22-year-old previously healthy male presented to the hospital with traumatic brain injury, open fracture of the right shoulder girdle, and compound fracture of the right femur shaft (all of which were treated during this encounter). The patient's injuries occurred in a deer versus motorcycle accident on the highway while the motorcycle was traveling at approximately 70 miles per hour. The patient was not wearing a helmet. The patient is now being brought to the operating room for decompressive craniectomy for the increasing mass effect due to the right frontal and right temporal intracranial contusions.

Procedure description:
The patient was brought to the operating room, and general anesthesia was initiated. Once adequate anesthesia was confirmed, the patient was prepped and draped in the usual sterile fashion. A craniotomy bone flap was created, removing a portion of the temporal bone using rongeurs. A #15 scalpel was used to open the dura over the temporal lobe. There was no gross herniation of the brain through this opening. A dural flap was made and clotted hematoma was evacuated. DuraGen graft matrix was applied. The galeal layer was closed with 2-0 sutures, and the skin was closed with staples.

Attention was then turned to the preservation of the bone flap for future replacement. A pocket was made within the subcutaneous tissue and fascia of the right periumbilical region. The bone flap was placed within this pocket, and the incision was closed with the 3-0 Prolene sutures in layers.

The patient tolerated the procedure well and was transferred to the neurological critical care unit still in critical condition.

Code all relevant ICD-10-CM diagnosis and ICD-10-PCS procedure codes in accordance with official guidelines and coding conventions.

Diagnosis Codes:

_____

_____

Procedure Codes:

_____

_____

MS-DRG:

_____

_____

Answers and Rationale

Preoperative diagnosis:
Traumatic brain injury

Postoperative diagnosis:
Same

Procedure performed:
Decompressive craniectomy with evacuation of hematoma

Indications:
A 22-year-old previously healthy male presented to the hospital with traumatic brain injury, open fracture of the right shoulder girdle[2] and compound fracture of the right femur shaft[3] (all of which were treated during this encounter). The patient's injuries occurred in a deer versus motorcycle accident[4] on the highway[5] while the motorcycle was traveling at approximately 70 miles per hour. The patient was not wearing a helmet. The patient is now being brought to the operating room for decompressive craniectomy for the increasing mass effect due to the right frontal and right temporal intracranial contusions.[1]

Procedure description:
The patient was brought to the operating room, and general anesthesia was initiated. Once adequate anesthesia was confirmed, the patient was prepped and draped in the usual sterile fashion. A craniotomy bone flap was created, removing a portion of the temporal bone using rongeurs.[7] A #15 scalpel was used to open the dura over the temporal lobe. [6] There was no gross herniation of the brain through this opening. A dural flap was made and clotted hematoma was evacuated.[6] DuraGen graft matrix was applied.[8] The galeal layer was closed with 2-0 sutures, and the skin was closed with staples.

Attention was then turned to the preservation of the bone flap for future replacement. A pocket was made within the subcutaneous tissue and fascia of the right periumbilical region. The bone flap was placed within this pocket, and the incision was closed with the 3-0 Prolene sutures in layers.

The patient tolerated the procedure well and was transferred to the neurological critical care unit still in critical condition.

Diagnosis Codes

S06.310A	Contusion and laceration of right cerebrum without loss of consciousness, initial encounter[1]
S42.91XB	Fracture of right shoulder girdle, part unspecified, initial encounter for open fracture[2]
S72.301B	Unspecified fracture of shaft of right femur, initial encounter for open fracture type I or II[3]
V20.9XXA	Unspecified motorcycle rider injured in collision with pedestrian or animal in traffic accident, initial encounter[4]
Y92.411	Interstate highway as the place of occurrence of the external cause[5]

Rationale for Diagnosis Codes

The terms "Injury, Brain, Traumatic" in the index instructs the coder to see category S06. The documentation specifies that the injuries are contusions of the frontal and temporal lobes. The terms for "Contusion, Brain" differentiate between focal and diffuse. In this case, the injuries are localized to two areas (the temporal and frontal lobes) making it most appropriate to "see Injury, Intracranial, Focal" in the index. When these instructions are followed, the coder is led *back* to "see Contusion, Cerebral," which direct the coder to assign a code from category S06.3 depending on the laterality of the injury. It is important to note that the indications section of the operative note mentions additional injuries that should be coded. This section is also where the external cause of injury documentation is found.

Procedure Codes

00C70ZZ	Extirpation of Cerebral Hemisphere, Open Approach[6]
00N00ZZ	Release of brain, Open Approach[7]
00U20JZ	Supplement Dura Mater with Synthetic Substitute, Open Approach[8]

Rationale for Procedure Codes

The craniectomy is reported separately although it is a part of the operative approach for the clot evacuation and graft, but it was not performed solely for that purpose. The actual intent of the bone removal was to avoid further damage to the brain tissue by "releasing" the brain and allowing it to swell without compression. The procedure therefore has its own objective and root procedure. The objective of creating the dural flap was to evacuate the hematoma. Since clotted hematoma is not liquid, the appropriate root operation is *Extirpation*—cutting or taking out solid matter from a body part. This is consistent with the advice given in *AHA Coding Clinic for ICD-10-CM and ICD-10-PCS*, second quarter, 2013, page 38. The dura was opened over the temporal lobe, which is coded to the cerebral hemisphere in accordance with the Body Part Key. The DuraGen synthetic graft material is placed to protect the brain from infection and foreign bodies "supplement" the remaining dura. The placement of the temporal bone into the subcutaneous tissue of the abdomen is inherent to the procedure and not coded separately.

MS-DRG

| 955 | Craniotomy for Multiple Significant Trauma | RW 5.6773 |

If the additional trauma diagnoses are not reported as secondary codes, the resulting MS-DRG would be lower-weighted 024 Craniotomy with Major Device Implant or Acute Complex CNS Principal Diagnosis without MCC (RW 3.7976).

Appendix A: Abbreviations

a.c.	before eating
a.d.	right ear/to, up to
a fib	atrial fibrillation
a flutter	atrial flutter
a.m.	morning
a.s.	left ear
a.u.	each ear, both ears
A&P	auscultation and percussion
A-P	anterior posterior
A-V	arteriovenous
AAL	anterior axillary line
ab	abortion
AB	blood type
abd	abdomen
ABE	acute bacterial endocarditis
ABO	referring to ABO incompatibility
abs. fev.	without fever
ACD	absolute cardiac dullness
ACL	anterior cruciate ligament
ACLS	advanced cardiac life support
ACVD	acute cardiovascular disease
ad lib	as desired, at pleasure
ad part. dolent.	to the aching parts
ad. us. ext.	for external use
AE	above the elbow
AGA	appropriate (average) for gestational age
AI	aortic insufficiency
AIDS	acquired immunodeficiency syndrome
AIH	artificial insemination by husband
AK	above the knee
AKA	above knee amputation
alb. (albus)	white
ALL	acute lymphocytic leukemia
ama	against medical advice
amb	ambulate
AMI	acute myocardial infarction
AML	acute myelogenous leukemia
AMML	acute myelomonocytic leukemia
ant	anterior
AOD	arterial occlusive disease
AODM	adult onset diabetes mellitus
AP	antepartum/anterior-posterior
Ap	apical
APM	arterial pressure monitoring
approx	approximately

aq.	water (aqua)
ARC	AIDS-related complex
ARD	acute respiratory disease
ARDS	adult respiratory distress syndrome
ARF	acute respiratory/renal failure
AROM	active range of motion/artificial rupture of membranes
AS	aortic stenosis/ arteriosclerosis
ASAP	as soon as possible
ASCVD	arteriosclerotic cardiovascular disease
ASHD	arteriosclerotic heart disease
AV	atrioventricular
AVF	arteriovenous fistula
ax	axillary
b.i.d.	two times a day
B&B	bowel and bladder
Ba	barium
BAL	blood alcohol level/bronchoalveolar lavage
BCC	basal cell carcinoma
BE	barium enema/below the elbow
BI	biopsy
BICROS	bilateral contralateral routing of signals
BK	below the knee
BKA	below knee amputation
BM	bowel movement
BMI	Body Mass Index
BMR	basal metabolic rate
BP	blood pressure
BPD	bronchopulmonary dysplasia
BPH	benign prostatic hypertrophy
Br	breastfeeding
BS	bachelor of surgery/breath sounds/bowel sounds
BSA	body surface area
BSD	bedside drainage
BUS	Bartholin, urethral, Skene's
bx	biopsy
C	centigrade/complements/cervical vertebrae
c	with
C-collar	cervical collar
c/m	counts per minute
c/o	complaints of
C/S	cesarean section
Ca	calcium/cancer
CA	cancer

CABG	coronary artery bypass graft		CTLSO	cervical-thoracic-lumbar-sacral-orthosis
CAD	coronary artery disease		CTZ	chemoreceptor trigger zone
CAPD	continuous ambulatory peritoneal dialysis		cu	cubic
CAT	computerized axial tomography		CV	cardiovascular
cath	catheterize		CVA	cerebral vascular accident/cerebrovascular accident/costovertebral angle
CBR	complete bed rest		CVD	cardiovascular disease
cc	chief complaint		CVL	central venous line
CCPD	continuous cycling peritoneal dialysis		CVMS	clean voided midstream urine
CCU	coronary care unit		CVP	central venous pressure
CDH	congenital dislocation of hip		CVU	cerebrovascular unit
CE	cardiac enlargement		CXR	chest x-ray
CF	cystic fibrosis		CXy	chest x-ray
CHD	congenital heart disease/congestive heart disease		cysto	cystoscopy
CHF	congestive heart failure		D	day/diopter
chgd	changed		D&C	dilation and curettage
chr.	chronic		D/C	discharge/discontinue
CIS	carcinoma in situ		dc	discontinue
cl liqs	clear liquids		DC'd	discharged/discontinued
CLD	chronic lung disease/chronic liver disease		DD	down drain
CLL	chronic lymphatic leukemia		DE	dose equivalent
cm	centimeter		decem	ten
cm2	square centimeters		decub.	decubitus ulcer/lying down
CMC	carpometacarpal		del	delivery
CMG	cystometrogram		det.	let it be given
CML	chronic myelogenous leukemia		dexter, dextra	the right
CMRI	cardiac magnetic resonance imaging		DIC	disseminated intravascular coagulopathy
CMV	cytomegalovirus		DIF	direct immunofluorescence
cn	cranial nerves		dim.	divide in half (dimidiate)
CNP	continuous negative airway pressure		Disp	disposition
CNS	central nervous system		DJD	degenerative joint disease
co	cardiac output		DM	diabetes mellitus
CO2	carbon dioxide		DNP	do not publish
COLD	chronic obstructive lung disease		DNR	do not resuscitate
conc.	concentration		DNS	do not show
cont.	continue		DOA	dead on arrival
COPD	chronic obstructive pulmonary disease		DOB	date of birth
CP	cerebral palsy		DOE	dyspnea on exertion
CPAP	continuous positive airway pressure		DR	delivery room
CPD	cephalopelvic disproportion		dr.	dram
CPM	continuous passive motion		Dsg	dressing
CPR	cardiopulmonary resuscitation		DTRs	deep tendon reflexes
CRF	chronic renal failure		DTs	delirium tremens
crit.	hematocrit		duo	two
CROS	contralateral routing of signals		duodecim.	twelve
CS	central service		dur. dolor.	while pain lasts
CSF	cerebrospinal fluid		DVT	deep vein thrombosis
CT	computerized tomography/corneal thickness/ carpal tunnel syndrome		dx	diagnosis
			e.m.p.	as directed

ead.	the same	**FB (fb)**	fingerbreadth
EBL	estimated blood loss	**FBR**	foreign body removal
EBV	Epstein-Barr virus	**FBS**	fasting blood sugar
ECG	electrocardiogram	**FDP**	fibrin degradation products
ECHO	enterocytopathogenic human orphan virus/echocardiogram	**Fe**	female/iron
ECMO	extracorporeal membrane oxygenation	**FEV**	forced expiratory volume
ECT	electro-convulsive therapy/emission computerized tomography	**FFP**	fresh frozen plasma
		FH	family history
ectopic	ectopic pregnancy (OB)	**FHT**	fetal heart tone
ED	emergency department/effective dose	**FI**	firm one finger down from umbilicus
EDC	estimated date of confinement/ expected date of confinement	**fl**	fluid
		fluoro	fluoroscopy
EEG	electroencephalogram	**FM**	face mask
EENT	eye, ear, nose, and throat	**FME**	full-mouth extraction
EGA	estimated gestational age	**FMG**	fine mesh gauze
EGD	esophagus, stomach and duodenum	**FOD**	free of disease
EKG	electrocardiogram	**fort.**	strong (fortis)
EMG	electromyogram	**FSE**	fetal scalp electrode
en	an enema, a clyster	**FTSG**	full thickness skin graft
eng.	engorged	**FTT**	failure to thrive
ENT	ear, nose, and throat	**FUDs**	follow-up days
EO	elbow orthosis	**FUO**	fever of unknown origin
EOG	electrooculography	**FVC**	forced vital capacity
EOM	extraocular motion	**fx**	fracture
EOMI	extraocular motion intact	**fxBB**	fracture, both bones
EOP	external occipital protuberance	**g**	gram
Epis.	episiotomy	**GA**	gastric analysis
EPO	erythropoietin	**gav.**	gavage
ER	emergency room	**GB**	gallbladder
ERCP	endoscopic retrograde cholangiopancreatography	**GI**	gastrointestinal
		GIFT	gamete intrafallopian transfer
ERG	electroretinogram	**Gly. supp.**	glycerin suppository
ESRD	end-stage renal disease	**gr.**	grain
EST	electroshock therapy	**grav**	number of pregnancies
ESWL	extracorporeal shockwave lithotripsy	**GSR**	galvanic skin response
et	and	**GSV**	greater saphenous vein
ET	endotracheal	**gsw**	gunshot wound
ETOH	alcohol	**gt./gtt.**	drop/drops
EVLT	endovenous laser treatment	**GU**	genitourinary
EVR	evoked visual response	**Gu**	guaiac
Ex	examination	**gyn**	gynecology
exc	excise	**h.d.**	at bedtime
ext.	extremity	**h**	hour
extr.	extract	**h.s.**	at bedtime
F	Fahrenheit/female	**H&P**	history and physical
F (on OB)	firm	**H2O2**	hydrogen peroxide
F/U	follow-up	**HA**	headache/hearing aide
FAS	fetal alcohol syndrome	**HAA**	hepatitis antigen B
FB	foreign body	**HAAb**	hepatitis antibody A

HaAg	hepatitis antigen A
HAV	hepatitis A virus
HB	headbox/hepatitis B
HBcAg	hepatitis antigen B
HBeAb	hepatitis antibody Be
HBeAg	hepatitis antigen Be
Hbg	hemoglobin
HBO	hyperbaric oxygen
HBP	high blood pressure
HBsAb	hepatitis antibody B
HBsAg	hepatitis antigen B
HBV	hepatitis B virus
HCl	hydrochloric acid
Hct	hematocrit
Hctz	hydrochlorothiazide
HCVD	hypertensive cardiovascular disease
HD	Hansen's disease
HD	hip disarticulation
HDL	high-density lipoproteins
HEENT	head, eyes, ears, nose, and throat
Hg/Hgb	hemoglobin
HH	hard of hearing
HIV	human immunodeficiency virus
HLV	herpes-like virus
HMD	hyaline membrane disease
HMS	hepatosplenomegaly
HOB	head of bed
hor. decub.	at bedtime
HORF	high output renal failure
HPI	history of present illness
HPL	human placental lactogen
HPV	human papilloma virus
HR	Harrington rod/heart rate/hour
HS	heelstick/hour of sleep
HSBG	heelstick blood gas
HSG	hysterosalpingogram
HSV	herpes simplex virus
ht.	height
HTLV/III	human T-cell lymphotropic virus– three
HTN	hypertension
Hx	history
hypo	hypodermic injection
I & D	incision and drainage
I & O	intake and output
IA	intra-arterial
IABP	intra-aortic balloon pump
IBW	ideal body weight
ICH	intracranial/cerebral hemorrhage
ICP	intracranial pressure
ICS	intercostal space
ICU	intensive care unit
ID	infective dose
Id31	radioactive iodine
IDDM	insulin dependent diabetis mellitis
Ig	immunoglobulin, gamma
IH	infectious hepatitis
IM	internal medicine/intramuscular/infectious mononucleosis
IMV	intermittent mandatory ventilation
indep	independent
INF	infusion
INJ	injection
instill	instillation
IOL	intraocular lens
IOP	intraoccular pressure
IP	intraperitoneal/interphalangeal
IPD	intermittent peritoneal dialysis
IPPB	intermittent positive pressure breathing
ISG	immune serum globulin
IT	intrathecal administration
IUD	intrauterine device
IV	intravenous
IVC	intravenous cholangiogram
IVF	in vitro fertilization
IVH	intraventricular hemorrhage
IVP	intravenous pyelogram
JODM	juvenile onset diabetes mellitus
JVD	jugular venous distention
K	potassium
KCL	potassium chloride
kg	kilogram
KI	potassium iodide
KJ	knee jerk
KO	keep open/knee orthosis
KUB	kidneys, ureters, bladder
KVO	keep vein open
L	left/lumbar vertebrae
L-S	lumbosacral
LA	left atrium
LAD	left anterior descending
LAT	lateral
LAV	lymphadenopathy associated virus
LAVH	laparascopic assisted vaginal hysterectomy
LBB	left bundle branch
LBP	lower back pain
LD	lethal dose
LDL	low-density lipoproteins

LE	lower extremity/lupus erythematosis
LEEP	loop electrocautery excision procedure
LGA	large for gestational age
LHR	leukocyte histamine release
lido	lidocaine
liq.	solution (liquor)
LKS	liver, kidneys, spleen
LLETZ	large loop excision of transformation zone of cervix of uterus
LLL	left lower lobe
LLQ	left lower quadrant
LML	left medio lateral position
LMN	lower motor neuron
LMP	last menstrual period
LMS	left mentum anterior position (chin)
LMT	left mentum transverse position
LOC	level of consciousness/loss of consciousness
LOM	limitation of motion
LOP	left occiput posterior position
LOT	left occiput transverse position
LP	lumbar puncture
LPM	liters per minute
LR	lactated Ringer's/log roll
LS fusion	lumbar sacral fusion
LSA	left sacrum anterior position
LSB	left sternal border
LSO	lumbar sacral orthosis
LT	left
lul	left upper lobe
luq	left upper quadrant
LUTS	lower urinary tract symptoms
LV	left ventricle
lymphs	lymphocytes
lytes	electrolytes
M	manifest refraction/male
M1	mitral first sound
M2	mitral second sound
MA1	volume respirator
man. prim.	first thing in the morning
MBD	minimal brain disfunction
mcg	microgram
MCL	midclavicular line
MCP	metacarpophalangeal
MCT	mediastinal chest tube
MD	muscular dystrophy/myocardial disease/manic depression
MDD	manic-depressive disorder
MED	minimal effective dose
meds	medications
mEq	milliequivalent
mEq/1	milliequivalent per liter
MFD	minimum fatal dose
mg	milligram
MI	myocardial infarction
min	minimum, minimal, minute
misce.	mix
ML	midline
ml	milliliter
mm	millimeter
mmHg	millimeters of mercury
mono	monocyte/mononucleosis
mor. dict.	in the manner directed
MPD	maximum permissible dose
MR	mental retardation
MRA	magnetic resonance angiography
MRI	magnetic resonance imaging
MS	morphine sulfate/multiple sclerosis
MTD	right eardrum
MTP	metatarsophalangeal
MTS	left eardrum
multip.	multipara - pregnant woman who has more than one child
MVP	mitral valve prolapse
MWS	Mickety-Wilson syndrome
n.p.o.	nothing by mouth
N&V	nausea and vomiting
N2O	nitrous oxide
Na	sodium
NaCl	sodium chloride (salt)
NAD	no appreciable disease
NAT	nonaccidental trauma
NCA	neurocirculatory asthenia
NCPR	no cardiopulmonary resuscitation
NCR	no cardiac resuscitation
NEC	necrotizing enterocolitis/not elsewhere classified
NG	nasogastric
NIDDM	non-insulin dependent diabetes mellitus
NJ	nasojejunal
NKA	no known allergies
NKMA	no known medical allergies
NNR	new and nonofficial remedies
noc.	night
NP-CPAP	nasopharyngeal continuous positive airway pressure
npt	normal pressure and temperature
NS	normal saline/not significant
NSAID	nonsteroidal anti-inflammatory drug
NSD	nominal standard dose

NSR	normal sinus rhythm		PCD	polycystic disease
NST	nonstress test		PCG	phonocardiogram
NSVB	normal spontaneous vaginal bleeding		PCN	penicillin
NT	nasotracheal/nontender		PCTA	percutaneous transluminal angioplasty
NTE	neutral thermal environment		PCV	packed cell volume
NTP	normal temperature and pressure		PD	postural drainage/Parkinson's disease
nyd	not yet diagnosed		PDA	patent ductus arteriosus
O	blood type/oxygen		PE	physical examination/pulmonary embolism/pulmonary edema
o	no information			
o.d.	right eye		Peds	pediatrics
o.m.	otitis media		PEG	percutaneous endoscopic gastrostomy
o.n.	every night		PEN	parenteral and enteral nutrition
o.s.	left eye		PENS	percutaneous electrical nerve stimulation
o.u.	each eye, both eyes		PERRLA	pupils equal, regular, reactive to light and accommodation
O2	oxygen			
OA	osteoarthritis		PET	positron emission tomography
OAG	open angle glaucoma		PH	past history
OB	obstetrics		PI	present illness
OB-GYN	obstetrics and gynecology		PID	pelvic inflammatory disease
OFC	occipitofrontal circumference		PKU	phenylketonuria
ONH	optic nerve head		PMHx	past medical history
ophth	ophthalmology		PMI	point of maximum intensity
OR	operating room		PNC	premature nodal contraction
ORIF	open reduction internal fixation		PND	paroxysmal nocturnal dyspnea/ post nasal drip
os, oris	mouth			
OTD	organ tolerance dose		PO	(per os) by mouth/post operative
OTH	other routes of administration		POD	post operative day
ov.	ovum/office visit		post. cib.	after meals
oz.	ounce		post or PM	postmortem exam or autopsy
P	plan/after/pulse		PP	postprandial
P& A	percussion and auscultation		PPD	percussion and postural drainage
p.c.	after eating		PPH	post partum hemorrhage
p.m.	after noon		pr	per return
P+PD	percussion & postural drainage		preg	pregnant
p.r.	through the rectum		previa	placenta previa
p.r.n.	as needed for		primip	primipara - a woman having her first child
p/o	by mouth		PROM	premature rupture of membranes
P2	pulmonic 2nd sound		PSA	prostate specific blood antigen
PAC	premature atrial contraction		Pt	patient/prothrombin time
PAD	pulmonary artery diastolic		PT	physical therapy/prothrombin time
PAP	Papanicolaou test or smear/pulmonary artery pressure		PTA	prior to admission/percutaneous transluminal angioplasty
PAR	post anesthesia recovery/parenteral		PTB	patellar tendon bearing (cast)
para	along side of/number of pregnancies, as para 1, 2, 3, etc		PTCA	percutaneous transluminal coronary angioplasty
part. vic.	in divided doses		PTT	partial thromboplastin time
PAT	paroxysmal atrial tachycardia		PUD	peptic ulcer disease
path	pathology		pulv.	powder
PBI	protein-bound iodine		PVC	premature ventricular contraction
PC	packed cells		PVD	premature ventricular depolerization
			PVL	paraventricular leukomalasia

Px	prognosis		**RTC**	return to clinic
Q.	every		**RUL**	right upper lobe
q.2h	every two hours		**ruq**	right upper quadrant
q.a.m.	every morning		**Rx**	take (prescription; treatment)
q.d.	every day		**RxN**	reaction
q.h.	every hour		**s**	without
q.h.s.	every night		**S& A**	sugar and acetone
q.i.d.	four times daily		**s.c.**	subcutaneous
q.n.	every night		**s.l.**	under the tongue, sublingual
q.o.d.	every other day		**S.O.S.**	if necessary (si opus sit)
q.q.h.	every four hours		**S-C disease**	sickle cell hemoglobin-c disease
qns	quantity not sufficient		**S/P**	status post
qs	quantity sufficient		**SAH**	subarachnoid hemorrhage
quattour	four		**SB**	sinus bradycardia
quicdecem	fifteen		**SBFT**	small bowel follow through
quinque	five		**SCI**	spinal cord injury
quotid	daily		**SEM**	systolic ejection murmur
R	respiration/right atrium		**septem**	seven
r	roentgen units (x-rays)		**sex**	six
R,R,& E	round, regular, and equal		**SG**	Swan-Ganz
R/O	rule out		**SGA**	small for gestational age
RA	rheumatoid arthritis		**SH**	social history
RATx	radiation therapy		**sine**	without
RBB	right bundle branch		**SLE**	systemic lupus erythematosus
RBC	red blood cell		**SOAP**	subjective objective assessment plan
RCD	relative cardiac dullness		**SOB**	shortness of breath
RDS	respiratory distress syndrome		**sol.**	solution
REM	rapid eye movement		**SOP**	standard operation procedure
resp	respiration, respiratory		**SQ**	status quo/subcutaneous
Rh	Rhesus		**SROM**	spontaneous rupture of membranes
Rh neg	Rhesus factor negative		**ss**	half
RHD	rheumatic heart disease		**SSV**	small saphenous vein
RL	Ringer's lactate		**ST**	sinus tachycardia
RLE	right lower extremity		**staph**	staphylococcus
RLF	rentrolental fibroplasia		**stat**	immediately
RLL	right lower lobe		**STD**	sexually transmitted disease
rlq	right lower quadrant		**strep**	streptococcus
RMA	right mentum anterior position		**STSG**	split thickness skin graft
RML	right middle lobe		**STU**	skin test unit
RMP	right mentum posterior position		**subcu**	subcutaneous
RMT	right mentum transverse position		**subind.**	immediately after
ROA	right occiput anterior position		**supp**	suppository
ROM	range of motion		**Sv**	scalp vein
ROP	right occiput posterior position		**Sx**	sign/symptom
ROS	review of systems		**T**	temperature/tender/thoracic vertebrae
RPG	retrograde pyelogram		**T& C**	type and crossmatch
RR	recovery room		**t.i.d.**	three times daily
RRR	regular rate and rhythm		**T&A**	tonsils and adenoids
RSV	respiratory syncytial virus		**TA**	tension by applanation/transactional analysis

TAH	total abdominal hysterectomy
TAHBSO	total abdominal hysterectomy, bilateral salpingo-oophorectomy
TAT	tetanus antitoxin
Tb	tubercule bacillus
TB	tuberculosis
TBA	to be arranged
TBSA	total body surface area
Td	tetanus
temp	temperature
TENS	transcutaneous electrical nerve stimulation
THA	total hip arthroplasty
Thal	thalassemia
TI	tricuspid insufficiency
TIA	transient ischemic attack
TIBC	total iron binding capacity
tinct	tincture
TKA	total knee arthroplasty
TM	tympanic membrane
TMJ	temporomandibular joint
TNS	transcutaneous nerve stimulator/stimulation
TOA	tubo-ovarian abcess
TPN	total parenteral nutrition
TPR	temperature, pulse, respiration
trans	transverse
tres	three
TSD	Tay-Sachs disease
TUR	transurethral resection
TURP	transurethral resection of prostate
Tx	treatment
U/A	urinalysis
UAC	umbilical artery catheter/catheterization
UE	upper extremity

UFR	uroflowmetry
UGI	upper gastrointestinal
UGS	ultrasound-guided sclerotherapy
UMN	upper motor neuron
UPP	urethra pressure profile
ur.	urine
URI	upper respiratory infection
US	unstable spine/ultrasound
UTI	urinary tract infection
UVC	umbilical vein catheter
V Fib	ventricular fibrillation
V tach	ventricular tachycardia
VCG	vectorcardiogram
VDH	valvular disease of the heart
VF	visual field/ventricular fibrillation
VO2	maximum oxygen consumption
VP	vasopressin/voiding pressure
VPC	ventricular premature contraction
VPRC	volume of packed red cells
VS	vital signs/vesicular sound
VSD	ventricular septal defect
vv	veins
W-D	wet to dry (dressings)
WAK	wearable artificial kidney
WB	whole blood
WBC	white blood count
WLS	wet lung syndrome
WN	well nourished
WNL	within normal limits
Wt	weight
x	except
XM	cross match
Y-O	year-old
ZIFT	zygote intrafallopian transfer

Appendix B: Glossary

abuse. In medical reimbursement, an incident that is inconsistent with accepted medical, business, or fiscal practices and directly or indirectly results in unnecessary costs to the Medicare program, improper reimbursement, or reimbursement for services that do not meet professionally recognized standards of care or which are medically unnecessary. Examples of abuse include excessive charges, improper billing practices, billing Medicare as primary instead of other third-party payers that are primary, and increasing charges for Medicare beneficiaries but not to other patients.

actinic keratosis. Flat, scaly precancerous lesions appearing on dry, sun-aged, and overexposed skin, including the eyelids.

alteration. ICD-10-PCS root operation value 0. Modifying the anatomic structure of a body part without affecting the function of the body part. Used for cosmetic or other procedures whose primary purpose is to improve appearance.

amblyopia. Diminished sight in one eye without alteration in structure.

atelectasis. Collapse of lung tissue affecting part or all of one lung, preventing normal oxygen absorption to healthy tissues.

BKA. Below-the-knee amputation.

blepharochalasis. Loss of elasticity and relaxation of skin of the eyelid, thickened or indurated skin on the eyelid associated with recurrent episodes of edema, and intracellular atrophy.

blepharoplasty. Plastic surgery of the eyelids to remove excess fat and redundant skin weighting down the lid. The eyelid is pulled tight and sutured to support sagging muscles.

BMI. Body mass index. Tool for calculating weight appropriateness in adults. The Centers for Disease Control and Prevention places adult BMIs in the following categories: below 18.5, underweight; 18.5-24.9, normal; 25.0-29.9 overweight; 30.0 and above, obese. BMI may be a factor in determining medical necessity for bariatric procedures.

bypass. ICD-10-PCS root operation value 1. Altering the route of passage of the contents of a tubular body part. Includes one or more anastomoses, with or without the use of a device.

change. ICD-10-PCS root operation value 2. Taking out or off a device from a body part and putting back an identical or similar device in or on the same body part without cutting or puncturing the skin or a mucous membrane. All "change" procedures are coded with the approach *External*.

CMS. Centers for Medicare and Medicaid Services. Federal agency that administers the public health programs.

comminuted. Fracture type in which the bone is splintered or crushed.

compliance program. Set of written policies and procedures related to the delivery of services and developed and monitored internally to ensure that the facility/business is providing high-quality services, while at the same time eliminating waste, fraud, and abuse.

concomitant. Occurring at the same time, accompanying.

congenital. Present at birth, occurring through heredity or an influence during gestation up to the moment of birth.

control. ICD-10-PCS root operation value 3. Stopping, or attempting to stop, postprocedural bleeding. The site of the bleeding is coded as an anatomical region and not to a specific body part.

creation. ICD-10-PCS root operation value 4. Making a new genital structure that does not take over the function of a body part. Used only for sex change operations.

cul-de-sac. Blind pouch, or cavity, such as the pouch of Douglas (retro uterine) or the conjunctival fornix, which is the loose pocket of conjunctiva between the eyelid and the eyeball that permits the eyeball to rotate freely.

data granularity. Degree or detail contained in data; the fineness in which data fields are subdivided.

destruction. ICD-10-PCS root operation value 5. Physical eradication of all or a portion of a body part by the direct use of energy, force, or a destructive agent. None of the body part is physically taken out.

detachment. ICD-10-PCS root operation value 6. Cutting off all or a portion of the upper or lower extremities. The body part value is the site of the detachment, with a qualifier, if applicable, to further specify the level where the extremity was detached.

dilation. ICD-10-PCS root operation value 7. Expanding an orifice or the lumen of a tubular body part. The orifice can be natural or artificially created. Accomplished by stretching a tubular body part using intraluminal pressure or by cutting part of the orifice or wall of the tubular body part.

division. ICD-10-PCS root operation value 8. Cutting into a body part, without draining fluids and/or gases from the body part, in order to separate or transect a body part. All or a portion of the body part is separated into two or more portions.

drainage. ICD-10-PCS root operation value 9. Taking or letting out fluids and/or gases from a body part. The qualifier "diagnostic" is used to identify drainage procedures that are biopsies.

epididymis. Coiled tube on the back of the testis that is the site of sperm maturation and storage and where spermatozoa are propelled into the vas deferens toward the ejaculatory duct by contraction of smooth muscle.

epiphora. Overflow of tears down the cheeks due to a stricture in the lacrimal passages.

ESWL. Extracorporeal shockwave lithotripsy. Destruction of calcified substances in the gallbladder or urinary system by means of directing shock waves at the calculus through a liquid medium to smash the concretion into small particles that can then be passed out of the body.

excision. ICD-10-PCS root operation value B. Cutting out or off, without replacement, a portion of a body part. The qualifier "diagnostic" is used to identify excision procedures that are biopsies.

external. ICD-10-PCS approach value X. Procedures performed directly on the skin or mucous membrane and procedures performed indirectly by the application of external force through the skin or mucous membrane.

extirpation. ICD-10-PCS root operation value C. Taking or cutting out solid matter from a body part. The solid matter may be an abnormal byproduct of a biological function or a foreign body; it may be imbedded in a body part or in the lumen of a tubular body part. The solid matter may or may not have been previously broken into pieces.

extraction. ICD-10-PCS root operation value D. Pulling or stripping out or off all or a portion of a body part by the use of force. The qualifier "diagnostic" is used to identify extraction procedures that are biopsies.

fibroadenoma. Benign neoplasm of glandular epithelium frequently found in the breast.

foreskin. Prepuce.

fragmentation. ICD-10-PCS root operation value F. Breaking solid matter in a body part into pieces. Physical force (e.g., manual, ultrasonic) applied directly or indirectly is used to break the solid matter into pieces. The solid matter may be an abnormal byproduct of a biological function or a foreign body. The pieces of solid matter are not taken out.

fraud. Intentional deception or misrepresentation that is known to be false and could result in an unauthorized benefit. Fraud arises from a false statement or misrepresentation that affects payments under the Medicare program. Examples include claiming costs for noncovered items and services disguised as covered items, incorrect reporting of diagnosis and procedures to maximize reimbursement, intentionally double billing for the same services, billing services that were not rendered, etc.

fusion. ICD-10-PCS root operation value G. Joining together portions of an articular body part, rendering the articular body part immobile. The body part is joined together by a fixation device, bone graft, or by other means.

imbricate. Process of building a surface of overlapping layers of apposing material, such as tissue, for closing a wound or other opening in a body part.

inguinal. Within the groin region.

inguinal hernia. Loop of intestine that protrudes through the abdominal peritoneum into the inguinal canal.

insertion. ICD-10-PCS root operation value H. Putting in a nonbiological appliance that monitors, assists, performs, or prevents a physiological function but does not physically take the place of a body part.

inspection. ICD-10-PCS root operation value J. Visually and/or manually exploring a body part. Visual exploration may be performed with or without optical instrumentation. Manual exploration may be performed directly or through intervening body layers.

irrigation. To wash out or cleanse a body cavity, wound, or tissue with water or other fluid.

lavage. Washing.

lazy eye. Decreased or impaired vision in one or both eyes without detectable anatomic damage to the retina or visual pathways, brought on by disuse, often as a result of esotropia. Lazy eye is usually not correctable by eyeglasses or contact lenses.

LUTS. Lower urinary tract symptoms.

lymphadenitis. Inflammation of the lymph nodes.

lymphoma. Tumors occurring in the lymphoid tissues that are most commonly malignant.

major diagnostic category. Classification of diagnoses typically grouped by body system. Used in diagnostic-related group (DRG) reimbursement.

map. ICD-10-PCS root operation value K. Locating the route of passage of electrical impulses and/or locating functional areas in a body part. Applicable only to the cardiac conduction mechanism and the central nervous system.

medical auditor. Professional who evaluates a provider's utilization, quality of care, or level of reimbursement.

medical necessity. Medically appropriate and necessary to meet basic health needs; consistent with the diagnosis or condition and national medical practice guidelines regarding type, frequency, and duration of treatment; rendered in a cost-effective manner.

melanoma. Highly metastatic malignant neoplasm composed of melanocytes that occur most often on the skin from a preexisting mole or nevus but may also occur in the mouth, esophagus, anal canal, or vagina.

mesentery. Two layers of peritoneum that fold to surround the organs and attach to the abdominal wall.

micturition. Urination.

missed abortion. Retention of a dead fetus within the uterus in cases where fetal demise occurred before the completion of 20 weeks gestation. Abortion in this context refers to retained products of conception from the death of a normal fetus that does not follow spontaneous or induced abortion, or missed delivery.

morbid obesity. Accumulation of excess fat in the subcutaneous connective tissue with increased weight beyond the limits of skeletal requirements, defined as 125 percent or more over the ideal body weight. It is often associated with serious conditions that can become life threatening, such as diabetes, hypertension, and arteriosclerosis.

morbidity. Diseased condition or state.

mortality. Condition of being mortal (subject to death).

myositis. Inflammation of a muscle with voluntary movement.

NCHS. National Center for Health Statistics. Division of the Centers for Disease Control and Prevention that compiles statistical information used to guide actions and policies to improve the public health of U.S. citizens. The NCHS maintains the ICD-9-CM and ICD-10-CM coding systems.

no needle anesthetic (nna). An air jet injector that delivers a spray of anesthetic under high pressure through the skin.

nosologist. Scientist who studies the classification of diseases.

occlusion. ICD-10-PCS root operation value L. Completely closing an orifice or the lumen of a tubular body part. The orifice can be natural or artificially created.

open. ICD-10-PCS approach value 0. Cutting through the skin or mucous membrane and any other body layers necessary to expose the site of the procedure.

PEG. Percutaneous endoscopic gastrostomy.

percutaneous. ICD-10-PCS approach value 3. Entry, by puncture or minor incision, of instrumentation through the skin or mucous membrane and/or any other body layers necessary to reach the site of the procedure.

percutaneous endoscopic. ICD-10-PCS approach value 4. Entry, by puncture or minor incision, of instrumentation through the skin or mucous membrane and/or any other body layers necessary to reach and visualize the site of the procedure.

Peyronie's disease. Development of fibrotic hardened tissue or plaque in the cavernosal sheaths in the penis. This causes pain and a severe chordee or curvature in the penis, typically during erection. Peyronie's disease may need to be treated by surgical excision of the plaques with grafting.

photocoagulation. Application of an intense laser beam of light to disrupt tissue and condense protein material to a residual mass, used especially for treating ocular conditions.

prepuce. Fold of penile skin covering the glans.

progress note. Providers documentation of the encounter, treatment, or interaction with the patient and caregiver and retained as part of the permanent medical record.

reattachment. ICD-10-PCS root operation value M. Putting back in or on all or a portion of a separated body part to its normal location or other suitable location. Vascular circulation and nervous pathways may or may not be reestablished.

release. ICD-10-PCS root operation value N. Freeing a body part from an abnormal physical constraint, by cutting or by the use of force. Some of the restraining tissue may be taken out but none of the body part is taken out.

removal. ICD-10-PCS root operation value P. Taking out or off a device from a body part. If a device is taken out and a similar device put in without cutting or puncturing the skin or mucous membrane, the procedure is coded to the root operation "change." Otherwise, the procedure for taking out a device is coded to the root operation "removal."

repair. ICD-10-PCS root operation value Q. Restoring, to the extent possible, a body part to its normal anatomic structure and function. Used only when the method to accomplish the repair is not one of the other root operations.

replacement. ICD-10-PCS root operation value R. Putting in or on biological or synthetic material that physically takes the place and/or function of all or a portion of a body part. The body part may have been taken out or replaced, or may be taken out, physically eradicated, or rendered nonfunctional during the "replacement" procedure. A "removal" procedure is coded for taking out the device used in a previous "replacement" procedure.

reposition. ICD-10-PCS root operation value S. Moving to its normal location, or other suitable location, all or a portion of a body part. The body part is moved to a new location from an abnormal location, or from a normal location where it is not functioning correctly. The body part may or may not be cut out or off to be moved to the new location.

resection. ICD-10-PCS root operation value T. Cutting out or off, without replacement, all of a body part.

restriction. ICD-10-PCS root operation value V. Partially closing an orifice or the lumen of a tubular body part. The orifice can be natural or artificially created.

revision. ICD-10-PCS root operation value W. Correcting, to the extent possible, a portion of a malfunctioning device or the position of a displaced device. Revision can include correcting a malfunctioning or displaced device by taking out and/or putting in components of the device, such as a screw or pin.

seton. Finely spun thread or other fine material for leading the passage of wider instruments through a fistula, canal, or sinus tract.

spermatocele. Noncancerous accumulation of fluid and dead sperm cells normally located at the head of the epididymis that exhibits itself as a hard, smooth scrotal mass and do not normally require treatment unless they become enlarged or cause pain.

staging. Determination of the course of a disease, as in the case of a malignancy, to determine whether the malignancy is confined to the primary tumor, has spread to one or more lymph nodes, or has metastasized.

stricture. Narrowing of an anatomical structure. *Synonym(s): STX.*

supplement. ICD-10-PCS root operation value U. Putting in or on biological or synthetic material that physically reinforces and/or augments the function of a portion of a body part. The biological material is nonliving, or is living and from the same individual. The body part may have been previously replaced, and the supplement procedure is performed to physically reinforce and/or augment the function of the replaced body part.

TAHBSO. Total abdominal hysterectomy, bilateral salpingo-oophorectomy.

thoracentesis. Surgical puncture of the chest cavity with a specialized needle or hollow tubing to aspirate fluid from within the pleural space for diagnostic or therapeutic reasons.

tracheostomy. Formation of a tracheal opening on the neck surface with tube insertion to allow for respiration in cases of obstruction or decreased patency. A tracheostomy may be planned or performed on an emergency basis for temporary or long-term use.

transfer. ICD-10-PCS root operation value X. Moving, without taking out, all or a portion of a body part to another location to take over the function of all or a portion of a body part. The body part transferred remains connected to its vascular and nervous supplies.

transplantation. ICD-10-PCS root operation value Y. Putting in or on all or a portion of a living body part taken from another individual or animal to physically take the place and/or function of all or a portion of a similar body part. The native body part may or may not be taken out, and the transplanted body part may take over all or a portion of its function.

via natural or artificial opening. ICD-10-PCS approach value 7. Entry of instrumentation through a natural or artificial external opening to reach the site of the procedure.

via natural or artificial opening endoscopic. ICD-10-PCS approach value 8. Entry of instrumentation through a natural or artificial external opening to reach and visualize the site of the procedure.

via natural or artificial opening endoscopic with percutaneous endoscopic assistance. ICD-10-PCS approach value F. Entry of instrumentation through a natural or artificial external opening to reach and visualize the site of the procedure, and entry, by puncture or minor incision, of instrumentation through the skin or mucous membrane and any other body layers necessary to aid in the performance of the procedure.

WHO. World Health Organization. International agency comprising UN members to promote the physical, mental, and emotional health of the people of the world and to track morbidity and mortality statistics worldwide. WHO maintains the International Classification of Diseases (ICD) medical code set.